Pocket Guide to Ocular Oncology and Pathology

Hans E. Grossniklaus
Editor

Pocket Guide to Ocular Oncology and Pathology

Springer

Editor
Hans E. Grossniklaus, M.D.
Emory University School of Medicine
Emory Eye Center
Department of Ophthalmology
Atlanta, GA
USA

ISBN 978-3-662-50828-2 ISBN 978-3-642-29782-3 (eBook)
DOI 10.1007/978-3-642-29782-3
Springer Heidelberg New York Dordrecht London

Softcover re-print of the Hardcover 1st edition 2012

Printed on acid-free paper

Springer is part of Springer Science+Business Media (www.springer.com)

Preface

We are pleased to present the *Pocket Guide to Ocular Oncology and Pathology*. This work is intended to be a general outline and guide to clinical ocular oncology with emphasis on the pathologic features of most ocular tumors that may be encountered in clinical practice. The guide is divided into seven parts. *Basic Principles and Techniques* covers general topics in ocular oncology, such as tumor classifications, imaging, transillumination, and others. The next six parts cover tumors specific for different ocular tissues, such as *conjunctiva/cornea*, *retina/RPE/ciliary epithelium*, *retina* (*retinoblastoma*), *uvea* (*nonmelanocytic uveal tumors*, *nevus*, *and melanoma*), and *optic nerve* (*phakomatoses*). This guide should be brought to the clinic and operating room for quick reference to the clinical features, diagnosis, pathology, and treatment of ocular tumors. We hope that this guide is extensively used and as the field evolves will be updated in future iterations. We acknowledge that this book was supported in part by the Emory University Teacher Scholar Award.

Hans E. Grossniklaus, M.D., M.B.A.
Chris Bergstrom, M.D., OD
G. Baker Hubbard, M.D.
Jill R. Wells, M.D.
Arun D. Singh, M.D.

Contents

Part III Retinal, RPE, and Ciliary Epithelial Tumors

Part IV Retinal Tumors: Retinoblastoma

Contributors

Carryn Anderson, M.D. Department of Radiation Oncology, University of Iowa, Iowa City, IA, USA

Chris Bergstrom, M.D. Department of Ophthalmology, Emory University School of Medicine, Atlanta, GA, USA

Harry H. Brown, M.D. Department of Pathology, Harvey and Bernice Jones Eye Institute, University of Arkansas for Medical Sciences, Little Rock, AR, USA

Guillermo L. Chantada, M.D. Hemato-oncology Service, Hospital JP Garrahan, Buenos Aires, Argentina

Aimee V. Chappelow, M.D. Department of Ophthalmology, Cole Eye Institute, Cleveland Clinic, Cleveland, OH, USA

Victoria M.L. Cohen Ocular Oncology Service, Moorfields Eye Hospital and St. Bartholomew's Hospital, London, UK

Jeffrey Yau Huei Chung, M.D. Department of Ophthalmology, Cole Eye Institute, Cleveland Clinic, Cleveland, OH, USA

Hajir Dadgostar, M.D., Ph.D. Valley Retina Associates Medical Group Encino, CA, USA

Matthew Emanuel, M.D. Department of Ophthalmology, Emory University School of Medicine, Atlanta, GA, USA

Paul T. Finger Department of Ophthalmology, New York Eye and Ear Infirmary, New York, NY, USA

Felicia Fountain, M.D. Department of Ophthalmology, Emory University School of Medicine, Atlanta, GA, USA

Evelyn X. Fu, M.D. Department of Ophthalmic Oncology, Cole Eye Institute, Cleveland Clinic Foundation, Cleveland, OH, USA

Jeffrey M. Goshe, M.D. Department of Ophthalmology, Cole Eye Institute, Cleveland Clinic, Cleveland, OH, USA

Emory Eye Center, Atlanta, GA, USA

Hans E. Grossniklaus, M.D. Emory University School of Medicine, Emory Eye Center, Departments of Ophthalmology, Atlanta, GA, USA

F. Lawson Grumbine, M.D. Department of Ophthalmology, Emory University, Atlanta, GA, USA

Brandy C. Hayden, BS Department of Diagnostic Imaging, Cole Eye Institute, Cleveland Clinic Foundation, Cleveland, OH, USA

Martina C. Herwig, M.D. Department of Ophthalmology, Emory University School of Medicine, Atlanta, GA, USA

Department of Ophthalmology, University of Bonn, Bonn, Germany

Santosh G. Honavar, M.D. Department of Ocular Oncology, LV Prasad Eye Institute, Hyderabad, Andhra Pradesh, India

Martin Heur, M.D., Ph.D. Department of Ophthalmology, University of Southern California Keck School of Medicine, Los Angeles, CA,, USA

G. Baker Hubbard III, M.D. Department of Ophthalmology, Emory University School of Medicine, Atlanta, GA, USA

The Emory Eye Center, Atlanta, GA, USA

Linda Janku, COA Department of Ophthalmic Oncology, Cole Eye Institute, Cleveland Clinic, Cleveland, OH, USA

Deval Joshi, M.D. Department of Ophthalmology, University of Florida, Gainesville, FL, USA

Sunir Joshi, M.D. Beraja Medical Institute, Coral Gables, FL, USA

Sumitra Khandewal, M.D. Department of Ophthalmology, Emory University School of Medicine, Atlanta, GA, USA

Emory Eye Center,Atlanta, GA, USA

Phillip Laird, M.D. Department of Ophthalmology, Emory University, Atlanta, GA, USA

Brian J. Lee, M.D. Department of Ophthalmology, Cole Eye Institute, Cleveland Clinic, Cleveland, OH, USA

Craig Lewis, M.D. Lansing Ophthalmology, East Lansing, MI, USA

Michael Levien, M.D. Department of Pediatric Oncology, Cleveland Clinic Children's Hospital, Cleveland, OH, USA

Karin U. Loeffler, M.D. Department of Ophthalmology, Emory University School of Medicine, Atlanta, GA, USA

Department of Ophthalmology, University of Bonn, Bonn, Germany

Curtis E. Margo, M.D., MPH Department of Ophthalmology, University of South Florida, Tampa, FL, USA

Ron Margolis, M.D. Department of Ophthalmic Oncology, Cole Eye Institute, Cleveland Clinic Foundation, Cleveland, OH, USA

Sonia Mehta, M.D. Department of Ophthalmology, Emory University School of Medicine, Atlanta, GA, USA

Masood Naseripour Eye Research Center, Iran University of Medical Sciences, Tehran, Iran

Claudia Perez-Straziota, M.D. Department of Ophthalmology, Emory University School of Medicine, Atlanta, GA, USA

Luke Peterson, M.D. Department of Ophthalmology, Emory University School of Medicine, Atlanta, GA, USA

Ying Qian, M.D. Department of Ophthalmology, Cole Eye Institute, Cleveland Clinic, Cleveland, OH, USA

Jerome C. Ramos-Esteban, M.D. Department of Ophthalmic Oncology, Cole Eye Institute, Cleveland Clinic Foundation, Cleveland, OH, USA

David Risner, M.D. Department of Ophthalmology, Emory University School of Medicine, Atlanta, GA, USA

Joshua Robinson, M.D. Department of Ophthalmology, Emory University Eye Center, Atlanta, GA, USA

Kaori Sayanagi, M.D. Department of Ophthalmology, Cole Eye Institute, Cleveland Clinic, Cleveland, OH, USA

Lynn Schoenfield Department of Pathology, Cleveland Clinic, Cleveland, OH, USA

Arun D. Singh, M.D. Department of Ophthalmic Oncology, Cole Eye Institute, Cleveland Clinic Foundation, Cleveland, OH, USA

Jim Sargent, M.D. Department of Ophthalmology, Emory Eye Center, Atlanta, GA, USA

Mehran Taban, M.D. Taban-Department of Ophthalmology, Cleveland Clinic, Cleveland, OH, USA

Mary E. Aronow, M.D. Department of Ophthalmic Oncology, Cole Eye Institute, Cleveland Clinic Foundation, Cleveland, OH, USA

Alexandre A.C.M. Ventura, M.D. Department of Ophthalmology, Cole Eye Institute, Cleveland Clinic, Cleveland, OH, USA

Harpreet Singh Walia, M.D. Department of Ophthalmology, Emory University School of Medicine, Atlanta, GA, USA

Werner Wackernagel, M.D. Department of Ophthalmology and Optometry, Medical University Graz, Graz, Austria

Jill R. Wells, M.D. Department of Ophthalmology, Emory University School of Medicine, Atlanta, GA, USA

Qing Zhang, M.D. Department of Ophthalmology, Emory University School of Medicine, Atlanta, GA, USA

Part I

Basic Principles and Techniques

AJCC-UICC Ophthalmic Oncology Task Force Definitions for Eye Cancer

1

Paul T. Finger

Synonyms

Eye Tumor Classification Systems

Definitions

The American Joint Committee on Cancer (AJCC) is a broadly supported organization established in 1959 to formulate and publish cancer classification systems. The International Union Against Cancer (UICC) complements the AJCC by incorporating cancer organizations from over 100 countries around the world. The AJCC Cancer Staging Manual is the gold standard for staging cancers throughout medicine, and the 7th edition of this manual was recently published. AJCC-UICC Ophthalmic Oncology Task Force is composed of an international committee of ophthalmic oncologists, ophthalmic pathologists, geneticists, molecular biologists, and statisticians who worked within a peer-review process to develop a tumor node metastasis (TNM)-based classification for eye cancer for inclusion in the AJCC 7th Edition *Cancer Staging Manual*. Each of the 46 participants was selected because of his or her experience with writing the 6th edition and/or specific published expertise. Chapters define clinically and histopathologically relevant features as well as methods used for diagnosis and treatment. New biomarkers and significant clinical factors were defined as "data points" to be collected by tumor registries.

P.T. Finger, M.D.
Ocular Tumor, Orbital Disease and Ophthalmic Radiation Therapy,
The New York Eye Cancer Center,
New York City, NY, USA
e-mail: pfinger@eyecancer.com

H.E. Grossniklaus (ed.), *Pocket Guide to Ocular Oncology and Pathology*,
DOI 10.1007/978-3-642-29782-3_1, © Springer-Verlag Berlin Heidelberg 2013

Aims

To develop and implement common definitions for ocular cancer. These definitions were designed to be relevant for clinical care and to conform to a standardized classification system used for all cancers throughout all of medicine. The AJCC-UICC eye cancer staging system was created by the ophthalmic community to perform as a scientific language that will enable research and improve clinical care.

Methods

The American Joint Committee on Cancer (AJCC)–International Union Against Cancer (UICC) have united to create a common terminology. In the past, this terminology system was anatomically based. However, in its current 7th revision, the AJCC-UICC chapters on ophthalmic tumors have evolved as to include known and proposed genetic, radiographic, and molecular biomarkers for metastasis.

The committee is comprised of specialists in ophthalmic oncology, ocular plastic surgery, pathology, and ophthalmic radiation therapy. There are contributors from the United States of America, England, Japan, India, Sweden, Finland, the Netherlands, Canada, France, Hungary, and Germany. The committee includes members with leadership positions in major ophthalmic journals and ophthalmic societies. Chapters were developed within an internal peer-review system. Each chapter was written and reviewed by teams of physicians with clinical and pathology training. Once initial "in-house" review and editing was completed, each chapter was sent out for multiple evaluations by outside reviewers. Final editorial revision was performed by the chair of the Task Force, the section editor within the AJCC-UICC, and the publisher (Springer).

Results

The 7th edition chapters included eyelid carcinoma, conjunctiva squamous carcinoma, conjunctival melanoma, uveal melanoma, retinoblastoma, lacrimal gland carcinoma, and orbital sarcoma. A new chapter has been added defining ocular adnexal lymphoma. In addition, each chapter includes a list of additional tumor types that can be classified using that specific classification system.

Each chapter was written to include clinically relevant anatomic definitions of tumor size and location as well as factors that could affect prognosis for life. They include methods for clinical diagnosis and pathology processing.

Diagnostics

Though not the primary goal of each chapter, methods of diagnosis and treatment are described. The committee agreed that certain methods would be required to use the classification system. Clinical methods typically include initial ophthalmic evaluation, metastatic surveys, and treatments that are commonly employed. The ophthalmic pathology component of each staging system describes the parameters used to diagnose these tumors, methods of tissue handling and processing, as well as findings thought to affect prognosis.

Differential Diagnosis

A list of differential diagnosis is contained in each chapter. However, the methods of differential diagnosis are not included. The purpose of the staging system is to define the size, location, and prognostic factors affecting eye cancers.

Biomarkers and Data Points

In an effort to extend prognostic factors beyond the classic anatomically based tumor node metastasis (TNM) classification, the AJCC-UICC challenged our committee to include evidence-based biomarkers for metastasis. Like prostate-specific antigen (PSA) for prostate, the committee included known biomarkers for metastasis of eye tumors in each chapter (as available). If there existed research suggesting that a genetic, molecular, or physiologic biomarker was promising but unproved, they were allowed to suggest that data be collected as a "data point."

Summary

The AJCC-UICC Ophthalmic Task Force has provided a unified system or common language to define almost all ocular malignancies. The 7th edition includes new sections on clinical diagnosis, pathology methods, and biomarkers for metastasis. Major peer-reviewed journals in ophthalmology have recently added the classification in their instructions for authors and require its use for publication. Standardization of methods and nomenclature facilitates research comparisons among defined groups of patients, tumors, and published studies.

The following are ophthalmic oncology headings in the AJCC-UICC TNM classification 7th edition:

- Adenoid Cystic Carcinoma (Cylindroma) of Eyelid General 00000 37/37
- Adenoid Cystic Carcinoma of Lacrimal Glands Disease 00000 38/38
- B-cell Lymphoma Marginal Zone (MALT) Pathology 00238 218/218
- Canthal Tumors General 00000 354/354
- Conjunctival Lymphoma Diagnosis and Treatment 01386 536/536
- Conjunctival Melanoma Diagnosis and Treatment 02496 537/537
- Conjunctival Tumors General 00000 539/539
- Corneal Tumors Pathology 00572 574/574
- Hemangiopericytoma, of Orbit Disease 00000 1058/1058
- Lacrimal Glands, Tumors General 00000 1265/1265
- Leiomyosarcoma, of Orbit Disease 00000 1307/1307
- Lymphoma Definition 00000 1373/1373
- Lymphomas General 00000 1377/1377

- Melanoma Disease 00000 1428/1428
- Melanoma Choroid Pathology 01443 1429/1429
- Melanoma Iris Pathology 01447 1430/1430
- Melanomas Ciliary Body Pathology 01444 1431/1431
- Melanomas, Conjunctival Disease 00000 1432/1432
- Mucoepidermoid Carcinoma Conjunctiva Pathology 01520 1506/1506
- Optic Nerve Glioblastoma (Malignant Optic Glioma) Disease 00000 1665/1665
- Optic Nerve Glioma Malignant Disease 00000 1666/1666
- Orbital Retinoblastoma Diagnosis and Treatment 02516 1692/1692
- Osteosarcoma, of Orbit Disease 00000 1700/1700
- Plasmacytoma, of Orbit Disease 00000 1822/1822
- REAL Classification for Lymphomas Major Studies and Classifications 02032 1955/1955
- Radiographic Techniques for Intraocular Tumors Diagnostic Procedure 02523 1946/1946
- Retinoblastoma Disease 00000 1997/1997
- Rhabdomyosarcoma, of Orbit Disease 00000 2018/2018
- Sarcoma, Orbital Disease 00000 2048/2048
- Sebaceous Gland Carcinoma Disease 00000 2076/2076
- Sebaceous Carcinoma/Adenocarcinoma Disease 00000 2075/2075
- Squamous Cell Carcinoma, of Eyelid Disease 00000 2144/2144
- Squamous Cell Carcinoma, of Conjunctiva Disease 00000 2145/2145
- Squamous Dysplasia, of Conjunctiva Disease 00000 2147/2147
- Tapioca Melanoma Iris Pathology 02249 2235/2235

The members of the 7th Edition, AJCC-UICC Ophthalmic Oncology Task Force include Col Darryl J. Ainbinder, MD; Daniel M. Albert, MD, MS; James O. Armitage, MD; James J. Augsburger, MD; Nikolas E. Bechrakis, MD; Maj John H. Boden, MD; Patricia Che´vez-Barrios, MD; Sarah E. Coupland, MBBS, PhD, FRCPath; Bertil Damato, MD, PhD; Laurence Desjardins, MD; Ralph C. Eagle, MD; Deepak P. Edward, MD; Bita Esmaeli, MD; Paul T. Finger, MD (Chair); James C. Fleming, MD; Brenda L. Gallie, MD; Dan S. Gombos, MD; Jean-Daniel Grange, MD; Hans E. Grossniklaus, MD, MBA; Barrett G. Haik, MD; Col John B. Halligan, MD; J. William Harbour, MD; George J. Harocopos, MD; Leonard M. Holbach, MD; John L. Hungerford, MD;Martine J. Jager, MD, PhD; Zeynel A. Karcioglu, MD; Tero Kivela, MD; Emma Kujala, MD; Ashwin C. Mallipatna, MBBS; Col Robert A Mazzoli, MD; Hugh McGowan, MD; Tatyana Milman, MD; A. Linn Murphree, MD; Tim G. Murray, MD, MBA; Jack Rootman, MD, FRCS; Didi de Wolff-Rouendaal, MD, PhD; Andrew P. Schachat, MD; Stefan Seregard, MD; E. Rand Simpson, MD; Arun D. Singh, MD; Valerie A. White, MD, MHSc; Matthew W. Wilson, MD; Christian W. Wittekind, MD; Guopei Yu, MD, MPH.

Further Reading

Ainbinder DJ, Esmaeli B, Groo SC, Finger PT, Brooks JP (2009) Introduction of the 7th edition eyelid carcinoma classification system from the American Joint Committee on Cancer – international union against cancer staging manual. Arch Pathol Lab Med 133:1256–1261

Coupland SE, White VA, Rootman J, Damato B, Finger PT (2009) A TNM-based clinical staging system for ocular adnexal lymphomas. Arch Pathol Lab Med 133:1262–1267

Finger PT (2003) Guest editorial: do you speak ocular tumor? Ophthalmology 110(1):13–14

Finger PT, 7th Edition, AJCC-UICC Ophthalmic Oncology Task Force (2009) The 7th edition AJCC staging system for eye cancer: an international language for ophthalmic oncology. Arch Pathol Lab Med 133:1197–1198

Rootman J, White VA (2009) Changes in the 7th edition of the AJCC TNM classification and recommendations for pathologic analysis of lacrimal gland tumors. Arch Pathol Lab Med 133:1268–1271

The AJCC-UICC Ophthalmic Oncology Task Force (2002) Ophthalmic sites. Part X. In: Greene FL, Page DL, Fleming ID, et al (eds) AJCC cancer staging manual, 6th edn. Springer, New York, pp 347–384

The AJCC-UICC Ophthalmic Oncology Task Force (2009) Ophthalmic sites. Part X. In: Edge SB, Byrd DR, Carducci MA, Compton CA, Fritz AG, Greene FL, Trotti A. (eds) AJCC cancer staging manual, 7th edn. Springer, New York, pp 523–589

Anatomic Considerations

2

Hans E. Grossniklaus

Overview

The eye (Fig. 2.1) is approximately 24 mm long and is composed of three layers (outer to inner): (1) cornea/sclera; (2) uveal tract consisting of choroid, ciliary body, and iris; and (3) neurosensory retina (contiguous with ciliary nonpigmented epithelium and posterior pigment epithelium of iris). The anterior chamber is filled with aqueous (1 cc), and the posterior compartment is filled with vitreous (4 cc) (volumes in adult eye).

Cornea

The cornea is the transparent outer layer of the anterior portion of the eye that measures 11 × 10 mm in adult. It is composed of five layers (outer to inner): (1) nonkeratinized stratified squamous epithelium, (2) Bowman's layer (collagenous layer), (3) stroma (parallel lamellae of collagen and keratocytes), (4) Descemet's membrane (basement membrane), and (5) endothelium monolayer of hexagonal cells that pump water out of stroma via Na/K ATPase pump. The cornea is avascular and receives nutrition from the tear film and aqueous. It is approximately 500 μ thick centrally and 700 μ thick peripherally. The epithelium may give rise to squamous neoplasia (dysplasia) arising in the limbus and extending onto the corneal surface. Corneal stromal tumors are rare.

H.E. Grossniklaus, M.D.
Emory University School of Medicine,
Emory Eye Center,
Department of Ophthalmology,
Atlanta, GA, USA
e-mail: ophtheg@emory.edu

H.E. Grossniklaus (ed.), *Pocket Guide to Ocular Oncology and Pathology*,
DOI 10.1007/978-3-642-29782-3_2, © Springer-Verlag Berlin Heidelberg 2013

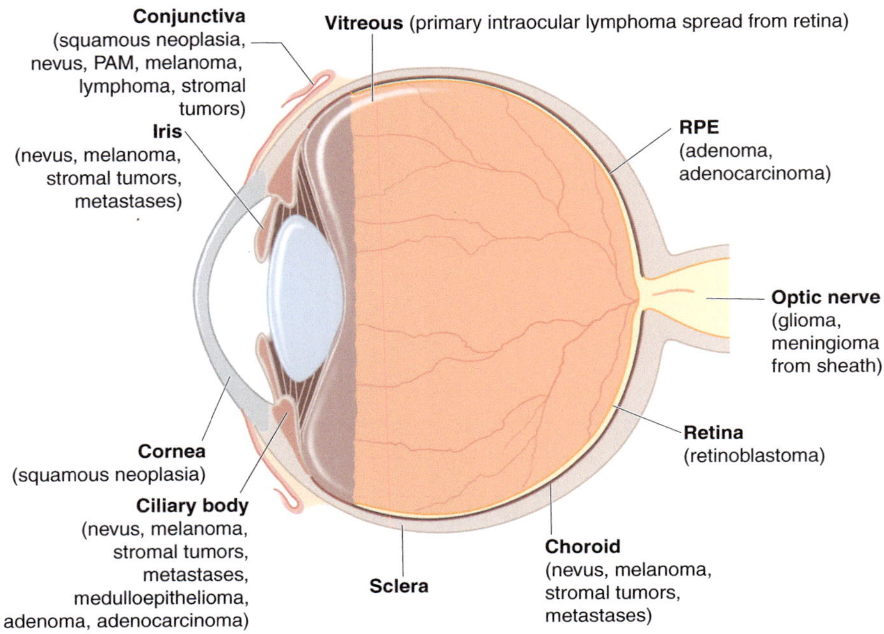

Fig. 2.1 Diagram of eye shows three coats: outer (cornea/sclera), middle (choroid, ciliary body, iris), and inner (retina). The types of tumors that may arise in these layers are indicated

Conjunctiva

The surface of the conjunctiva is composed of nonkeratinized stratified squamous epithelium with goblet cells. The substantia propria underlying epithelium is composed of fibrovascular tissue with occasional interspersed lymphocytes. The palpebral conjunctiva lines the inner surface of eyelids. The bulbar conjunctiva covers the exposed sclera. The fornix is where palpebral and bulbar conjunctivas meet. Goblet cells provide the mucinous component of tear film and increase in density further from the limbus. The conjunctiva receives its nutrition from the vascular supply in substantia propria. Conjunctival epithelium may give rise to squamous neoplasia. Conjunctival melanocytes may give rise to nevus, PAM, and melanoma. The substantia propria may give rise to a variety of tumors including hematopoietic (lymphoma), neural (schwannoma, neurofibroma), fibrocytic (fibrous histiocytoma), vascular (hemangioma), and others.

Lens

The lens is of surface ectodermal origin. It is composed of a capsule, cortex, and nucleus. The lens epithelium is inside the capsule and divides at the equator (lens bow), and the more mature lens cells toward the center of the lens are anucleate.

Lens cells contain proteins known as lens crystallins. The lens is suspended by zonular fibers (suspensory ligament) from the pars plicata of ciliary body. There is no known primary neoplasia of the lens in humans. The lens may become cataractous secondary to irradiation and/or intraocular surgery for ocular tumors. In general, it is safe to perform cataract surgery on an eye treated for an intraocular malignancy 6 months after the tumor has favorably responded to therapy.

Uveal Tract

The uveal tract is composed of the choroid, ciliary body, and iris. It contains an anterior opening (pupil) and a posterior opening through which the optic nerve fibers pass. The venous drainage of the uveal tract is via vortex veins—avoid these during brachytherapy. The choroid consists of fibrocytes, melanocytes, and vascular channels, larger vessels in outer layer (Sattler's layer), medium-sized vessels in middle (Haller's layer), and capillaries in inner layer (choriocapillaris). The ciliary body consists of two regions—pars plicata anteriorly and pars plana posteriorly; it is also consists of five layers—(outer to inner) supraciliary space, muscular layer (longitudinal, circular, and transverse smooth muscles), stroma (fibrovascular tissue including melanocytes), pigment epithelium, and nonpigmented epithelium (produces aqueous). The iris is composed of five layers—(anterior to posterior) anterior border layer, stroma (fibrovascular tissue including melanocytes), muscular layer (sphincter and dilator muscles), anterior pigment epithelium, and posterior pigment epithelium. A uveal melanoma arises from melanocytes in choroid, ciliary body, or iris. Other uveal tumors may occur—smooth muscle tumors (leiomyoma, leiomyosarcoma), neural tumors (schwannoma, neurofibroma), vascular tumors (hemangioma), neuroepithelial tumors (ciliary body adenoma/adenocarcinoma, medulloepithelioma), and metastases.

Neurosensory Retina

The neurosensory retina has nine layers—internal limiting membrane, nerve fiber layer, ganglion cell layer, inner plexiform layer, inner nuclear layer, outer plexiform layer, outer nuclear layer, photoreceptor cell layer, and external limiting membrane. Retinoblastoma is the most common primary intraocular tumor of childhood; heritable form due to 13q14 mutation arises from cells in inner or outer nuclear layer of retina. Retinocytoma is the benign variant of retinoblastoma.

Retinal Pigment Epithelium (RPE)

The RPE is a monolayer of pigmented hexagonal cells overlying Bruch's membrane. The RPE often contains lipofuscin and gives the red/orange color to fundus. These cells are very metabolically active and supply vitamin A to photoreceptors. RPE tumors include pseudoadenomatous hyperplasia, adenoma, and low-grade adenocarcinoma.

Vitreous

The vitreous occupies 4/5 of the eye, is 4 cc in volume, and is 4 g in weight. It is composed of water, collagen, and hyaluronic acid. Primary intraocular lymphoma (PIOL) seeds into vitreous from retinal blood vessels. Metastatic tumors rarely present in vitreous, such as melanoma, lung, and breast carcinoma.

Sclera

The sclera is the white part of eye composed of episclera, stroma, and lamina fusca. Vascular channels, nerves, and accompanying cells may pass through holes in sclera (i.e., Axenfeld's loop—not to be confused with a tumor). Calcific plaques may occur anterior to the insertions of recti muscles.

Optic Nerve

The optic nerve is 40 mm long and contains nerve fibers that arise from ganglion cell layer of retina. Nerve fiber bundles in the optic nerve head pass through holes in sclera (lamina cribrosa). Fibrovascular pial septa supply nutrition to the optic nerve. Glial cells are present in nerve fiber bundles. The optic nerve is surrounded by arachnoid, pia mater, and dura mater (meninges). Primary optic nerve tumors include astrocytoma (pilocytic astrocytoma) which arises from glial cells and meningioma which arises from the arachnoid layer of the meninges.

Angiographic Techniques for Intraocular Tumors

3

Kaori Sayanagi and Arun D. Singh

Synonyms

Fluorescein angiography, indocyanine angiography, autofluorescence

Definition

Angiography involves injection of an intravenous dye (fluorescein or indocyanine green) followed by fundus photography either with a fundus camera or a scanning laser ophthalmoscope (SLO).

Purpose

To visualize retinal and choroidal vasculature and to assess integrity of the blood retinal barrier.

Principle

Fluorescein is 80% bound to protein after intravenous injection, and it is eliminated by the liver and kidney within 24 h. The peak excitation is at 465–590 nm. Indocyanine green is highly protein bound (98%) and eliminated by the liver via bile. The peak excitation is at 790–805 nm.

K. Sayanagi, M.D.
Department of Ophthalmology, Cole Eye Institute,
Cleveland Clinic Foundation, Cleveland, OH, USA

A.D. Singh, M.D. (✉)
Department of Ophthalmic Oncology, Cole Eye Institute, Cleveland Clinic Foundation,
9500 Euclid Ave, Desk i-329, Cleveland, OH 44195, USA
e-mail: singha@ccf.org

H.E. Grossniklaus (ed.), *Pocket Guide to Ocular Oncology and Pathology*,
DOI 10.1007/978-3-642-29782-3_3, © Springer-Verlag Berlin Heidelberg 2013

Indication

Fluorescein angiography and indocyanine green angiography are useful tools for the diagnosis of the various retinal and choroidal diseases including intraocular tumors. Because of the characteristics of the dye, indocyanine green angiography is superior to fluorescein in visualizing choroidal circulation, whereas the fluorescein is superior to indocyanine green angiography in visualizing retinal circulation. Several intraocular tumors, such as melanoma, hemangioma, and metastasis, have characteristic angiographic patterns (Fig. 3.1). For angiography, patient cooperation

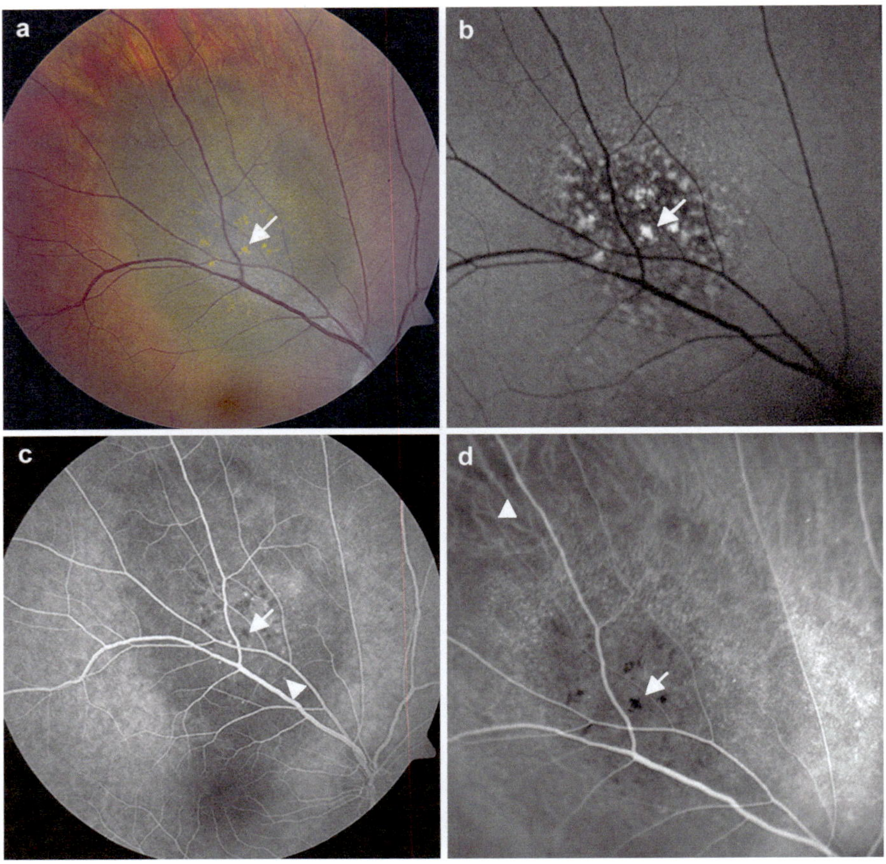

Fig. 3.1 Fundus photograph of a choroidal melanoma with shallow subretinal fluid and orange pigmentation (*arrow*) overlying the central portion of the tumor (**a**). On autofluorescence, the orange pigmentation (lipofuscin) appears bright (**b**, *arrow*). Fluorescein angiogram in the venous phase shows circumscribed hypofluorescence outlining the tumor margin (**c**). Note the patches of the hypofluorescence corresponding to the orange pigmentation (**c**, *arrow*) and pinpoint leakage at the level of the retinal pigment epithelium (**c**, *arrow head*). Indocyanine angiogram demonstrates choroidal vasculature in greater detail than fluorescein (**d**, *arrow head*). Orange pigmentation appears as dark patches (**d**, *arrow*)

is essential. A detailed explanation about the procedure, side effects, and what is expected of the patient is necessary. Simultaneously, confirmation of pupillary dilation and the visibility of the fixation light are also necessary. If the lesion is at the posterior pole, the internal fixation is sufficient. If the lesion is located at the midperipheral retina, an external fixation light is useful. Changing the camera angle is required for peripheral lesions. Images should be taken every 1–3 s from the dye-arrival time until the vein is filled with the dye. Delayed images of the lesion are also taken at 3, 5, and 10 (and 15) min.

The recently developed commercially available confocal SLO, the Heidelberg Retina Angiograph 2 (HRA2), provides three types of images: FA, ICG, and infrared reflectance images. Furthermore, it offers the fundus autofluorescence images, simultaneous images in several combinations, and wide-field images. The fundus autofluorescence image indicates the metabolism of retinal pigment epithelium and therefore provides useful additional information. In simultaneous image display mode, the point-to-point comparison of the images between FA and ICG is possible, facilitating improved understanding of the pathology. It is important to note that there is difference in the focus and brightness of the images between FA and ICG. The slight displacement of the camera back and forth allows finding the optimal focus point. In addition, the ICG images sometimes are overexposed especially in the early phase. This overexposure can be corrected either by decreasing the amount of indocyanine green dye injected or by reducing the sensitivity of the camera. The wide-field image is useful to document the full extent and margins of the lesion.

Contraindication

Side effects such as focal skin irritation and nausea are usually mild. Anaphylactic reaction is extremely rare and can lead to shock, laryngeal edema, and death. The risk of death following fluorescein angiography and indocyanine green angiography is estimated to be 1:222,000 and 1:333,333, respectively. There is contraindication to indocyanine green angiography in patients with allergy to iodine.

Further Reading

Hope-Ross M, Yannuzzi LA, Gragoudas ES et al (1994) Adverse reactions due to indocyanine green. Ophthalmology 101:529–533

Jorzik JJ, Bindewald A, Dithmar S, Holz FG (2005) Digital simultaneous fluorescein and indocyanine green angiography, autofluorescence, and red-free imaging with a solid-state laser-based confocal scanning laser ophthalmoscope. Retina 25:405–416

Yannuzzi LA, Rohrer KT, Tindel LJ et al (1986) Fluorescein angiography complication survey. Ophthalmology 93:611–617

Callender Classification of Uveal Melanomas

4

Martina C. Herwig and Hans E. Grossniklaus

Synonyms

N/A

Definition

The "Callender classification" was named after George R. Callender, who described different subtypes of uveal melanomas based on histologic criteria of 110 tumors in 1931. He identified three main cell types (spindle cell subtype A, spindle cell subtype B, and epithelioid cell). Based on the cytologic composition and pattern of the tumor, five different subtypes were distinguished: spindle cell subtype A, spindle cell subtype B, epithelioid type, fascicular type (Fig. 4.1), and mixed-cell type (consisting of mixtures of spindle and epithelioid cells). A correlation between the histologic cell type and clinical outcome resulted in the conclusion that "patients with melanotic tumors of the eye consisting of spindle cells unmixed with other types have a more favorable outlook than those with epithelioid, fascicular, or mixed-cell types." Addressing the disagreement about the interpretation and application of Callender

M.C. Herwig, M.D. (✉)
Department of Ophthalmology, Emory University School of Medicine,
Atlanta, GA, USA

Department of Ophthalmology, University of Bonn,
Bonn, Germany
e-mail: martina.herwig@ukb.uni-bonn.de

H.E. Grossniklaus, M.D.
Emory University School of Medicine,
Emory Eye Center,
Department of Ophthalmology,
Atlanta, GA, USA
e-mail: ophtheg@emory.edu

H.E. Grossniklaus (ed.), *Pocket Guide to Ocular Oncology and Pathology*,
DOI 10.1007/978-3-642-29782-3_4,

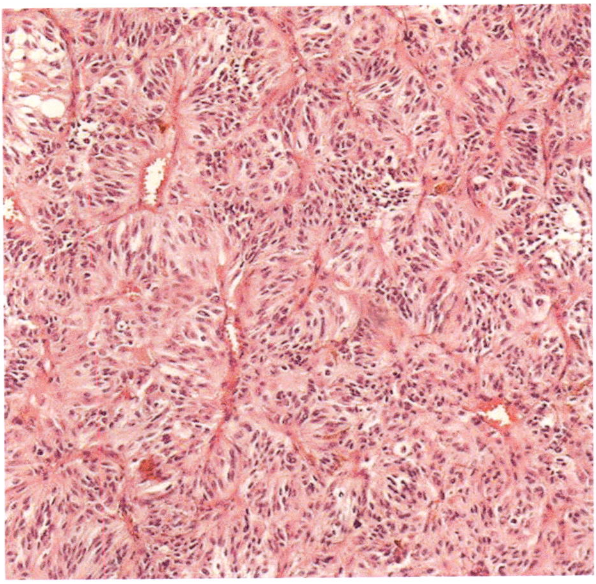

Fig. 4.1 Fascicular pattern of uveal melanoma with tumor cells arranges in fascicles (hematoxylin and eosin, ×10)

classification, a "modified Callender classification" was introduced by McLean and associates in 1983. They distinguished between three different types of uveal melanoma based on cell morphology: spindle cell melanoma (composed of spindle B cells), epithelioid cell melanoma, and melanoma of mixed-cell type. Spindle A cells were no longer regarded as malignant cells but benign nevus cells. In addition, a new cell type was introduced, the small epithelioid cell (intermediate cell), that was smaller than Callender epithelioid cell and exhibited features intermediate between spindle B and epithelioid cells. The classification of uveal melanomas into spindle cell melanoma (composed of spindle B cells), mixed-cell type melanoma, or epithelioid cell melanoma is still widely accepted as it is a relevant prognostic factor of patients' survival. While the mixed-cell type melanoma is the most common form, the epithelioid cell melanoma has generally the worst outcome.

Pathology

The main cell types are depicted as follows (Fig. 4.2):

- *Spindle A cells* are fusiform, cohesive cells with poorly defined cell borders. The nucleus is also spindle-shaped, and sometimes its central fold can be seen light microscopically as dark stripe. This cell type is regarded as a benign nevus cell and can therefore be observed in uveal melanomas arising from a nevus.
- *Spindle B cells* are also fusiform and cohesive with poorly defined cell borders but plumper than spindle A cells. Prominent nucleoli are detected in the spindle-shaped nucleus. This is the most common cell type in choroidal melanoma.

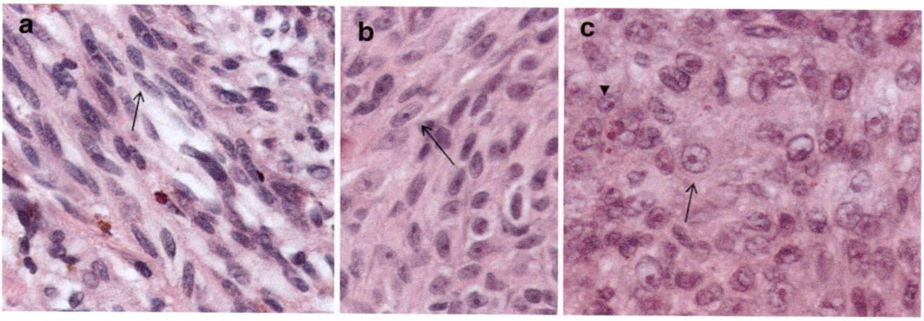

Fig. 4.2 Hematoxylin-eosin (H&E) stain showing spindle A cells (**a**, *arrow*), spindle B cells with a prominent nucleolus (**b**, *arrow*), large epithelioid cells (**c**, *arrow*), and intermediate cells (**c**, *arrowhead*) (hematoxylin and eosin, ×100)

- *Epithelioid cells* are non-cohesive cells with defined cell borders. The round, large nucleus contains a prominent nucleolus. This cell type is associated with a poor outcome.
- *Intermediate cells* (small epithelioid cells) are a frequent cell type intermediate between spindle B cells and epithelioid cells.

Cross-References

Choroidal melanoma, ciliary body melanoma, iris melanoma

Further Reading

Callender GR (1931) Malignant melanotic tumors of the eye: a study of histologic types in 111 cases. Trans Am Acad Ophthalmol Otolaryngol 36:131–142

Herwig MC, Grossniklaus HE (2012) Pathology of choroidal melanoma. In: Ryan SJ (ed) Retina, 5th edn. Elsevier Mosby, Philadelphia

Iwamoto T, Jones IS, Howard GM (1972) Ultrastructural comparison of spindle A, spindle B, and epithelioid-type cells in uveal malignant melanoma. Invest Ophthalmol 11:873–889

McLean IW, Foster WD, Zimmerman LE, Gamal JW (1983) Modifications of Callender's classification of uveal melanoma at the Armed Forces Institute of Pathology. Am J Ophthalmol 96:502–509

Yanoff M, Sassani JW (2009) Ocular melanocytic tumors. In: Yanoff M, Sassani JW (eds) Ocular pathology, 6th edn. Mosby, St. Louis, pp 707–714

Collaborative Ocular Melanoma Study (COMS)

5

David Risner and Hans E. Grossniklaus

Synonyms

COMS

Definition

The Collaborative Ocular Melanoma Study (COMS) was a prospective, multicenter, NIH-sponsored clinical trial. There were two randomized trials, one each for medium and large tumors. There are two observational studies for small tumors.

Aims

The aim of the COMS was to compare outcomes in the medium and large melanoma trials. The main outcome was all-cause mortality. The aim of the observational studies was to determine the proportion of small melanomas that grew and the mortality associated with small choroidal melanomas.

D. Risner, M.D. (✉)
Department of Ophthalmology,
Emory University School of Medicine, Atlanta, GA, USA
e-mail: david.risner@emory.edu

H.E. Grossniklaus, M.D.
Emory University School of Medicine,
Emory Eye Center,
Department of Ophthalmology,
Atlanta, GA, USA
e-mail: ophtheg@emory.edu

H.E. Grossniklaus (ed.), *Pocket Guide to Ocular Oncology and Pathology*,
DOI 10.1007/978-3-642-29782-3_5, © Springer-Verlag Berlin Heidelberg 2013

Methods

Small Melanoma Trial

The small melanoma trial was for uveal melanomas that measured 1.5–2.4 mm in height and 5–16 mm in basal diameter. The recommended treatment in this multicenter trial was observation. There were 204 patients enrolled.

Medium Melanoma Trial

The medium melanoma trial was for patients with uveal melanomas that measured 2.5–10 mm in height and less than 16 mm in basal diameter. Patients were randomized to plaque brachytherapy or enucleation. In iodine-125 plaque brachytherapy, for choroidal melanoma 5 mm or greater in apical height, the dose was prescribed to the apex of the tumor; for tumors 2.5–4.9 mm high at the apex, the prescription point was 5 mm from the interior surface of the sclera. The protocol dose to the prescription point was 85 Gy.

Large Melanoma Trial

This trial was for patients with uveal melanomas that measured greater than 10 mm in apical height and greater than 16 mm in basal diameter. Patients were randomized to radiation prior to enucleation or plaque brachytherapy. In the radiation prior to enucleation group, an average of 20 Gy (18–23 Gy) was to be delivered in five daily fractions of 4 Gy each. Radiotherapy was to be completed within a maximum of 8 days, and the eyes were enucleated on the day the last fraction was delivered whenever possible but no more than 80 h later.

Results

Small Melanoma Trial

The estimated proportion of small tumors that grew was 11%, 21%, and 31% at 1, 2, and 5 years of enrollment. The 5-year tumor-related mortality was 6 of the 204 patients, and the all-cause mortality was 27 of the 204 patients.

Medium Melanoma Trial

Morbidity was as follows: 49% of treated eyes had substantial impairment in visual acuity by 3 years after brachytherapy, defined as a loss of six or more lines of visual acuity from the pretreatment level or visual acuity of 20/200 or worse; 57 eyes of 657 (9%) failed local treatment and required enucleation. The Kaplan-Meier estimate of 5-year all-cause mortality was 19% for enucleation and 18% for brachytherapy. The Kaplan-Meier estimate of 5-year melanoma-related mortality was 11% for enucleation and 9% for brachytherapy. Melanoma-related mortality at 10 years was 21% for brachytherapy and 22% for enucleation.

Large Melanoma Trial

The estimated 5-year survival rate was 57% for all-cause mortality in the enucleation alone group and 62% for pre-enucleation radiation. The estimated survival rate from melanoma-related mortality was 72% for the enucleation alone group and 74% for pre-enucleation radiation group. The 10-year melanoma-related death rates were 45% for the pre-enucleation radiation group and 40% for enucleation alone.

Conclusions

1. The small melanoma observation study showed that most small tumors do not grow within 5 years and there is a low risk of dying from a small choroidal melanoma within 5 years.
2. The medium tumor trial demonstrated there is no statistically significant difference in mortality if tumors are treated with brachytherapy or enucleation.
3. The large tumor trial confirmed there is no survival benefit from pre-enucleation irradiation.

Further Reading

Collaborative Ocular Melanoma Study Group (1997) Mortality in patients with small choroidal melanoma. COMS report no. 4. Arch Ophthalmol 115:886–893

Collaborative Ocular Melanoma Study Group (1998a) The collaborative ocular melanoma study (COMS) randomized trial of pre-enucleation radiation of large choroidal melanoma. I: characteristics of patients enrolled and not enrolled. COMS report no. 9. Am J Ophthalmol 125:767–778

Collaborative Ocular Melanoma Study Group (1998b) The collaborative ocular melanoma study (COMS) randomized trial of pre-enucleation radiation of large choroidal melanoma. II. Initial mortality findings. COMS report no. 10. Am J Ophthalmol 125:779–796

Collaborative Ocular Melanoma Study Group (1998c) The collaborative ocular melanoma study (COMS) randomized trial of pre-enucleation radiation of large choroidal melanoma. III. Local complications and observations following enucleation. COMS report no. 11. Am J Ophthalmol 126:362–372

Collaborative Ocular Melanoma Study Group (2001a) Collaborative ocular melanoma study (COMS) randomized trial of I-125 brachytherapy for medium choroidal melanoma. I. Visual acuity after 3 years. COMS report no. 16. Ophthalmology 108(2):348–366

Collaborative Ocular Melanoma Study Group (2001b) The COMS randomized trial of iodine 125 brachytherapy for choroidal melanoma. III. Initial mortality findings. COMS report no. 18. Arch Ophthalmol 119:969–982

Collaborative Ocular Melanoma Study Group (2002) The COMS randomized trial of iodine 125 brachytherapy for choroidal melanoma. Local treatment failure and enucleation in the first 5 years after brachytherapy. COMS report no. 19. Ophthalmology 198:2197–2206

Collaborative Ocular Melanoma Study Group (2004) The collaborative ocular melanoma study (COMS) randomized trial of pre-enucleation radiation of large choroidal melanoma. IV. Ten-year mortality findings and prognostic factors. COMS report no. 24. Am J Ophthalmol 138:936–951

Collaborative Ocular Melanoma Study Group (2006) The COMS randomized trial of iodine 125 brachytherapy for choroidal melanoma. V. Twelve-year mortality rates and prognostic factors. COMS report no. 28. Arch Ophthalmol 124:1684–1693

Fine-Needle Aspiration Biopsy (FNAB)

6

Harry H. Brown and Chris Bergstrom

Synonyms

Fine-needle aspiration (FNA), fine-needle aspiration cytology, "skinny needle" biopsy

Purpose

Fine-needle aspiration biopsy is a relatively noninjurious and well-tolerated method of obtaining a tissue sample for pathological examination that is efficient, timely, cost-effective, and safe when properly performed.

Principle

A relatively thin (23–27 gauge) needle, attached to a syringe in a specially designed handle, is inserted into a palpable mass and vacuum pressure is then applied while moving the needle back and forth ("passes") at different angles and locations within the mass. Masses deeper in the body may be sampled under ultrasound or CT-directed guidance. Pressure is then released and the needle is withdrawn from the tissue. The material obtained in the needle is expelled onto glass slides for

H.H. Brown, M.D. (✉)
Department of Pathology, Harvey and Bernice Jones Eye Institute,
Universitiy of Arkansas School of Medicine, Little Rock, AR, USA
e-mail: brownharryh@uams.edu

C. Bergstrom, M.D.
Department of Ophthalmology,
Emory University School of Medicine, Atlanta, GA, USA
e-mail: cbergs2@emory.edu

H.E. Grossniklaus (ed.), *Pocket Guide to Ocular Oncology and Pathology*,
DOI 10.1007/978-3-642-29782-3_6, © Springer-Verlag Berlin Heidelberg 2013

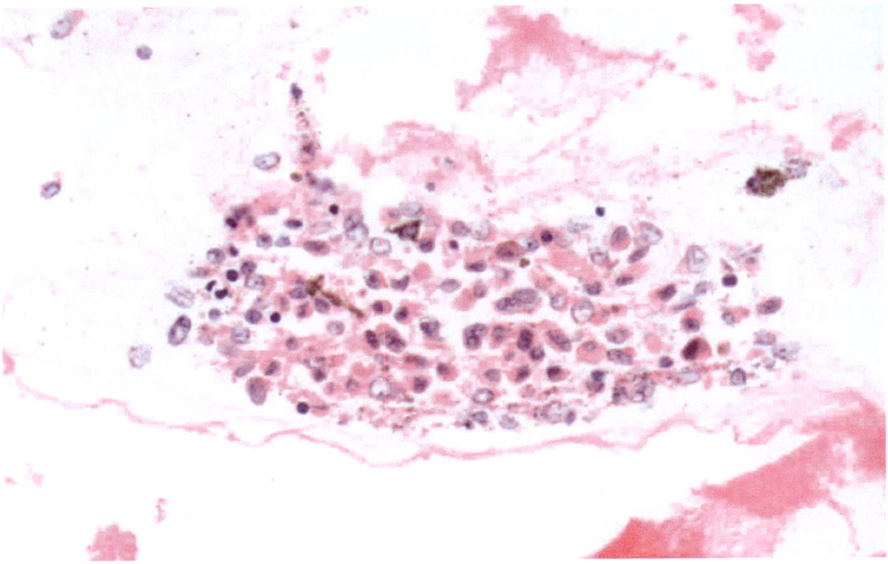

Fig. 6.1 Fine-needle aspiration of a choroidal melanoma shows numerous spindle and epithelioid melanoma cells (hematoxylin and eosin, ×100)

preparation of direct smears which may either be air dried or alcohol fixed and subsequently stained (Fig. 6.1). Immediate cytopathological evaluation may be performed to determine the adequacy of the specimen obtained and the possible need for additional passes to be performed. Additionally, material from the needle or syringe may be placed in formalin fixative, spun down by centrifugation, and the pellet formed submitted for histological processing in the same fashion as a solid tissue sample.

Indications/Contraindications

In ophthalmology, FNAB may be employed for the diagnosis of ocular adnexal masses and intraocular masses, although the latter requires technical expertise both clinically and in pathological interpretation and is restricted primarily to certain academic centers. The technique and cytopathological interpretation is within the purview of most anatomic pathologists, although usage for ocular adnexal masses is not as nearly as common as for other body sites. The ability to perform immunophenotypic studies (either by flow cytometry or immunohistochemistry) has improved the ability to render definitive diagnoses in cases where cytological features may be difficult to interpret, such as for small lymphocyte cell populations. FNA has been employed to determine the etiology of mass lesions of the eyelid, conjunctiva, orbit (Fig. 6.1), and intraocular tissue, primarily the uveal tract. A growing indication for biopsy of uveal melanoma is to determine prognostic information. Contraindications

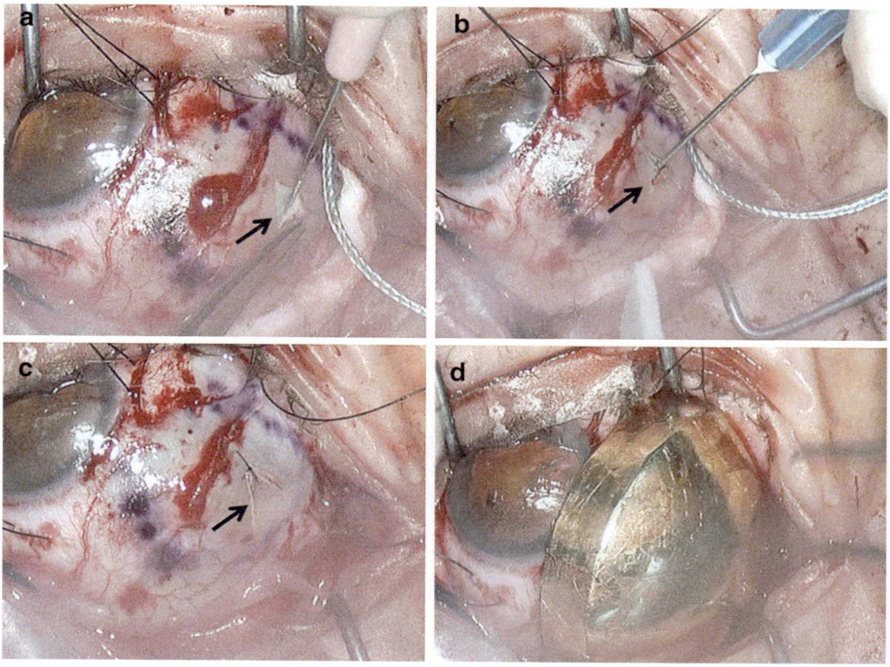

Fig. 6.2 The tumor margins have been marked and the rectus muscle disinserted. A partial thickness scleral flap is made over the tumor (**a**). A needle is passed through the lamellar bed into the tumor (**b**). The flap is closed and cryotherapy applied to the biopsy site (**c**). A radioactive plaque is fixated over the biopsy site and tumor (**d**). (Note—the tumor demarcation is indicated by the *blue dots*, and the scleral flap/biopsy site is indicated by the *arrow*)

are few; one significant contraindication is intraocular FNA where retinoblastoma is suspected clinically; such tumors are often friable and may readily seed the needle tract and become implanted extraocularly.

Technique

In general, FNAB of tumors anterior to the equator of the eye are biopsied through the sclera and tumors posterior to the equator are biopsied transvitreally. To biopsy a tumor transsclerally, the tumor margins are marked using transillumination and the rectus muscle disinserted if necessary. A 50% scleral thickness flap is created over the dome of the tumor (Fig. 6.2a). A needle is passed through the scleral lamellar bed into the tumor, and suction is applied as "passes" are made into the tumor (Fig. 6.2b). Care must be taken not to pass the needle too deep so as to perforate the retina. The scleral flap is closed with a preplaced 8-0 nylon suture (Fig. 6.2c). Cryotherapy is applied to the biopsy site. A radioactive plaque is anchored to the episclera (Fig. 6.2d) if brachytherapy is required. Posterior tumors are biopsied transvitreally through the pars plana with a 25- or 27-gauge needle using indirect

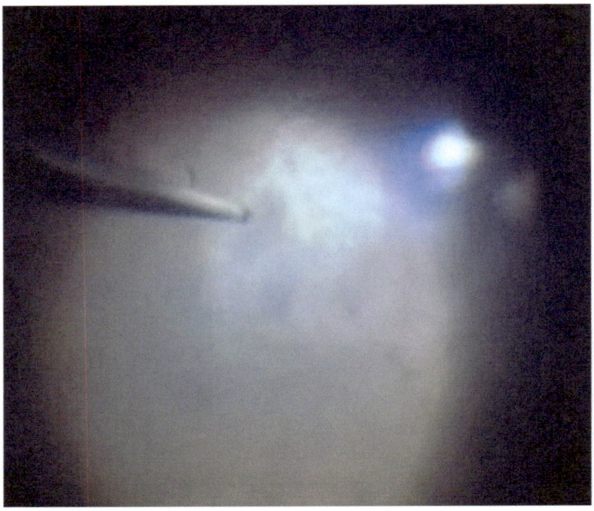

Fig. 6.3 A 25-gauge vitrector is passed through the retina into the tumor

ophthalmoscopy. This approach is technically challenging. Another technique is to use a 25-gauge vitrectomy set up using the operating microscope and BIOM viewing system (Fig. 6.3).

Advantages/Disadvantages

Advantages to the use of FNA for orbital masses include possibly sparing the patient a surgical procedure for a benign process not requiring extirpation; saving the patient time, expense, and morbidity from an open biopsy; and guiding the clinician to the correct surgical procedure when one is indicated. Disadvantages are that pathological evaluation is largely cytomorphological (examination of individual cells and small clusters of cells) rather than the additional architectural clues gained on solid tissue histological examination. Sampling of fibrous masses may not yield diagnostic material. Differentiation of benign from low-grade malignant processes may not be possible, particularly in regard to spindle cell melanocytic proliferations. Technical complications include hemorrhage, optic nerve injury, retinal detachment, and unintended puncture of the eye.

Cross-References

Uveal melanoma brachytherapy, surgical techniques

Further Reading

Glasgow BJ, Foos RY (1993) Ocular cytopathology. Butterworth-Heinemann, Stoneham
Singhal N, Mundi IK, Handa U et al (2011) FNA in diagnosis of orbital lesions causing proptosis in adults. Diagn Cytopathol. doi: 10.1002/dc.21649
Sturgis CD, Silverman JF, Kennerdell JS et al (2001) Fine-needle aspiration for the diagnosis of primary epithelial tumors of the lacrimal gland and ocular adnexa. Diagn Cytopathol 24:86–89
Tani E, Seregard S, Rupp G et al (2006) Fine-needle aspiration cytology and immunocytochemistry of orbital masses. Diagn Cytopathol 34:1–5

Ocular Oncology Service Overview

7

Hans E. Grossniklaus

Synonyms

Ocular oncology department, ocular oncology section

Definition

An ocular oncology service should offer a full range of clinical diagnostic tests, imaging, pathology support, and treatment options for patients with ocular malignancies. The following is a summary of some of the key elements of an ocular oncology service.

Mission

There should be an overall mission for the service. In addition to providing the best ocular oncology diagnosis and treatment available, the service should strive to develop and gain new information that will ultimately help patients with ocular tumors. An example of a mission statement is to have a team approach, utilize evidence-based medicine, and perform translational research. It is helpful to keep the mission statement in the forefront, including mentioning the mission at oncology service retreats.

H.E. Grossniklaus, M.D.
Emory University School of Medicine,
Emory Eye Center,
Department of Ophthalmology,
Atlanta, GA, USA
e-mail: ophtheg@emory.edu

H.E. Grossniklaus (ed.), *Pocket Guide to Ocular Oncology and Pathology*,
DOI 10.1007/978-3-642-29782-3_7, © Springer-Verlag Berlin Heidelberg 2013

Tumor Board

A regularly scheduled tumor board or conference is a key feature of an ocular oncology service. In this era of cancer centers that offer a full range of diagnostic and treatment options, difficult and unusual cases should be presented at the tumor board for group discussion and input. Ocular oncologists, pathologists, medical oncologists, radiation oncologists, ultrasonographers, as well as residents, fellows, and students should attend the tumor board. A consensus opinion should be reached for each case presented. In order for the tumor board to be successful, it is important to include several ocular oncologists who may have different approaches to a given tumor in order to generate meaningful discussion.

Journal Club

A regularly scheduled journal club is very useful for an ocular oncology service. Contemporary articles from other institutes should be critically evaluated at the journal clubs. These articles should span the spectrum of new techniques, collaborative prospective trials, review articles, and basic science articles related to ocular oncology. Participants should actively discuss and critique the article including comments from their own experiences.

Tissue Bank

An ocular tumor tissue bank is important for an ocular oncology service. The tissue bank will require Institutional Review Board (IRB) approval including informed consent from the patient. Tissues usually include a portion of the tumor, most often uveal melanoma or retinoblastoma, which are obtained under sterile conditions in the surgical suite after enucleation. A patient's blood may also be stored in the tissue bank, as in some instances relative's blood. These tissues may be used for experimental protocols, such as genetic tests for oncogenes. The tissue should be stored in a dedicated, secure −80°C freezer.

Database

A database is often part of an ocular oncology service. The database should be broad and include numerous datapoints, including patients' age, sex, eye involved, clinical features, pathology features, treatment, outcome, and all other pertinent information. Like the tissue bank, the database requires IRB approval. These data may be used for future clinical studies.

Meetings

It is important that the ocular oncology service hosts and/or participates in ocular oncology meetings in order to interact with ocular oncologists, pathologists, and researchers at other institutions. There is a range of clinical and research experience at geographically diverse institutes which should be shared in an open, collegial format.

Summary

In our current era of sophisticated molecular diagnostic techniques, imaging, radiation therapy, chemotherapy, and microsurgery, it is important for ocular oncology to participate and be part of mainstream oncology. This may be accomplished in part with the establishment of a formal ocular oncology service with set criteria for the service, including membership, participation, mission, and various components that lead to discovery, dissemination of information, and highest quality patient care.

Radiographic Techniques for Intraocular Tumors

8

Craig Lewis and Arun D. Singh

Computed Tomography (CT)

Synonyms

CT scan, Computed axial tomography (CAT) scan

Principle

X-rays are emitted from a source rotated around the patient with sensors on the opposite side. The data from the sensors is combined by tomographic reconstruction into two- or three-dimensional images.

Indication

CT scans are rarely indicated in the routine evaluation of intraocular tumors. In cases where the clinical examination and ultrasound findings are inconclusive, orbital CT scans may aid in characterizing lesions, especially if calcification is in question (Table 8.1).

C. Lewis, M.D.
Lansing Ophthalmology,
East Lansing, MI, USA

A.D. Singh, M.D. (✉)
Department of Ophthalmic Oncology, Cole Eye Institute, Cleveland Clinic Foundation,
9500 Euclid Ave, Desk i-329, Cleveland, OH 44195, USA
e-mail: singha@ccf.org

H.E. Grossniklaus (ed.), *Pocket Guide to Ocular Oncology and Pathology*,
DOI 10.1007/978-3-642-29782-3_8, © Springer-Verlag Berlin Heidelberg 2013

Table 8.1 Differential diagnosis of intraocular calcification

Neoplastic	Retinoblastoma Astrocytoma Retinocytoma Choroidal osteoma
Metaplastic	Phthisis bulbi
Degenerative, or metabolic (hypercalcemia)	Sclerochoroidal calcification

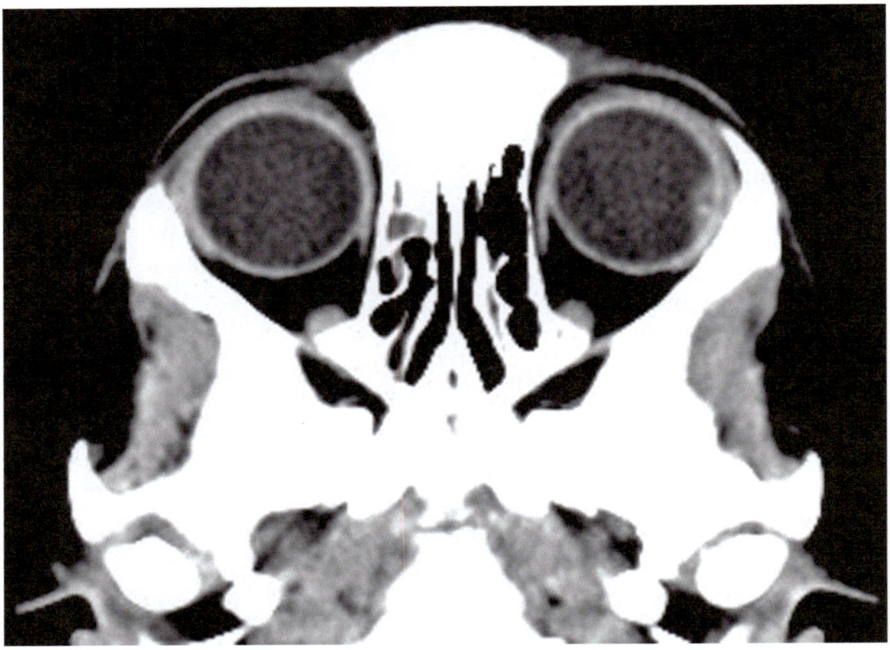

Fig. 8.1 CT scan of the orbit showing a calcified mass within left eyeball

Contraindications

Contrast dye allergy, pregnancy

Advantages

Superior bony detail and visualization of calcification (Fig. 8.1), and fast acquisition time and lower cost versus magnetic resonance imaging (MRI).

Disadvantages

Inferior soft tissue and orbital apex detail versus MRI, exposes patient to radiation, and pediatric and uncooperative patients may require sedation.

Magnetic Resonance Imaging (MRI)

Synonyms

Nuclear magnetic resonance imaging (NMRI)

Principle

A powerful magnetic field aligns primarily the hydrogen atoms in water in the body. Radio frequency pulses perturb the alignment of the hydrogen nuclei, and as the nuclei return to alignment, they produce a small signal detectable by the sensor. The data is converted into a two-dimensional image. Surface coils may be used to increase the local magnetic field and image resolution.

Indication

MRI scans are rarely indicated in the routine evaluation of intraocular tumors. In cases where the clinical examination and ultrasound findings are inconclusive, orbital MRI scans may aid in characterizing lesions including cases of suspected extension of intraocular tumors extrasclerally or along the optic nerve (Fig. 8.2), although there is poor correlation between MRI and histologic optic nerve extension.

Contraindications

Implanted ferromagnetic objects (cochlear implants, some metal implants, and cardiac pacemakers) and claustrophobia.

Advantages

Superior soft tissue and orbital apex detail and no exposure to ionizing radiation.

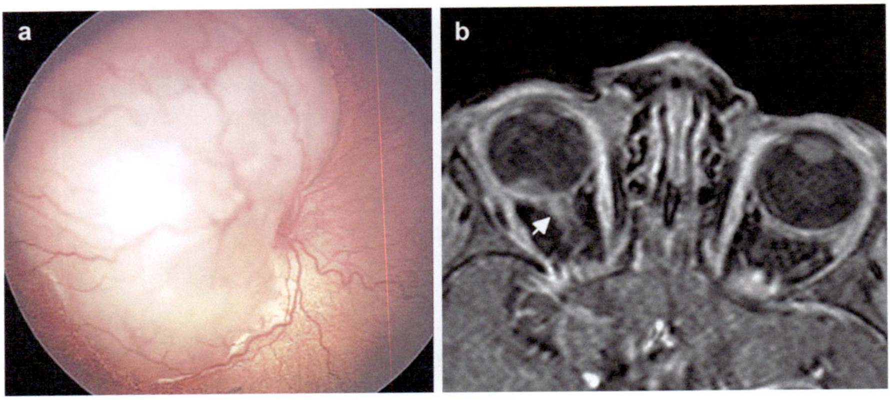

Fig. 8.2 Retinoblastoma in the right eye with partial obscuration of the disc and congestion of the visibly remaining disc margin (**a**). The tumor showed heterogeneous intense enhancement with gadolinium. The optic nerve showed enhancement (*arrow*) suggesting transuveal extension but no mass was seen within the optic nerve itself, and the sheath was preserved on the dedicated MRI of orbits (**b**, enhanced axial view)

Disadvantages

Higher cost versus CT imaging, longer acquisition times versus CT imaging, inferior bony detail versus CT imaging, and pediatric and uncooperative patients may require sedation.

Magnetic Resonance Spectroscopy (MRS)

Synonyms

Nuclear magnetic resonance spectroscopy (NMRS), chemical shift NMR microscopy, MR in vivo spectroscopy

Principle

A powerful magnetic field aligns susceptible nuclei in the target tissues. Radio frequency pulses perturb this alignment, and as the nuclei return to alignment, they produce a small signal detectable by the sensor. Each individual nucleus resonates at a characteristic frequency that is dependent upon the immediate chemical environment (the chemical shift). The resulting resonance spectra (signal power versus frequency) yield information about the biochemical composition of the tissue. Choroidal melanomas and other choroidal tumors contain an unusually high concentration of phosphodiesterase, detectable on phosphorous-31 MRS.

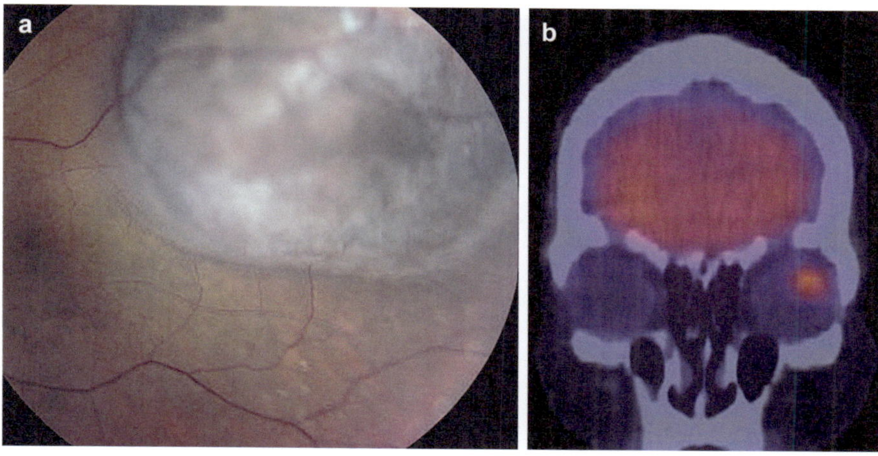

Fig. 8.3 Choroidal melanoma of the left eye. Fundus appearance (**a**). The tumor (13 mm in base and 6 mm in height) could be visualized by PET scan (maximum SUV of 8.6) and a CT scan. Fused image of PET/CT scan localizes hypermetabolic activity to the intraocular tumor (**b**)

Indication

MRS is currently a research tool.

Positron Emission Tomography (PET)

Synonyms

PET scan, fluorodeoxyglucose (FDG)-PET, PET/CT scan

Principle

Cells with higher rates of glucose metabolism (especially malignant cells) have an increased uptake of intravenous radiolabeled fluorine-18 FDG. Sensors detect the location of the fluorine-18 FDG, and the PET scanner creates a map of the tracer concentration in the body, often with a simultaneous CT scan for localization (PET/CT scan).

Indication

PET/CT scans are being investigated to assess choroidal melanoma viability after conservative treatment (Fig. 8.3). Whole body PET/CT scans are being investigated to improve detection of early metastatic disease in newly diagnosed choroidal melanomas.

Cross-References

AJCC-UICC ophthalmic oncology task force definitions of ocular tumors, angiographic techniques for intraocular tumors, and ultrasonography techniques.

Further Reading

Adam A, Dixon A (2008) Grainger & Allison's diagnostic radiology, 5th edn. Churchill Livingstone-Elsevier, Philadelphia

Singh AD, Damato BE, Pe'er J, Murphree AL, Perry JD (eds) (2007) Clinical ophthalmic oncology. Saunders-Elsevier, Philadelphia

Wilson MW, Rodriguez-Galindo C, Billups C, Haik BG, Laningham F, Patay Z (2009) Lack of correlation between the histologic and magnetic resonance imaging results of optic nerve involvement in eyes primarily enucleated for retinoblastoma. Ophthalmology 116(8):1558–1563

REAL and WHO Classification for Lymphomas

9

Harry H. Brown and Jill R. Wells

Definition

Unifying classification schemes of lymphoid neoplasms incorporating clinical, histopathological, immunophenotypic, and genetic characteristics

REAL (Revised European American Lymphoma) Classification

The REAL classification of lymphoid neoplasms was the result of collaboration between leading European and American scholars and practitioners as part of the International Lymphoma Study Group and published in 1994. Its aim was to introduce a classification scheme for global use in order to advance the understanding, diagnosis, and treatment of malignant lymphoma and facilitate communication and interaction among pathologists and clinicians worldwide. Prior to the REAL classification, American hematopathologists adhered to the Lukes-Collins and subsequently the Working Formulation classification schemes, while Europeans utilized the Kiel classification. The International Lymphoma Study Group, a group of 19 European and American experts in the field, met in Berlin in April 1993 to review and come to a consensus on categorization of lymphoid neoplasms. Hodgkin's disease, non-Hodgkin's lymphoma, and lymphoid leukemia were included. A list of disease entities was formulated by three members and submitted to 19 hematopathologists

H.H. Brown, M.D. (✉)
Department of Pathology, Harvey and Bernice Jones Eye Institute,
University of Arkansas School of Medicine, Little Rock, AR, USA
e-mail: brownharryh@uams.edu

J.R. Wells, M.D.
Department of Ophthalmology,
Emory University School of Medicine, Atlanta, GA, USA
e-mail: wells4@emory.edu

H.E. Grossniklaus (ed.), *Pocket Guide to Ocular Oncology and Pathology*,
DOI 10.1007/978-3-642-29782-3_9, © Springer-Verlag Berlin Heidelberg 2013

prior to the meeting; each was to review one or more topics and determine whether the entity was sufficiently characterized to be included, what necessary diagnostic criteria were applicable, and whether subgroups or grading within the entity was recognizable. The entities were then presented and discussed by open forum at the meeting. The final consensus by a majority of the participants was produced in a tabular form and a manuscript including the table and descriptions of the entities agreed upon. Those in which agreement was not reached by a majority were not included. The general principles reached included three major categories of disease: B-cell lymphoma, T-cell lymphoma, and Hodgkin's disease, with definite, provisional, and unclassifiable major categories in each. Standardized nomenclature was introduced for each entity. The definitions of the clinical entities as agreed upon in the REAL classification have been subsequently widely accepted and utilized and now form the basis of the World Health Organization (WHO) classification, the currently used terminology for hematopoietic neoplasia.

WHO (World Health Organization) Classification

In 2008, the International Agency for Research on Cancer published the 4th edition of the WHO Classification of Tumors of Hematopoietic and Lymphoid tissues. Changes in the classification of lymphomas resulted from new insights derived from clinical and laboratory research to better define heterogeneous or ambiguous categories. The areas of change relate to a greater appreciation of early lesions that challenge us to define the earliest steps in neoplastic transformation, the recognition of age as a defining feature of some diseases, further appreciation of site-specific impact on disease definitions, and a recognition of borderline categories in which current morphological, immunophenotypic, and genetic criteria do not permit sharp delineations into existing disease categories. Table 9.1 lists the B- and T-cell neoplasms.

The most common lymphomas to affect the ocular adnexa include extranodal marginal zone B-cell lymphoma of mucosa-associated lymphoid tissue (MALT lymphoma), follicular lymphoma, mantle cell lymphoma, and diffuse large B-cell lymphoma. The most common conjunctival lymphoma, the marginal zone lymphoma of mucosa-associated lymphoid tissue (MALT lymphoma), is an indolent B-cell non-Hodgkin lymphoma arising from the lymphoid tissue at extranodal sites. It is genetically characterized by different, usually mutually exclusive, genetic abnormalities that lead to activation of the nuclear factor kappa B (NF-kappaB) pathway. These lymphomas can arise in any extranodal organ or tissue; however, the stomach—where MALT lymphoma development has been strongly linked to chronic Helicobacter pylori infection—is the most common site. Treatment of non-gastric MALT lymphomas usually consists of radiotherapy. Systemic therapy (with chemotherapy and/or rituximab [Rituxan]) can be effective, while antibiotic therapies (e.g., doxycycline) should still be considered investigational. Less common ocular adnexal lymphomas include follicular, mantle cell, and diffuse large B cell. These are not as radiosensitive as MALT lymphomas and may require chemotherapy in addition to radiation. According to one study, 25% of ocular adnexal

Table 9.1 WHO Classification of Lymphomas

Mature B-cell neoplasms
Chronic lymphocytic leukemia/small lymphocytic lymphoma
B-cell prolymphocytic leukemia
Splenic marginal zone lymphoma
Hairy cell leukemia
Splenic lymphoma/leukemia, unclassifiable
Splenic diffuse red pulp small B-cell lymphoma*
Hairy cell leukemia-variant*
Lymphoplasmacytic lymphoma
Waldenström macroglobulinemia
Heavy chain diseases
Alpha heavy chain disease
Gamma heavy chain disease
Mu heavy chain disease plasma cell myeloma
Solitary plasmacytoma of bone
Extraosseous plasmacytoma
Extranodal marginal zone B-cell lymphoma of mucosa-associated lymphoid tissue (MALT lymphoma)
Nodal marginal zone B-cell lymphoma (MZL)
Pediatric type nodal MZL
Follicular lymphoma
Pediatric type follicular lymphoma
Primary cutaneous follicle center lymphoma
Mantle cell lymphoma
Diffuse large B-cell lymphoma (DLBCL), not otherwise specified
T-cell/histiocyte-rich large B-cell lymphoma
DLBCL associated with chronic inflammation
Epstein-Barr virus (EBV) + DLBCL of the elderly
Lymphomatoid granulomatosis
Primary mediastinal (thymic) large B-cell lymphoma
Intravascular large B-cell lymphoma
Primary cutaneous DLBCL, leg type
ALK⁺ large B-cell lymphoma
Plasmablastic lymphoma
Primary effusion lymphoma
Large B-cell lymphoma arising in HHV8-associated multicentric Castleman disease
Burkitt lymphoma
B-cell lymphoma, unclassifiable, with features intermediate between diffuse large B-cell lymphoma and Burkitt lymphoma
B-cell lymphoma, unclassifiable, with features intermediate between diffuse large B-cell lymphoma and classical Hodgkin lymphoma
Hodgkin Lymphoma
Nodular lymphocyte-predominant Hodgkin lymphoma
Classical Hodgkin lymphoma

(continued)

Table 9.1 (continued)

Nodular sclerosis classical Hodgkin lymphoma
Lymphocyte-rich classical Hodgkin lymphoma
Mixed cellularity classical Hodgkin lymphoma
Lymphocyte-depleted classical Hodgkin lymphoma
Mature T-cell neoplasms
T-cell prolymphocytic leukemia
T-cell large granular lymphocytic leukemia
Chronic lymphoproliferative disorder of NK cells*
Aggressive NK cell leukemia Systemic EBV + T-cell lymphoproliferative disease of childhood (associated with chronic active EBV infection)
Hydroa vacciniforme-like lymphoma
Adult T-cell leukemia/lymphoma
Extranodal NK/T-cell lymphoma, nasal type
Enteropathy-associated T-cell lymphoma
Hepatosplenic T-cell lymphoma
Subcutaneous panniculitis-like T-cell lymphoma
Mycosis fungoides Sézary syndrome
Primary cutaneous CD30+ T-cell lymphoproliferative disorder
Lymphomatoid papulosis
Primary cutaneous anaplastic large-cell lymphoma
*Primary cutaneous aggressive epidermotropic CD8+ cytotoxic T-cell lymphoma**
Primary cutaneous gamma-delta T-cell lymphoma
*Primary cutaneous small/medium CD4+ T-cell lymphoma**
Peripheral T-cell lymphoma, not otherwise specified
Angioimmunoblastic T-cell lymphoma
Anaplastic large-cell lymphoma (ALCL)
*ALK^+ Anaplastic large-cell lymphoma (ALCL), ALK^-**

*Provisional diagnosis or provisional subtypes of other neoplasms

lymphoma patients died because of their lymphoma. Lymphoma-related death was significantly associated on multivariable analysis with advanced clinical stage, age greater than 60 years, and large tumor growth fractions. Subtyping ocular adnexal lymphoma according to the WHO lymphoma classification, the stage of disease, and tumor cell growth fraction aided in prediction of tumor relapse, development of systemic disease, and lymphoma-related death.

Cross-References

Conjunctival lymphoma

Further Reading

Bertoni F, Coiffier B, Salles G, Stathis A, Traverse-Glehen A, Thieblemont C, Zucca E (2011) MALT lymphomas: pathogenesis can drive treatment. Oncology (Williston Park) 25(12):1134–1142

Cogliatti SB (2002) Who is WHO and what was REAL? Swiss Med Wkly 132:607–617

Coupland SE, Hellmich M, Au-Haedrich C et al (2004) Prognostic value of cell-cycle markers in ocular adnexal lymphoma: an assessment of 230 cases. Graefes Arch Clin Exp Ophthalmol 242:130–145

Harris NL, Jaffe ES, Stein H et al (1994) A revised European-American classification of lymphoid neoplasms: a proposal from the International Lymphoma Study Group. Blood 84:1361–1392

Jaffe ES (2009) The 2008 WHO classification of lymphomas; implications for clinical practice and translational research. Hematology Am Soc Hematol Educ Program 2009:523–531

O'Keefe JS, Sippy BD, Grossniklaus HE et al (2002) Anterior chamber infiltrate associated with systemic lymphoma. Ophthalmology 109:253–257

Pileri SA, Agostinelli C, Sabattini E et al (2011) Lymphoma classification: the quiet after the storm. Semin Diagn Pathol 28:113–123

Swerdlow SH, Campo E, Harris NL, Jaffe ES, Pileri SA, Stein H, Thiele J, Vardiman JW (eds) (2008) WHO classification of tumours of haematopoietic and lymphoid tissues, 4th edn. IARC Press, Lyon

Jaffe ES (2008) The 2008 WHO classification of lymphomas: implications for clinical practice and translational research. Hematology 2009:523–531

Surgical Techniques 10

Hans E. Grossniklaus, Chris Bergstrom,
G. Baker Hubbard III, and Jill R. Wells

Overview

There are numerous surgical techniques, including laser surgery and radiation, that are utilized in ocular oncology. These procedures may be used to biopsy and/or treat ocular tumors. The following is a brief overview of some techniques utilized for specific tumor types.

Conjunctival Tumors

Map biopsies: sebaceous carcinoma, PAM, melanoma

Multiple biopsies are obtained of the bulbar and tarsal conjunctiva in the map biopsy technique. They may be one per quadrant of the bulbar conjunctiva and three per tarsal conjunctiva as depicted (Fig. 10.1). This may be done in a minor procedure

H.E. Grossniklaus, M.D. (✉)
Emory University School of Medicine, Emory Eye Center,
Department of Ophthalmology,
Atlanta, GA, USA
e-mail: ophtheg@emory.edu

C. Bergstrom, M.D. • J.R. Wells, M.D.
Department of Ophthalmology, Emory University School of Medicine,
Atlanta, GA, USA
e-mail: cbergs2@emory.edu; jwells4@emory.edu

G.B. Hubbard III, M.D.
Department of Ophthalmology, Emory University School of Medicine,
Atlanta, GA, USA

The Emory Eye Center, Atlanta, GA, USA
e-mail: ghubba2@emory.edu

H.E. Grossniklaus (ed.), *Pocket Guide to Ocular Oncology and Pathology*,
DOI 10.1007/978-3-642-29782-3_10, © Springer-Verlag Berlin Heidelberg 2013

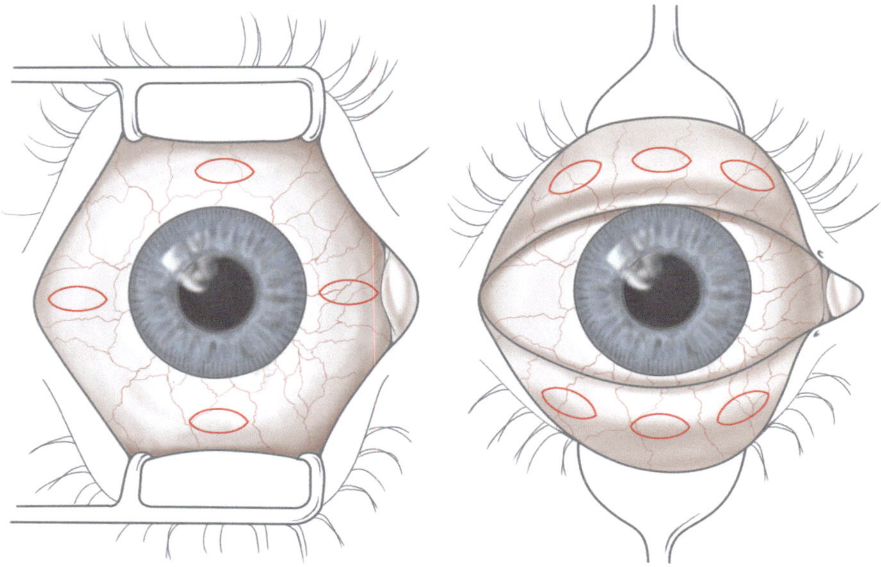

Fig. 10.1 Map biopsies of conjunctiva

room using local anesthesia, .12 forceps, and Westcott scissors. The biopsies are approximately 1–2 mm in diameter, and often no closure of the conjunctiva is required. The biopsies should be labeled regarding the site and submitted in separate cassettes for processing. A diagram of where the biopsies are obtained should be made, placed in the patient's chart, and accompany the cassettes to the pathology lab.

Resection: dysplasia, squamous cell carcinoma, PAM, melanoma, vascular tumors, peripheral nerve sheath tumors

The technique for resection of conjunctival tumors and cryotherapy is shown in Fig. 10.2. 2–3 mm external to the periphery of the tumor is marked with a marking pen. Debridement of involved cornea in cases of epithelial (dysplasia, squamous cell carcinoma) and melanocytic (PAM, melanoma) tumors is carried out with Weck cell sponges and absolute ethyl alcohol. In those tumors, hemostasis is obtained during resection with single use Weck cell sponges without cautery (dry field technique: no balance salt solution is used). The tumor is excised with .12 forceps and Westcott scissors using a no-touch technique. A superficial sclerectomy may be performed using a crescent blade. Double freeze-thaw cryotherapy is applied to the lateral and deep margins of excision for epithelial and melanocytic tumors.

Resection with sclerectomy: squamous cell carcinoma, melanoma, mucoepidermoid carcinoma, spindle cell carcinoma

In cases of extension of the tumor into the deep sclera, the tumor may be excised with a partial sclerectomy and patch graft application (Fig. 10.3). The tumor is resected as described above with the addition of a partial-thickness sclerectomy. A patch graft may be placed with interrupted 8-0 nylon sutures.

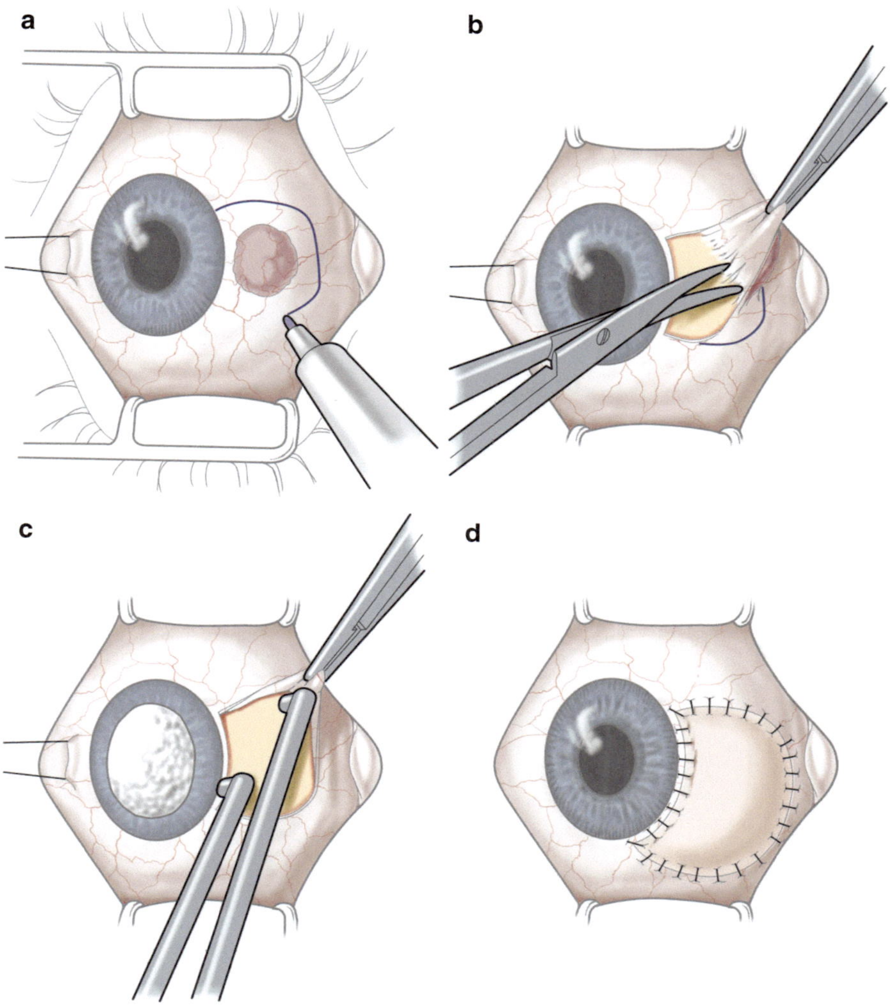

Fig. 10.2 Resection of conjunctival tumor with amniotic membrane graft placement

Brachytherapy: squamous cell carcinoma, melanoma, fibrous histiocytoma

In cases of deep extension where an eye wall resection cannot be performed, plaque brachytherapy (Fig. 10.4) may be applied using COMS dosing. The conjunctival tumor is outlined with a marking pen. A plaque is placed directly over the conjunctival tumor with care not to cover the insertion of an extraocular muscle. The plaque often straddles the limbus and extends onto the cornea. The plaque is sewn into place on the sclera using interrupted 5-0 nylon sutures through 3–4 islets. A tarsorrhaphy may be utilized.

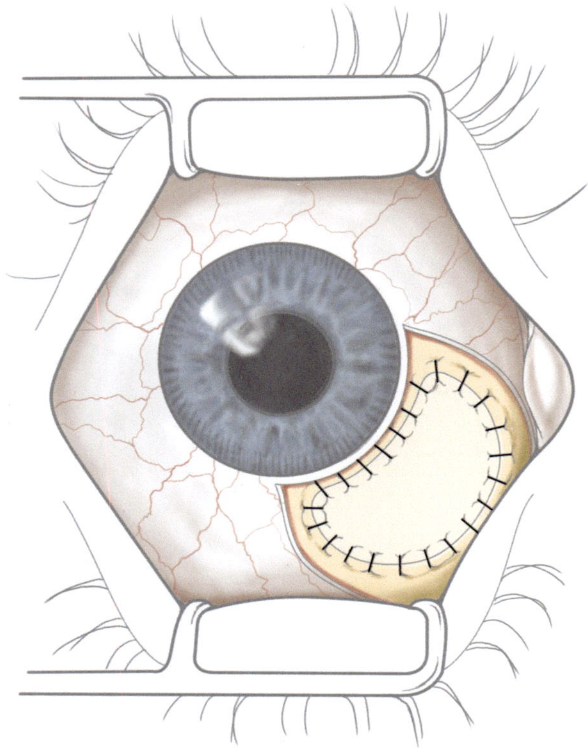

Fig. 10.3 Scleral patch graft after conjunctival tumor resection with partial lamellar sclerectomy

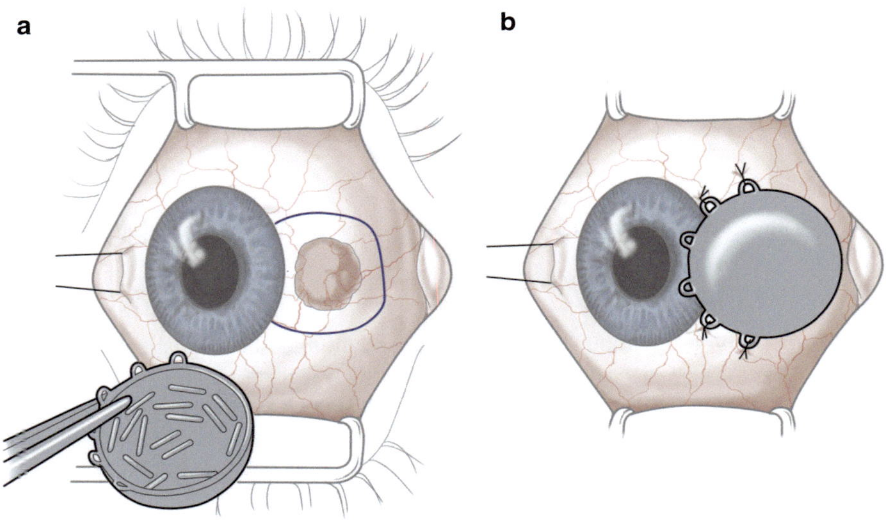

Fig. 10.4 Brachytherapy for conjunctival tumor

Iris/Ciliary Body Tumors

Fine-needle aspiration biopsy (FNAB): melanoma, metastasis

This technique may be performed at the slit lamp using topical anesthesia, including a 4% lidocaine pledget. A 1-cc syringe primed with BSS (not artificial tears) is used. A 27-gauge bevel down needle is inserted into the cornea near the limbus (Fig. 10.5) parallel and tangential to the tumor. Tumor cells may be aspirated using a vacuum cleaner technique, and the tumor may be impaled. The syringe is capped and submitted immediately for cytologic evaluation.

Iridectomy: melanoma

An iridectomy may be performed for iris melanocytic tumors confined to the iris leaflet without extension into the iridocorneal angle or ciliary body. This procedure is accomplished using a Weck blade to enter the anterior chamber at the limbus (Fig. 10.6). The wound may be enlarged to the left and right with the blade or corneoscleral scissors. Jeweler's forceps are utilized to lift the involved portion of iris, and DeWecker or Vannas scissors are used to excise the tumor. This may be accomplished using a peripheral or sector iridectomy. The corneal/limbal wound is then closed with interrupted 10-0 nylon sutures.

Iridocyclectomy/eye wall resection: melanoma, leiomyoma

A Flieringa ring may be place at the beginning of the procedure (Fig. 10.7). Transillumination and a marking pen are used to delineate the extent of the tumor.

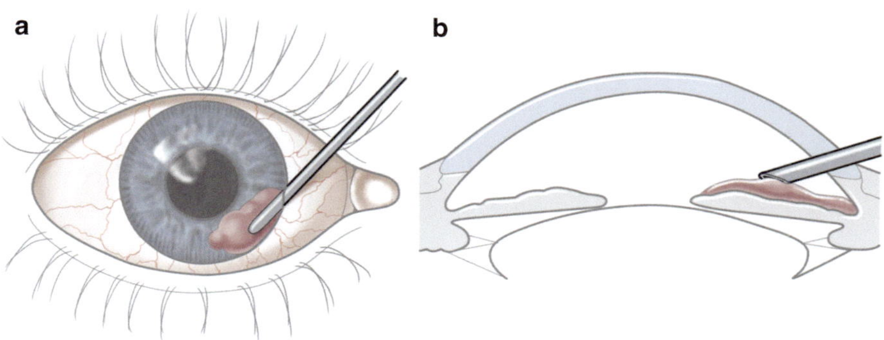

Fig. 10.5 Fine needle aspiration biopsy (FNAB) of iris lesion

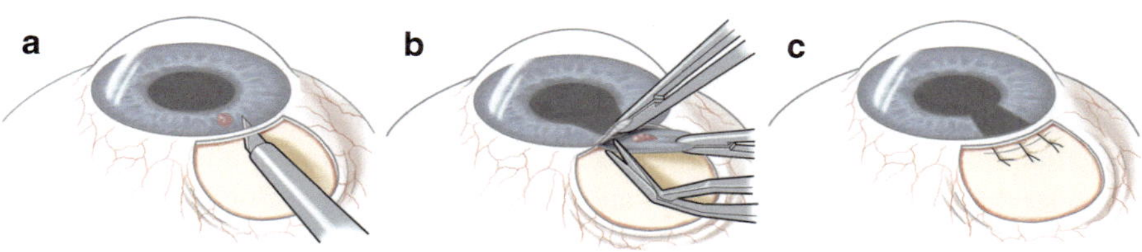

Fig. 10.6 Iridectomy

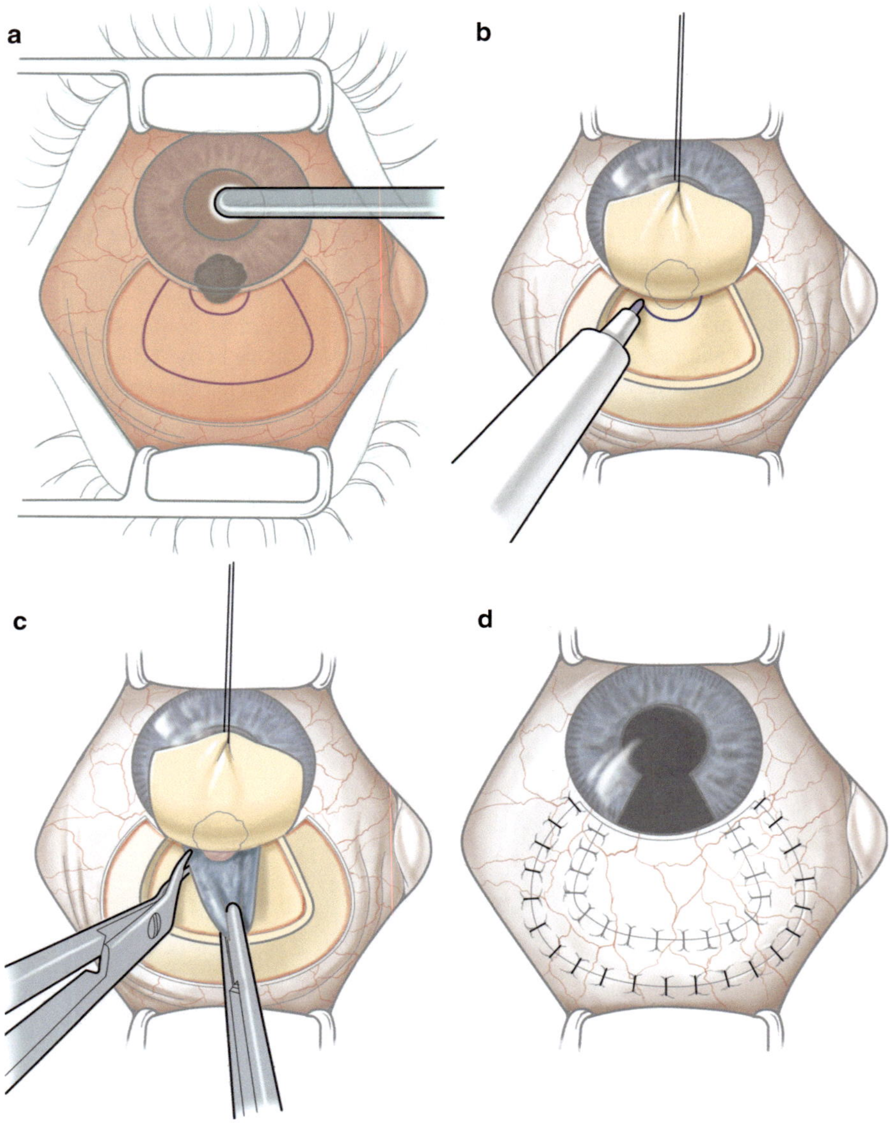

Fig. 10.7 Iridocylcectomy with partial lamellar sclerectomy

A partial-thickness limbal-based scleral flap is raised with a crescent blade, and the transillumination blockage caused by the tumor is outlined with a marking pen in the scleral bed. Dissecting scissors are used to perform a sector iridectomy and excise the sclera/underlying tumor including ciliary body component. The scleral bed flap is closed with interrupted sutures, and the conjunctiva is closed.

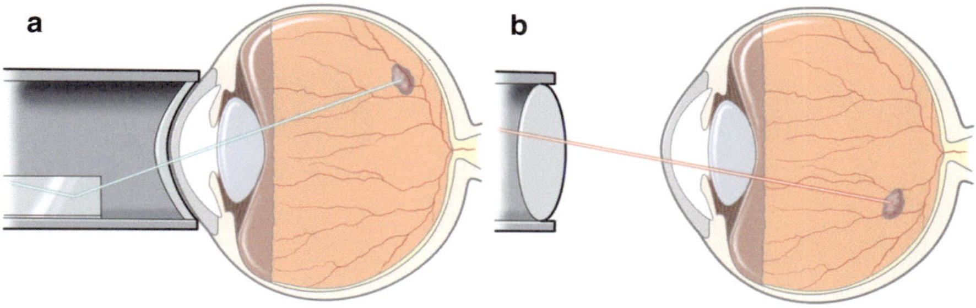

Fig. 10.8 Laser photocoagulation of retinal tumors

Brachytherapy: melanoma

For focal and localized peripheral iris tumors, a plaque covering the tumor and partially covering the cornea is utilized similar to what is shown in Fig. 4. For diffuse iris tumors, the plaque may entirely cover the cornea. A plaque containing I^{125} or Pd^{103} seeds is sewn to the sclera immediately posterior to the limbus for 360° so it directly covers the entire corneal surface. This is accomplished with approximately six interrupted 5-0 nylon sutures. There should be COMS dosing delivered. A tarsorrhaphy should be placed.

Retinal Tumors

Laser photocoagulation: hemangioblastoma, focal retinoblastoma

General techniques for laser photocoagulation are depicted utilizing a contact lens and indirect ophthalmoscope (Fig. 10.8). Laser photocoagulation may be performed in the clinic using local anesthesia (a retrobulbar block). The laser used (diode, argon) and laser power are dependent on the technique and tumor being treated. Examples are as follows. Photodynamic therapy (PDT) may be used for hemangioblastoma using a contact lens to deliver argon laser for 83 s after intravenous verteporfin injection. The argon green laser spot size is 6,000 μm, and half (300 mW/cm^2) or full (600 mW/cm^2) is utilized. For transpupillary thermotherapy (TTT) for retinoblastoma, an 810-nm diode laser is used, usually via indirect ophthalmoscopic delivery in the operating room under mask anesthesia. Doses range from 500–1,000 mW for several seconds to several minutes duration, depending on the size of the tumor. This technique may be used at the slit lamp in some instances for choroidal melanoma.

Choroidal Tumors

Fine-needle aspiration biopsy (*FNAB*): melanoma, metastasis

An FNAB may be performed via transvitreal or transscleral approaches (Fig. 10.9). Transvitreal FNAB may be accomplished in the operating room after a retrobulbar

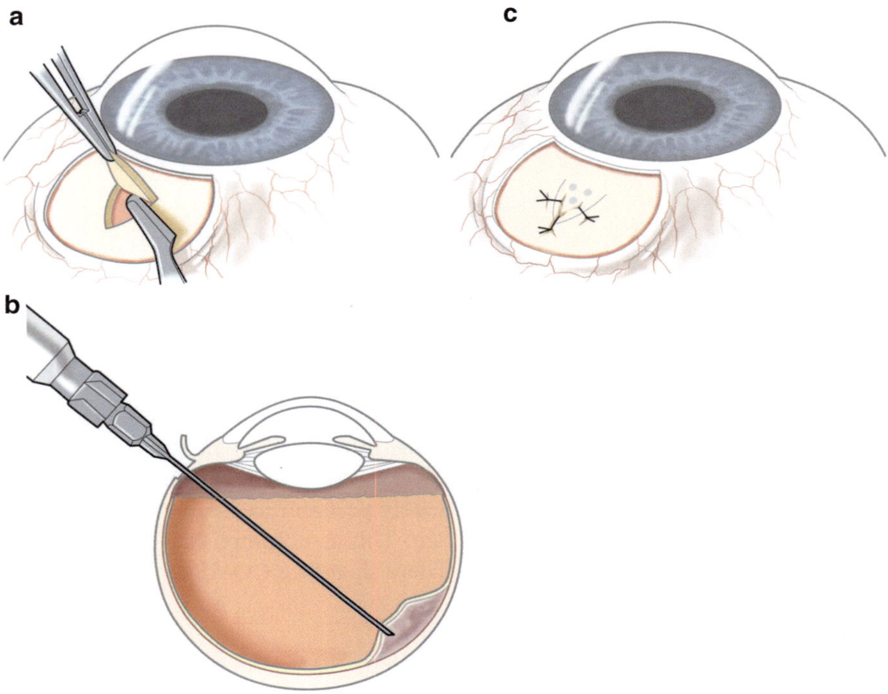

Fig. 10.9 Transcleral and transvitreal fine needle aspiration biopsy (FNAB)

block. A 27-gauge 1 ½-in. needle is inserted posterior to the limbus 3.5 (pseudophakic) or 4.0 (phakic) and directed toward the tumor under indirect ophthalmoscopic visualization. The needle is attached to a connector and syringe, and the syringe is aspirated. The transcleral approach is accomplished in the operating room using an operating microscope. After the conjunctiva is dissected, the tumor is localized by transillumination and outlined on the sclera with a marking pen. A partial-thickness scleral flap is made using a #15 blade, and a 27-gauge ½-in. needle on a connector is inserted into the tumor. The syringe is aspirated, and the needle is removed and capped. The scleral bed is then treated with cryotherapy. The scleral flap is closed with interrupted 8-0 nylon sutures, and the conjunctiva is closed with interrupted 6-0 plain gut sutures.

Brachytherapy: melanoma, some metastases

The technique for plaque brachytherapy for choroidal tumors is shown in Fig. 10.10. This is performed in the operating room under retrobulbar block or general anesthesia, depending on the condition of the patient and whether extraocular muscles will be disinserted. A conjunctival limbal peritomy is performed over the quadrant or quadrants occupied by the tumor. The conjunctiva is bluntly dissected, and the extraocular muscles surrounding and overlying the tumor are isolated with 2-0 silk sutures. Up to two extraocular muscles are disinserted as needed for exposure using Jameson muscle hooks, double-armed 6-0 Vicryl suture including the

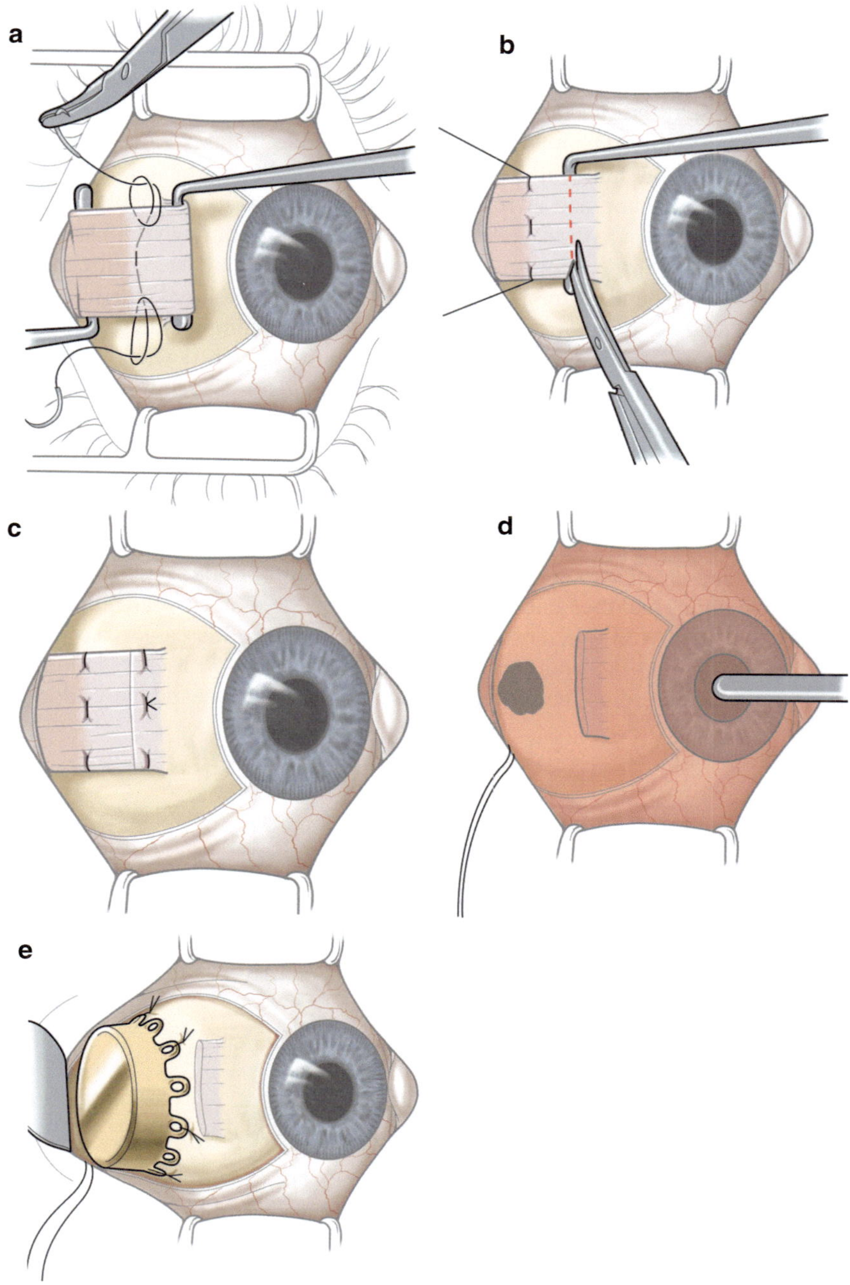

Fig. 10.10 Brachytherapy for choroidal tumor

quick stitch technique. The needles are cut from the suture, and the suture is taped to the patient's cheek/forehead at the end of the surgery in order to locate the extraocular muscle. After the plaque is removed approximately 1 week after placement, the extraocular muscles are located with the suture, and the suture is replaced with a fresh 6-0 Vicryl suture. The muscle is then reattached to its insertion as shown. For plaque placement, the tumor is identified by transillumination or indirect ophthalmoscopy/scleral indentor, and its margins are outlined on the sclera with a marking pen. The plaque is sewn to the sclera using 5-0 nylon sutures through the islets. There are typically two to three sutures used. Plaque placement may be confirmed using intraoperative ultrasound. After placement, the conjunctiva is closed with interrupted 6-0 plain gut sutures. A tarsorrhaphy may be placed depending on the size and location of the plaque. The plaque is then removed approximately 1 week after placement, depending on the radiation oncology dosing protocol.

Enucleation: melanoma, retinoblastoma, medulloepithelioma

An enucleation technique is shown in Fig. 10.11. A 360° limbal peritomy is performed with Westcott scissors and blunt dissection. The extraocular recti muscles are isolated with muscle hooks and 4-0 silk traction sutures and are disinserted as needed for exposure using Jameson muscle hooks and double-armed 6-0 Vicryl suture including the quick stitch technique. The superior oblique tendon is isolated with muscle hooks and then cut. The inferior oblique tendon is isolated with muscle hook, clamped with a hemostat, cut, and the distal end is cauterized prior to removing the clamp. The optic nerve is strummed and cut with enucleation scissors. Pressure is placed on the posterior orbit using a gauze soaked with lidocaine/

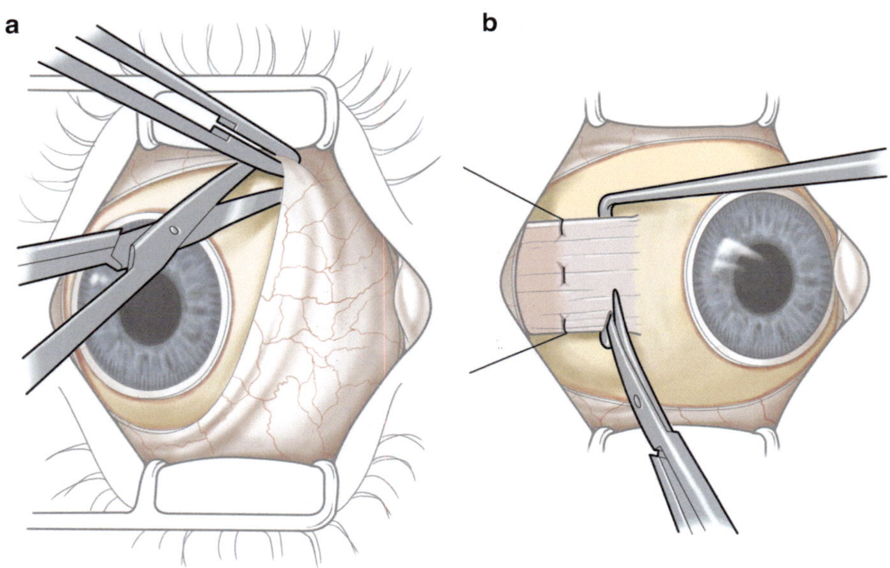

Fig. 10.11 Enucleationa

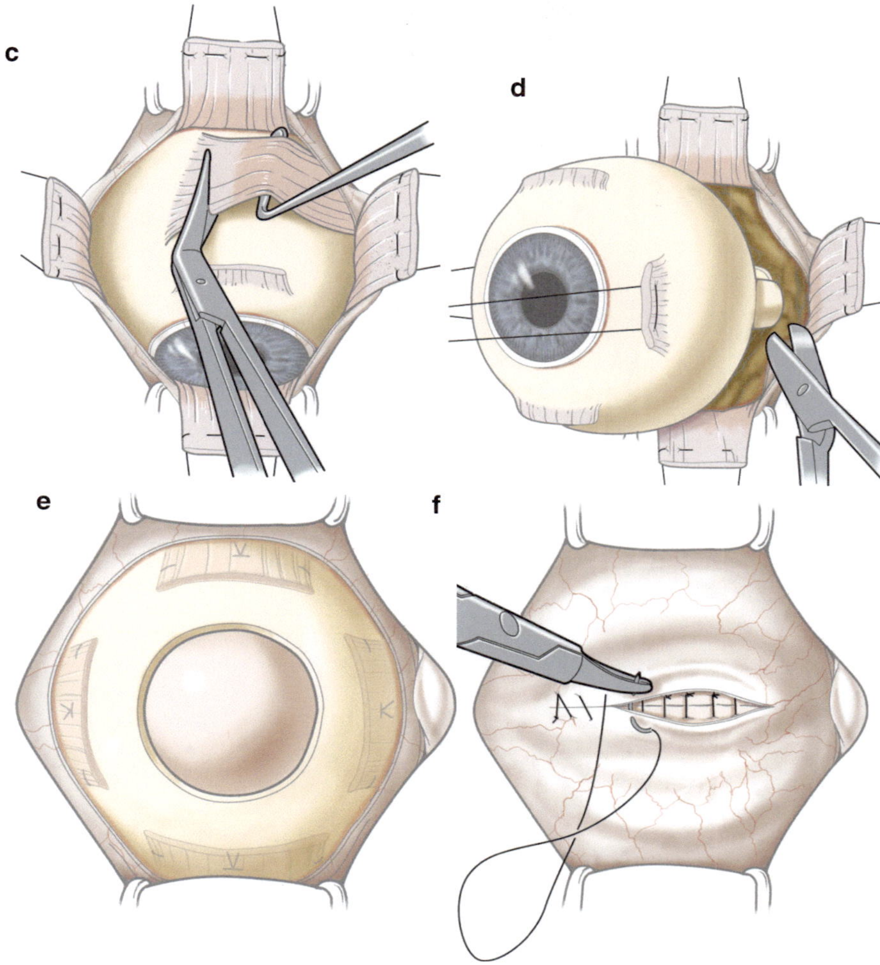

Fig. 10.11 (continued)

marcaine/epinephrine. In cases of an acrylic implant, the implant may be covered with donor sclera sewn in place with a purse-string 5-0 Vicryl or mersilene suture. The implant is placed in the orbit. Approximate locations of the extraocular muscle insertions are marked with a marking pen, and the muscles are attached as shown. Alternatively, the muscles may be directly attached to hydroxyapatite and Medpor implants. Tenon's capsule is closed with interrupted 5-0 Vicryl suture, and the conjunctiva is closed with 6-0 plain gut suture. A conformer and pressure patch are placed.

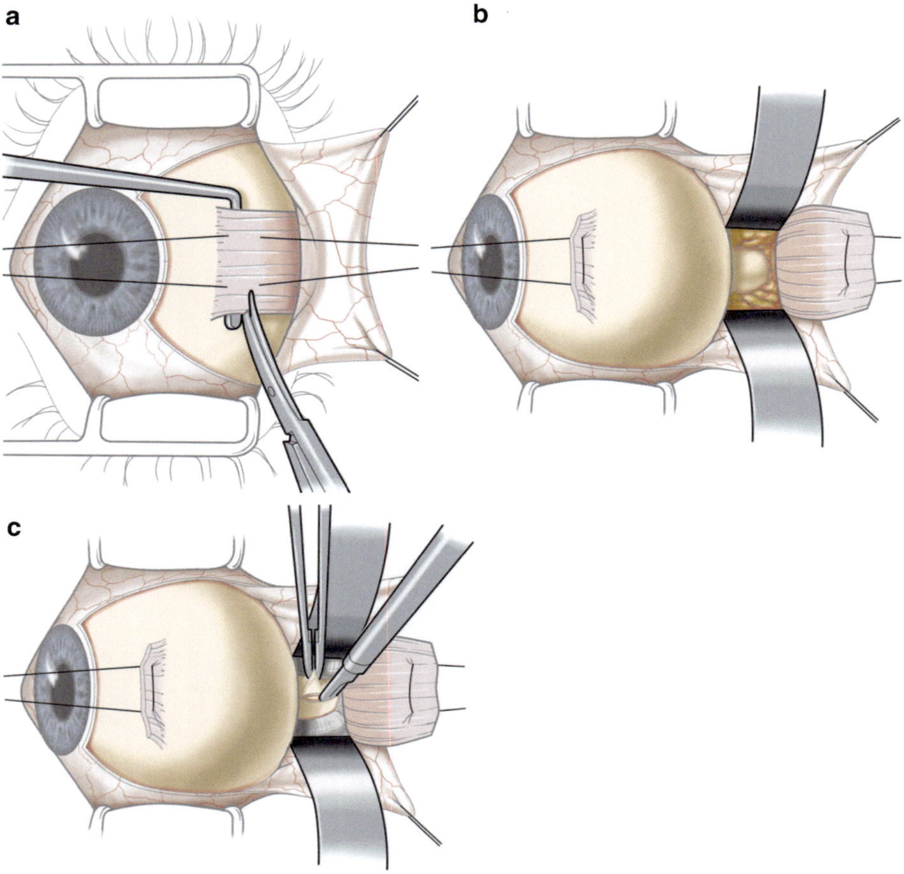

Fig. 10.12 Optic nerve biopsy

Optic Nerve Tumors

Optic nerve tumors: glioma, meningioma, metastasis

Biopsy

An optic nerve biopsy technique, generally performed by an oculoplastic surgeon, is shown in Fig. 10.12. A medial fornix approach may be utilized to expose the optic nerve just posterior to the globe. Top: A peritomy is performed along the nasal limbus with wing incision. The conjunctiva is tagged with 7-0 plain gut sutures. Double-armed 6-0 Vicryl sutures are place in the medial rectus, and a single 5-0 nylon suture is passed near the limbus for retraction. Middle: The medial rectus is disinserted, the globe is abducted, retractors are placed, and the nerve is exposed with gentle retraction of the neighboring orbital fat. Cottonoids are placed around the nerve. Bottom: The nerve sheath, perineural tissue, and nerve may be biopsied. The medial rectus is reattached, and the conjunctiva is closed after the biopsy.

Further Reading

Damato B (2000) Ocular tumors: diagnosis and treatment. Butterworth-Heinemann, Oxford

Shields JA, Shields CL (2007) Intraocular tumors. An atlas and text. Lippincott & Williams, Philadelphia

Singh AD (2007) Clinical ophthalmic oncology. Elsevier, Saunders, Philadelphia

Tissue Preparation for Pathological Examination

11

Harry H. Brown, Jill R. Wells, and Hans E. Grossniklaus

Synonyms

None.

Basic Characteristics

Tissue Fixation

Unless special procedures are necessary, tissue excised in the clinic or operating room should be placed in fixative immediately to avoid autolysis. 10% neutral buffered formalin is the standard fixative used in surgical pathology. Tissue may be submitted in the fresh state when intraoperative consultation is desired or if studies requiring fresh tissue (lymphoma workup) are indicated; prior communication with the pathologist is critical to achieve optimal utilization of the available tissue. Transport media may be necessary for immunofluorescence studies, flow cytometry,

H.H. Brown, M.D. (✉)
Department of Pathology, Harvey and Bernice Jones Eye Institute,
University of Arkansas School of Medicine, Little Rock, AR, USA
e-mail: brownharryh@uams.edu

J.R. Wells, M.D.
Department of Ophthalmology,
Emory University School of Medicine, Atlanta, GA, USA
e-mail: jwells4@emory.edu

H.E. Grossniklaus, M.D.
Emory University School of Medicine,
Emory Eye Center,
Department of Ophthalmology,
Atlanta, GA, USA
e-mail: ophtheg@emory.edu

H.E. Grossniklaus (ed.), *Pocket Guide to Ocular Oncology and Pathology*,
DOI 10.1007/978-3-642-29782-3_11,

and cytogenetic analysis. In such special situations, transportation of the unfixed tissue must be done quickly and handled immediately upon receipt; again, prior communication with the pathologist is required.

Gross Examination

Once accessioned, the tissue specimen must undergo gross examination by a pathologist or pathology assistant, who will describe the characteristics of the tissue, dissect the specimen, and submit some or all of the specimen for histological examination by placing selected tissue portions into labeled cassettes. Specimens harboring malignancy will have ink applied to the surgical margin(s) prior to sectioning; this ink will remain through tissue processing and sectioning and be visible on microscopic examination. Determining how the specimen is sectioned, such as a conjunctival tumor, will depend on the size of the lesion (Fig. 11.1).

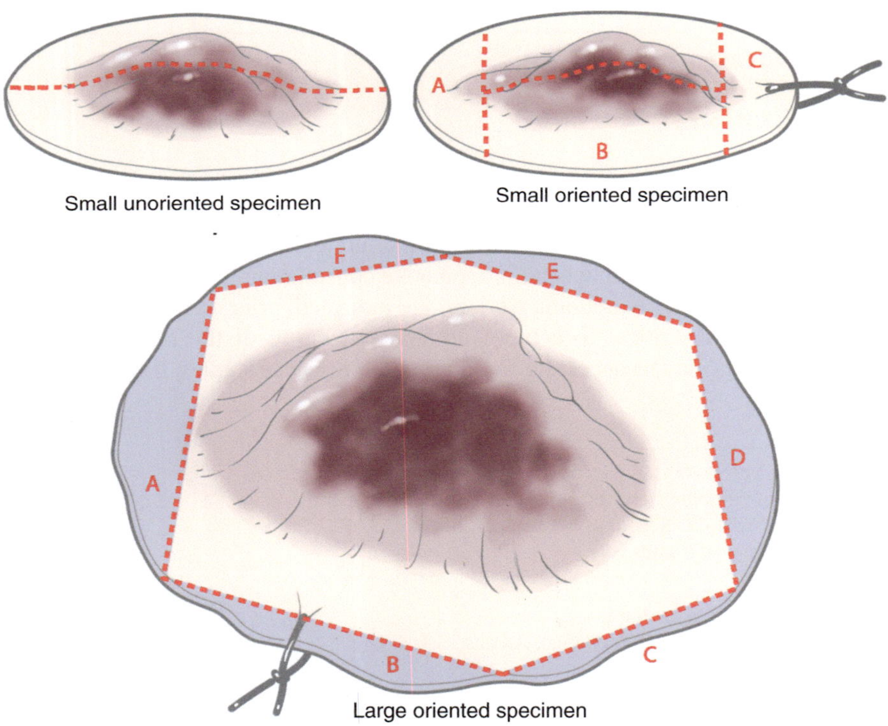

Fig. 11.1 The extent of the tumor in a conjunctiva or intraocular tumor resection should be determined at the dissecting microscope. Small unoriented specimens may be bisected. Small specimens that have been oriented by the surgeon should be cut and submitted in such a way as to be able to evaluate the center of the tumor and margins of resection. Large specimens should include the center of the tumor in a cassette and may have their margins inked and submitted in separate cassettes

Tissue Processing

Automated tissue processors are employed, typically overnight, to infiltrate the tissue with molten paraffin which can then be cooled and solidified. In order to achieve this, the tissue must first be dehydrated by passing through a series of graded alcohols, ending in absolute alcohol. The alcohol that has replaced the water in the tissue must then be removed and replaced with a clearing agent, an organic solvent that is miscible with paraffin; most laboratories use xylene for this procedure. Finally, the xylene-saturated tissue is placed in molten paraffin which supports the tissue structure when chilled. The entire processing typically takes 10–12 h.

Tissue Embedding, Cutting, and Staining

The tissue sections from the tissue processor are then embedded in a paraffin block for mounting on a microtome, a machine capable of slicing thin (2–5-μm) sections of the tissue. These are floated on a warm water bath to eliminate wrinkles and then picked up by a glass slide. The glass slides are then stained, routinely with hematoxylin and eosin, and coverslipped. The end result is a histological section of the submitted tissue, now ready for microscopic examination.

Special Procedures

Frozen Sectioning

For intraoperative consultation, time is of the essence. Thus, the fixation and processing steps above must be replaced by a procedure capable of rapid production of a stained histological section. Frozen sectioning takes the tissue from the gross bench, and by placing the tissue in a cutting medium and mounting it on a chuck and rapidly freezing it to −25°F or so, the tissue can be sectioned in a cryostat within minutes of receipt.

Immunofluorescence and Immunohistochemistry

Using fluorescein-labeled antibodies to highlight immunoglobulin deposition along the epidermal basement membrane in ocular cicatricial pemphigoid requires fresh tissue and frozen sectioning as described above. Immunohistochemistry may be performed on formalin-fixed, paraffin-embedded material.

Flow Cytometry

Flow cytometry is the method of analyzing individual cells suspended in a fluid and requires fresh tissue. It is most commonly employed in the evaluation of lymphoproliferative processes by fluorochrome labeling the cells with various antibodies against surface molecules specific to lymphocyte subsets and to other cell types and then passing the cells single file through an exciting light source and amplifying light emissions with a photodetector. The results are analyzed by computer, and scatter plots are generated.

Molecular Pathology

Examination of DNA and RNA is possible by using amplification techniques (polymerase chain reaction [PCR]) with specifically developed primers to detect genetic mutations or alterations. The procedure can be performed on fixed nucleic acid retrieved from paraffin-embedded tissue.

Special Considerations

Conjunctival Biopsy Specimens

Conjunctiva tends to roll up on itself while in fixative, making it difficult to assess the margins. It is therefore helpful to gently spread the specimen epithelial side up on pieces of heavy paper or cardboard prior to fixation. Surgeons should consider submitting smaller margins as separate specimens in different labeled containers.

Enucleated Eyes Harboring Melanoma

These eyes are transilluminated prior to dissection to be sure the PO (pupil-optic nerve) section also contains the melanoma. A sample of fresh tumor for genetic and other testing may be obtained prior to fixation as shown in Fig. 11.2. The eye is held directly in front of a bright light source, and the eye is rotated on the surface of the light until the tumor shadow is prominent. The outline is traced with a marking device. A razor blade is then used to make two parallel slices through the eye, creating a PO section which includes the tumor (Fig. 11.3).

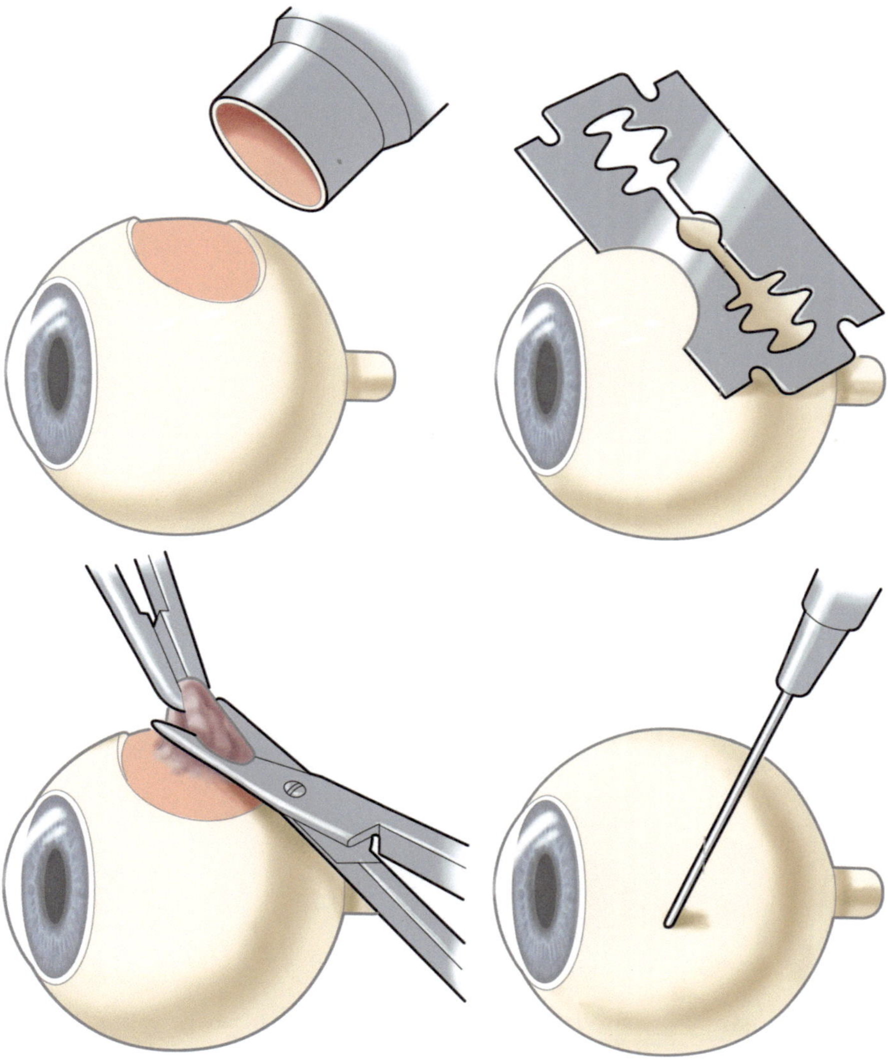

Fig. 11.2 There are several methods of obtaining fresh tumor in the operating room under sterile conditions. These include obtaining a section of sclera and tumor with a trephine, making a cut with a razor blade into the eye and removing tumor with forceps, and transscleral aspiration of a tumor using a 23-gauge needle

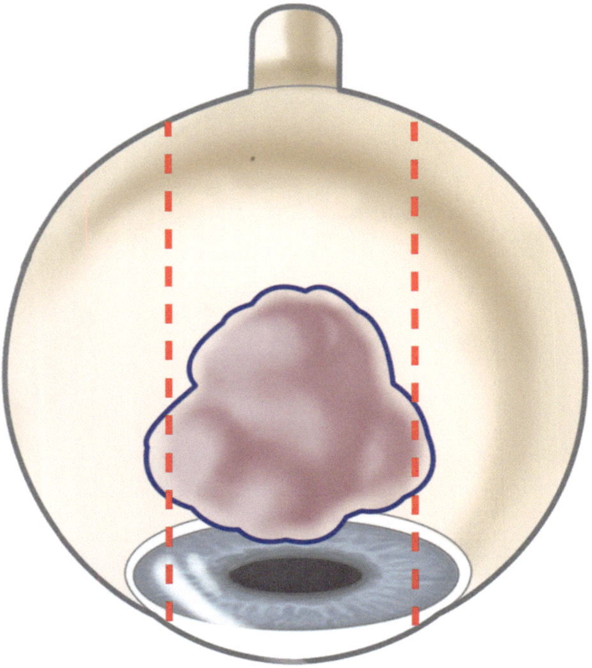

Fig. 11.3 After transillumination and marking outline of the tumor in the sclera, a pupil-optic nerve (PO) section containing the center of the tumor is created by removing the calottes as shown

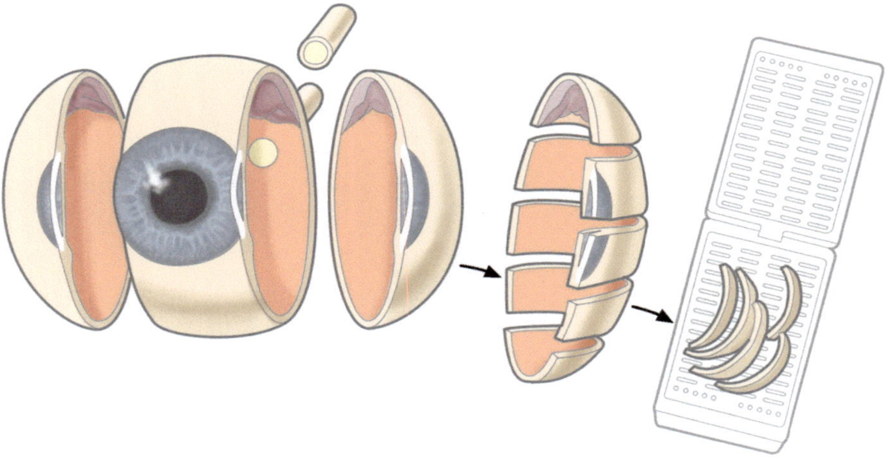

Fig. 11.4 When an eye with a retinoblastoma is sectioned, the PO section and calottes should be submitted for processing as shown. Each calotte may be bread-loafed and submitted in a separate cassette. The distal end of the optic nerve should also be submitted in a separate cassette for processing

Enucleated Eyes Harboring Retinoblastoma

The eye should be submitted in four blocks. One block is the central PO section containing the optic nerve, tumor, and anterior chamber structures. Two blocks will contain the calottes in anterior-posterior segments embedded on edge to examine more choroidal surface. The last block contains the cross section of the margin of the optic nerve (Fig. 11.4).

Further Reading

Eagle RC (1995) Specimen handling in the ophthalmic pathology laboratory. Ophthalmol Clin North Am 8(1):1–15

Folberg R, Salomao D, Grossniklaus HE, Proia AD, Rao NA, Cameron JD (2003) Recommendations for the reporting of tissues removed as part of the surgical treatment of common malignancies of the eye and its adnexa. Am J Surg Path 27:999–1004

Rosa Jr RH, Gombos DS, Harocopos G, Kivela TT, Kramer TR, Milman T (2011) Ophthalmic pathology and intraocular tumors; Section 4, basic and clinical science course. American Academy of Ophthalmology, San Francisco, CA

Xavier S, Chantada GL, François D, Wilson MW, de Davila MTG, Carlos RG, Murali C, Patricia CB (2009) Proceedings of the consensus meetings from the International Retinoblastoma Staging Working Group on the pathology guidelines for the examination of enucleated eyes and evaluation of prognostic risk factors in retinoblastoma. Arch Pathol Lab Med 133(8):1199–1202

Transillumination

12

Linda Janku and Arun D. Singh

Definition

Transillumination, or diaphanography, is the process of passing light through an opaque object and illuminating all the irregularities within the object. Clinical applications of transillumination date back to 1905 due to its simplicity and, in fact, were one of the first imaging modalities.

Purpose

In order to effectively assess a patient with transillumination, absolute darkness is necessary. A very bright light is transmitted through a fiber optic probe, which is placed against the anesthetized eye (Fig. 12.1).

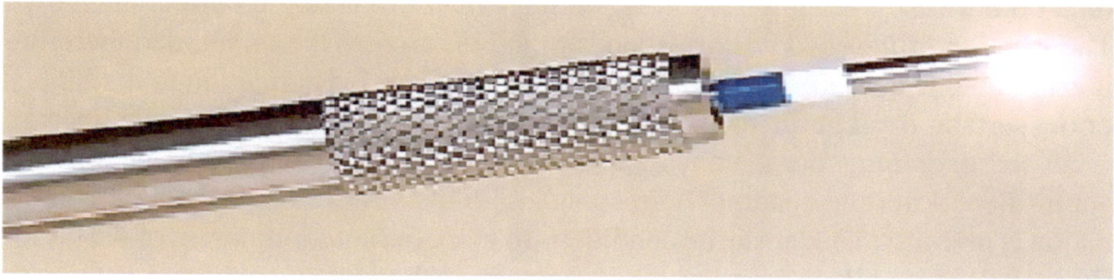

Fig. 12.1 Transillumination probe

L. Janku, COA
Department of Ophthalmic Oncology, Cole Eye Institute, Cleveland Clinic, Cleveland, OH, USA

A.D. Singh, M.D. (✉)
Department of Ophthalmic Oncology, Cole Eye Institute, Cleveland Clinic Foundation, 9500 Euclid Avenue, Desk i-329, Cleveland, OH 44195, USA
e-mail: singha@ccf.org

H.E. Grossniklaus (ed.), *Pocket Guide to Ocular Oncology and Pathology*, DOI 10.1007/978-3-642-29782-3_12, © Springer-Verlag Berlin Heidelberg 2013

Principle

Transillumination may be done transpupillarly (across the pupil) or transocularly (across the globe). Transpupillary transillumination is accomplished by placing the illuminator on the cornea. Transocular transillumination is achieved by placing the fiber optic probe directly opposite to the tumor.

Indications

Transillumination is a supplementary test to indirect ophthalmoscopy, ultrasonography, and ultrasound biomicroscopy. It is often used in the office setting to detect, differentiate, locate, and measure the size of the tumor. In presence of opaque media, transillumination may reveal a shadow indicating presence of an intraocular tumor.

Contraindications

A patient must be able to cooperate and has to respond to the examiner's request of maintaining gaze in a particular direction. The bright light can also be uncomfortable to some patients. In Blacks and patients with ocular melanocytosis, transillumination may not be revealing due to the increased uveal pigmentation.

Advantages/Disadvantages

As uveal melanoma is usually pigmented, it will cast a shadow on transillumination (Fig. 12.2). Other choroidal tumors such as hemangioma, metastasis, and leiomyoma do not cast a shadow, and these findings help in making a correct diagnosis. The location of the shadow corresponds to the location of the tumor, and therefore it is possible to determine the anterior or posterior margins in relation to the limbus or ora serrata. In addition, the size of the shadow can be measured using calipers.

In the operating room, transillumination is an integral part of brachytherapy application. After the quadrant corresponding to the tumor is exposed, transillumination is performed under sterile conditions to mark the anterior margin of the tumor (Fig. 12.2). This allows appropriate placement of the plaque anchoring sutures to the sclera.

Cross-References

Ultrasonography, brachytherapy

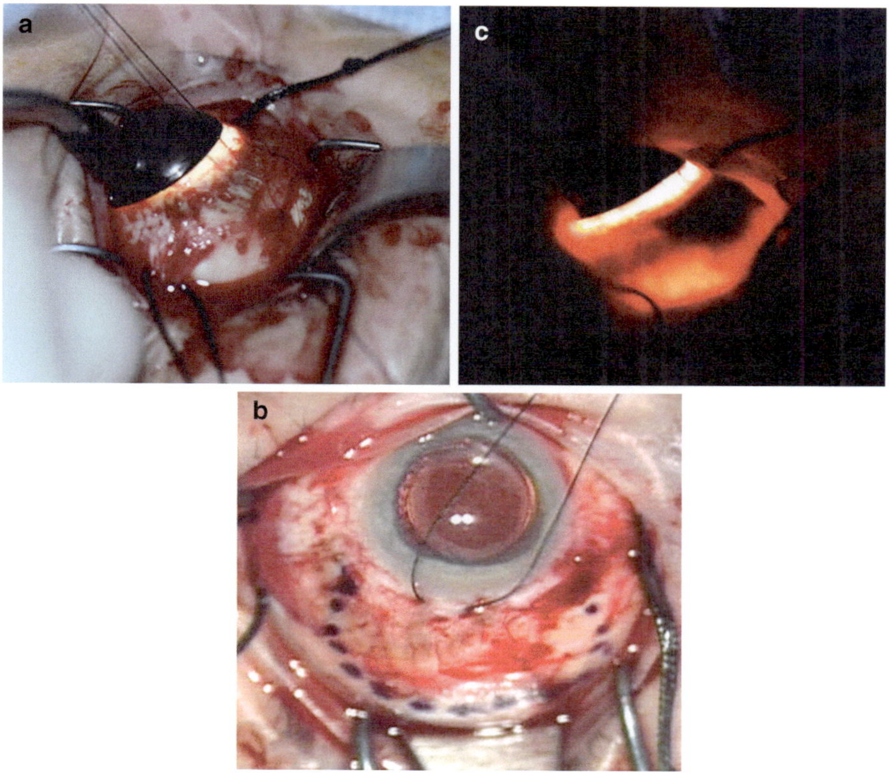

Fig. 12.2 Intraoperative photos of transillumination. The quadrant containing the tumor is exposed, and the transilluminator is placed over the cornea (**a**). The room lights are turned off and the tumor shadow is visible (**b**). The tumor margins are marked for plaque placement (**c**)

Further Reading

Thompson ES (1905) Instruments and methods of examination. The Sachs lamp for transillumination of the eye. Trans Am Ophthalmol Soc 10:456–460

Trichopoulos N, Damato BE (2007) Examination techniques. In: Singh AD, Damato BE, Pe'er J, Murphree AL, Perry JD (eds) Clinical ophthalmic oncology, 1st edn. Saunders-Elsevier, Philadelphia, pp 171–174

Ultrasound Techniques

13

Brandy C. Hayden and Arun D. Singh

Synonyms

Echographic techniques, Ultrasonographic techniques

Definition

Ultrasonography of the eye is a diagnostic technique wherein high-frequency sound waves are used to examine and measure ophthalmic structures.

Purpose

Ophthalmic ultrasonography is used to evaluate a large range of ophthalmic disorders and pathology using a safe, noninvasive diagnostic tool that provides real-time images.

Principle

Ultrasonography of the eye uses a transducer that emits high-frequency acoustic waves ranging from 8 to 80 MHz. During the evaluation, the eye is anesthetized with a topical anesthetic. A coupling agent is applied to the transducer before placing it on

B.C. Hayden, BS (✉)
Department of Diagnostic Imaging, Cole Eye Institute, Cleveland Clinic Foundation, Cleveland, OH, USA
e-mail: haydenb@ccf.org

A.D. Singh, M.D.
Department of Ophthalmic Oncology, Cole Eye Institute, Cleveland Clinic Foundation, 9500 Euclid Avenue, Desk i-329, Cleveland, OH 44195, USA
e-mail: singha@ccf.org

H.E. Grossniklaus (ed.), *Pocket Guide to Ocular Oncology and Pathology*,
DOI 10.1007/978-3-642-29782-3_13,

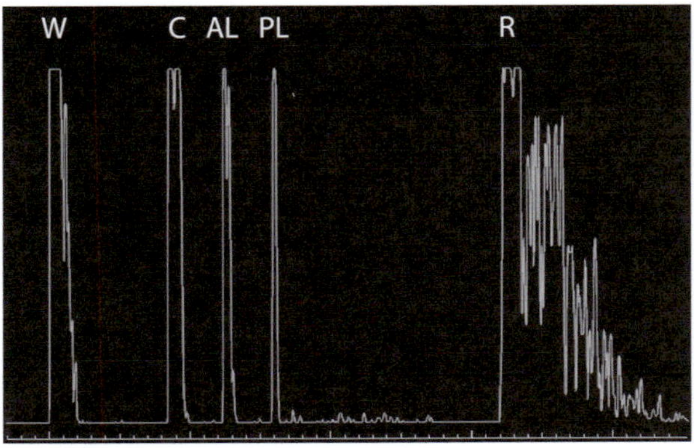

Fig. 13.1 Immersion biometric A-scan of a normal phakic eye. The spikes correspond to water bath (*W*), anterior and posterior cornea surface (*C*), anterior (*AL*) and posterior lens capsule (*PL*), and retina (*R*)

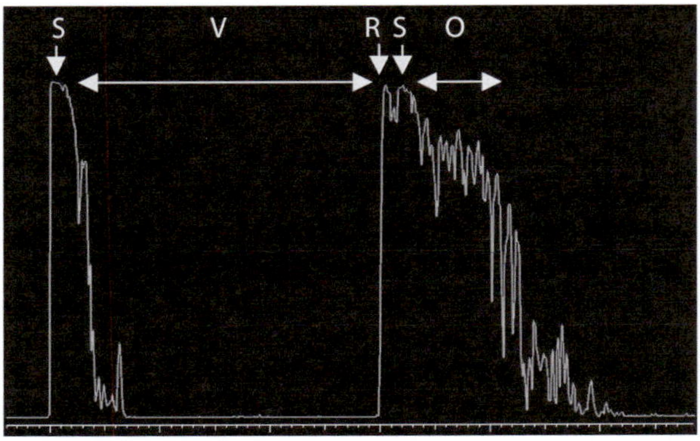

Fig. 13.2 Diagnostic A-scan in a normal eye. Echo showing transscleral A-scan produced by placing the probe against the sclera and directing the sound beam perpendicular to the retina. *S* sclera, *V* vitreous, *R* retina, *O* orbital tissue

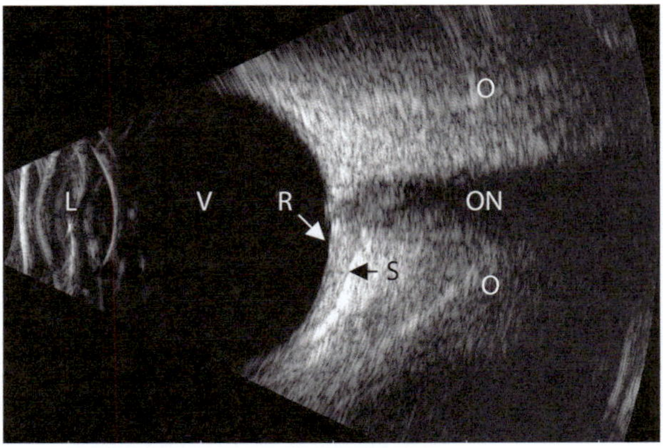

Fig. 13.3 Contact B-scan in a normal eye shows a cross section of the posterior segment. Axial scan obtained by directing the sound beam across the visual axis through the cornea and lens. *L* lens, *V* vitreous, *R* retina, *S* sclera, *ON* optic nerve, *O* orbital tissue

the eye. Echoes, or reflections of the sound waves, are produced at each interface of different materials having different acoustic impedances. The echoes are processed resulting in a picture representing structures of the eye.

The most frequently used ophthalmic ultrasound instrumentation includes biometry (Fig. 13.1), diagnostic A-scan (Fig. 13.2), B-scan (Fig. 13.3), and ultrasound biomicroscopy (UBM) (Fig. 13.4). A-scan is a one-dimensional display of echo strength over time utilizing frequencies in the range of 8–12 MHz. Biometric A-scan

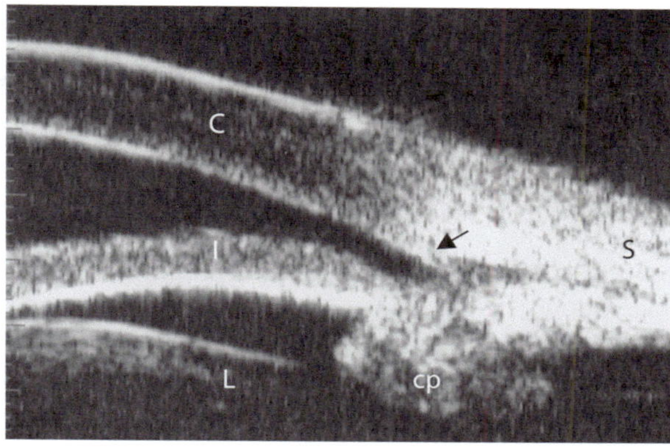

Fig. 13.4 UBM of the angle region. *Arrow* scleral spur (*arrow*), *cp* ciliary processes, *C* cornea, *L* lens, *I* iris, *S* sclera

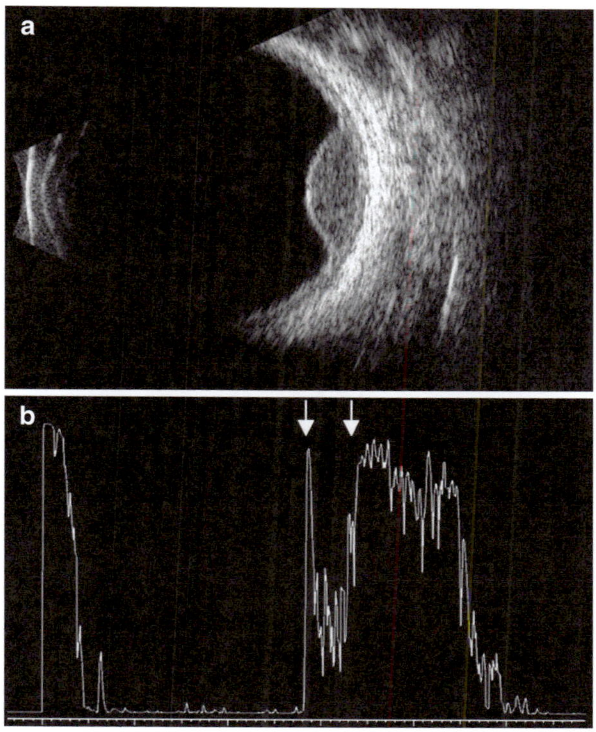

Fig. 13.5 Choroidal melanoma. Transverse B-scan demonstrates a dome-shaped lesion (**a**). Diagnostic A-scan directed perpendicular to the lesion shows the lesion is regularly structured and low reflective (**b**, *arrows*)

is used to determine axial eye lengths, most commonly prior to cataract surgery and intraocular lens implantation. Diagnostic A-scan allows for the detection and differentiation of abnormal intraocular tissues.

B-scan and UBM are two-dimensional displays of echoes utilizing frequencies in the range of 10–20 MHz and 35–80 MHz, respectively. B-scan is used to evaluate topographic features to assess shape, location, and extension of ocular structures and to evaluate retinal detachment, retinal tear, choroidal detachment, intraocular tumor, and orbital inflammation (Fig. 13.5). Ultrasound biomicroscopy allows evaluation of the anterior segment of the eye including anterior chamber, anterior chamber angle, and ciliary body. Color Doppler, which utilizes two-dimensional ultrasound combined with the evaluation of blood flow, and 3-D ultrasonography have limited applications in ophthalmology.

Indications

Ophthalmic ultrasonography is most frequently indicated for evaluation when media opacities, including corneal opacities, anterior chamber opacities, cataracts, vitreous hemorrhage, or inflammatory opacities, preclude ophthalmoscopic evaluation. It is also valuable for the documentation, measurement, and differentiation of intraocular tumors and the evaluation of anterior and orbital structures in the presence of clear media.

Contraindication

None.

Advantages

The superficial location of the eye and its primary aqueous-based structures make the use of high-frequency ultrasonography an ideal diagnostic tool. Ophthalmic ultrasound is noninvasive and well tolerated.

Disadvantages

Ocular structures and lesions in the posterior segment that are less than 0.5 mm in height cannot be clearly delineated with current ophthalmic ultrasonographic instruments.

Cross-References

Anatomic considerations, choroidal melanoma

Further Reading

Bryne S, Green R (2002) Ultrasound of the eye and orbit, 2nd edn. Mosby, St. Louis
Ossoinig KC (1979) Standardized echography- the basis of tissue differentiation. J Clin Ultrasound 19:127–210
Pavlin CJ, Foster FS (1995) Ultrasound biomicroscopy of the eye. Springer, New York
Singh AD, Hayden BH, Pavlin CJ (2008) Ophthalmic ultrasound. Ultrasound Clin 3:179–276

Part II

Conjunctival and Corneal Tumors

Conjunctival Carcinoma: Squamous Cell 14

Philip Laird and Hans E. Grossniklaus

Synonyms

There are no synonyms for this condition.

Definition

Invasive squamous cell carcinomas have features similar to dysplasias, but the basement membrane of the epithelium is violated, and the subepithelial tissue is invaded.

Etiology

Risk factors for conjunctival carcinoma include UVB exposure, HPV, advanced age, tobacco smoke, and occupational exposure to petroleum products. Conjunctival dysplasia is a precursor to conjunctival squamous cell carcinoma.

P. Laird, M.D. (✉)
Department of Ophthalmology, Emory Eye Center,
Atlanta, GA, USA
e-mail: plaird@emory.edu

H.E. Grossniklaus, M.D.
Emory University School of Medicine,
Emory Eye Center,
Department of Ophthalmology,
Atlanta, GA, USA
e-mail: ophtheg@emory.edu

H.E. Grossniklaus (ed.), *Pocket Guide to Ocular Oncology and Pathology*,
DOI 10.1007/978-3-642-29782-3_14, © Springer-Verlag Berlin Heidelberg 2013

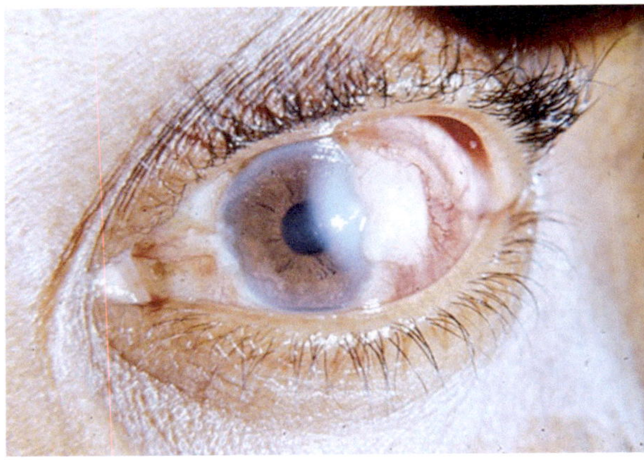

Fig. 14.1 Clinical appearance of conjunctival squamous cell carcinoma appearing as white nodule at the limbus

Clinical Presentation

Conjunctival squamous cell carcinoma may appear as a gelatinous mass, white plaque or mimic a diffuse inflammatory process (Fig. 14.1).

Diagnosis

The diagnosis is based on histopathologic examination of a surgically excised specimen.

Pathology

Histopathologic examination demonstrates infiltrating nests that have penetrated the epithelial basement membrane and spread into the conjunctival stroma (Fig. 14.2). Tumor cells may be well differentiated and easily recognizable as squamous, moderately differentiated, or poorly differentiated.

Differential Diagnosis

The clinical differential diagnosis includes papilloma, conjunctival dysplasia, amelanotic melanoma, and pyogenic granuloma. There are two variants of squamous cell carcinoma (spindle cell and mucoepidermoid) discussed elsewhere.

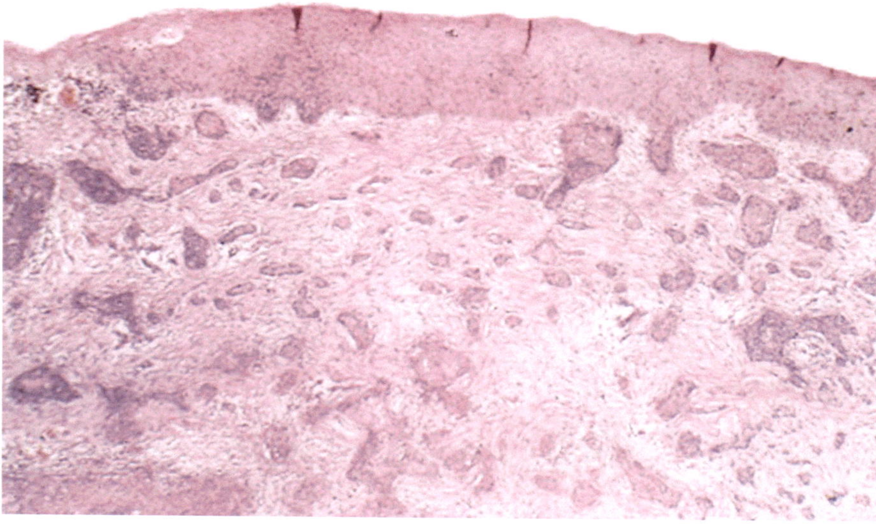

Fig. 14.2 The histopathologic appearance of the excised lesion shown in Fig. 14.1 demonstrates tongues of tumor cells invading the substantia propria

Prophylaxis

Excision or topical therapy of dysplasia, usually with mitomycin C.

Therapy

The treatment of choice is surgical excision with adjuvant cryotherapy of the margins of the lesion at the time of surgery. Additional postoperative adjuvant therapy, especially if the surgical margins of excision are positive, may include topical mitomycin C, interferon alpha-2b, 5-fuorouracil, or cidofovir. Intralesional interferon alpha-2b has also been used effectively. Ten million IU/1 cc of interferon alpha-2b may be injected into the lesion and/or around the lesion in refractory cases. These injections may be given every other week and repeated four to six times until resolution. Lesions that invade the sclera may be treated with excision including a partial lamellar sclerectomy. An alternative is plaque brachytherapy. If the lesion invades into the eye, enucleation may be required.

Prognosis

Recurrence rates as high as 30% have been reported for squamous cell carcinoma. Most tumors tend to recur within 2 years, but late recurrences have been reported. Metastasis is extremely rare. Sites of metastasis include preauricular, submandibular, and cervical lymph nodes, parotid gland, lungs, and bones. Lymph nodes should be evaluated at every examination.

Epidemiology

This lesion usually arises in adults, age 15–82 (mean 55), more commonly in men (67%) than women (33%). It usually occurs in the sun-exposed area of the conjunctiva (interpalpebral fissure) near the limbus and is associated with outdoor work in the sun.

Cross-References

Conjunctiva mucoepidermoid carcinoma, spindle cell carcinoma, surgical techniques

Further Reading

American Academy of Ophthalmology (2006–2007) Ophthalmic pathology and intraocular tumors. American Academy of Ophthalmology Basic and Clinical Science Course. 655 Beach Street Box 7424 San Francisco, CA 94120-7424, p51–54

Goehm M, Huang A (2004) Treatment of recurrent corneal and conjunctival intraepithelial neoplasia with topical interferon alpha 2b. Ophthalmology 111(9):1755–1761

Kemp E, Harnett AN, Chatterjee S (2002) Preoperative topical and intraoperative local mitomycin C adjuvant therapy in the management of ocular surface neoplasias. Br J Ophthalmol 86:31–34

Pe'er J (2005) Ocular surface squamous neoplasia. Ophthalmol Clin North Am 18(1):1–13

Peksayar G, Onal S (2003) Excision and cryosurgery in the treatment of conjunctival malignant epithelial tumors. Eye 17(2):228–332

Sherman MD, Feldman KA, Farahmand SM, Margolis TP (2002) Treatment of conjunctival squamous cell carcinoma with topical cidofovir. Am J Ophthalmol 134(3):432–433

Singh AD (2007) Clinical ophthalmic oncology. WB Saunders Company, Philadelphia, pp 136–140

Sturges A, Butt AL, Lai JE, Chodosh J (2008) Topical interferon or surgical excision for the management of primary ocular surface squamous neoplasia. Ophthalmology 115(8):1297–1302

Yeatts RP, Engelbrecht NE, Curry CD, Ford JG, Walter KA (2000) 5-Fluorouracil for the treatment of intraepithelial neoplasia of the conjunctiva and cornea. Ophthalmology 107:2190–2195

Conjunctiva: Mucoepidermoid Carcinoma

15

Jill R. Wells, F. Lawson Grumbine, and Hans E. Grossniklaus

Synonyms

Mucoepidermoid carcinoma is a variant of squamous cell carcinoma.

Definition

Mucoepidermoid carcinoma arises in the squamous mucosa, in this case, conjunctiva, and is composed of epithelial cells, some of which secrete mucin.

Etiology

There is no known etiology for conjunctival mucoepidermoid carcinoma.

J.R. Wells, M.D. (✉)
Department of Ophthalmology, Emory University School of Medicine,
Atlanta, GA, USA
e-mail: jwells4@emory.edu

F.L. Grumbine, M.D.
Department of Ophthalmology, Emory University School of Medicine,
Atlanta, GA, USA

Emory Eye Center,
Atlanta, GA, USA
e-mail: francis.lawson.grumbine@emory.edu

H.E. Grossniklaus, M.D.
Emory University School of Medicine,
Emory Eye Center,
Department of Ophthalmology,
Atlanta, GA, USA
e-mail: ophtheg@emory.edu

H.E. Grossniklaus (ed.), *Pocket Guide to Ocular Oncology and Pathology*,
DOI 10.1007/978-3-642-29782-3_15, © Springer-Verlag Berlin Heidelberg 2013

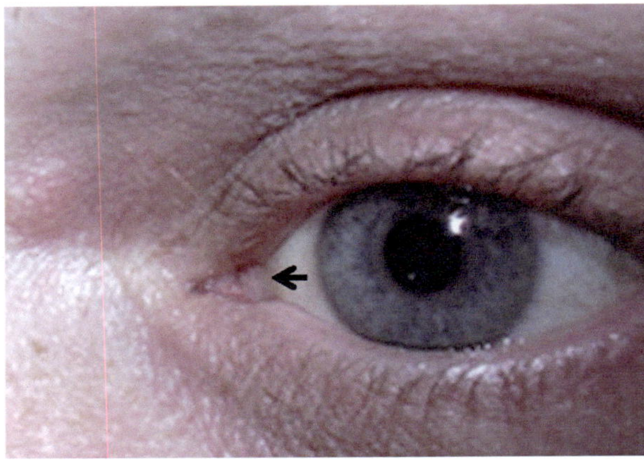

Fig. 15.1 An inconspicuous fleshy lesion is located in the conjunctiva near the left medial canthus (*arrow*)

Clinical Presentation

Conjunctival mucoepidermoid carcinoma may present as a fleshy nodule or plaque on the bulbar or palpebral conjunctiva. It may be inconspicuous (Fig. 15.1).

Diagnosis

A biopsy with special stains for mucin is required to establish the diagnosis.

Pathology

The tumor is composed of tongues, chords, and glandular configurations of cells (Fig. 15.2) with pleomorphic vesiculated nuclei, prominent nucleoli, and abundant acidophilic cytoplasm. Special stains for mucin will be positive in the mucin of occasional tumor cells. This tumor may exhibit intraocular invasion from the ocular surface. It may invade into the anterior chamber, trabecular meshwork, or suprachoroidal space.

Differential Diagnosis

The main entity in the differential diagnosis is squamous cell carcinoma. Mucoepidermoid carcinoma is an aggressive variant of squamous cell carcinoma that is more likely to invade intraocular structures or the orbit than conjunctival squamous cell carcinoma.

Prophylaxis

There is no known prophylaxis for mucoepidermoid carcinoma of the conjunctiva.

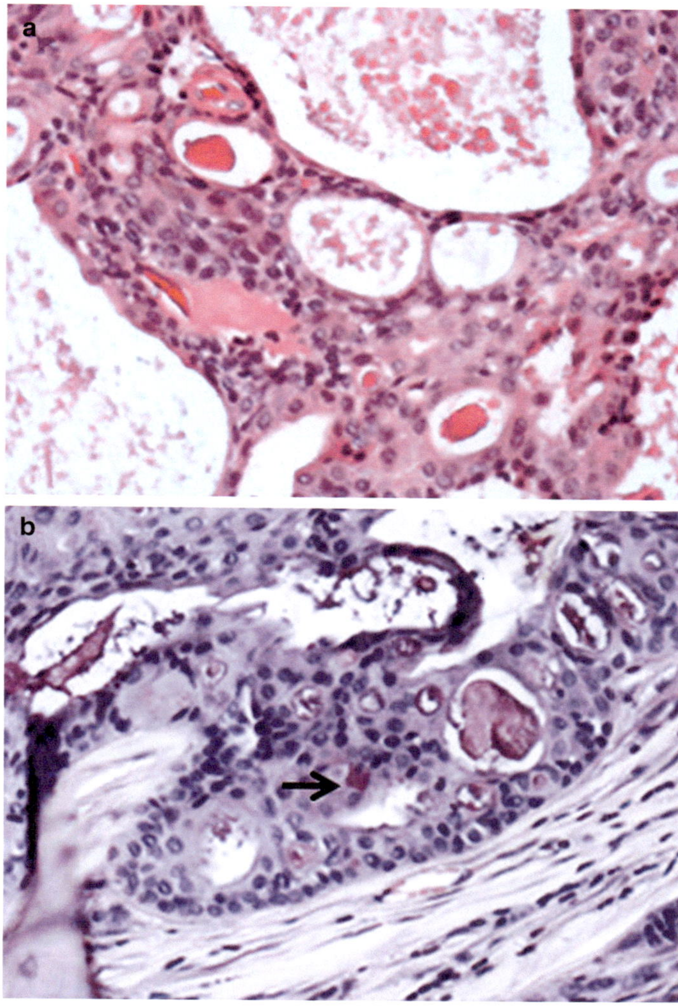

Fig. 15.2 (**a**). The tumor is composed of glandular configurations of cells with vesiculated nuclei and abundant cytoplasm. (**b**). Special stains for mucin show intracytoplasmic mucin (*arrow*) in tumor cells. (**a**. hematoxylin and eosin, 100×; **b**. mucicarmine, 100×)

Therapy

Complete surgical excision is recommended. In recurrent cases with intraocular or orbital invasion, enucleation or exenteration may be required. It may be possible to treat recurrent cases with plaque brachytherapy in select cases. It is possible that regional lymphatic spread may require a radical neck dissection.

Prognosis

The prognosis for mucoepidermoid carcinoma is guarded for retention of the globe, although if completely excised, the prognosis for life is good. The recurrence rate is high, and these patients need extended follow-up because distant metastases can occur late.

Epidemiology

Conjunctival mucoepidermoid carcinoma is rare and occurs in the same frequency in males and females.

Cross-References

Conjunctival squamous cell carcinoma, conjunctival spindle cell carcinoma, surgical techniques

Further Reading

Brownstein S (1981) Mucoepidermoid carcinoma of the conjunctiva with intraocular invasion. Ophthalmology 88(12):1226–1230

Carrau RL, Stillman E, Canaan RE (1994) Mucoepidermoid carcinoma of the conjunctiva. Ophthal Plast Reconstr Surg 10(3):163–168

Gamel JW, Eiferman RA, Guibor P (1984) Mucoepidermoid carcinoma of the conjunctiva. Arch Ophthalmol 102(5):730–731

Gunduz K, Shields CL, Shields JA et al (1998) Intraocular neoplastic cyst from mucoepidermoid carcinoma of the conjunctiva. Arch Ophthalmol 116:1521–1523

Herschorn BJ, Jakobiec FA, Hornblass A et al (1983) Mucoepidermoid carcinoma of the palpebral mucocutaneous junction. A clinical, light microscopic and electron microscopic study of an unusual tubular variant. Ophthalmology 90(12):1437–1446

Hwang IP, Jordan DR, Brownstein S et al (2000) Mucoepidermoid carcinoma of the conjunctiva: a series of three cases. Ophthalmology 107(4):801–805

Margo CE, Groden LR (1989) Intraepithelial neoplasia of the conjunctiva with mucoepidermoid differentiation. Am J Ophthalmol 108(5):600–601

Panda A, Sharma N, Seema S, Manotosh R (2003) Mucoepidermoid carcinoma of the conjunctiva managed by frozen section-guided excision and lamellar keratoplasty. Clin Experiment Ophthalmol 31(3):275–277

Rao NA, Font RL (1976) Mucoepidermoid carcinoma of the conjunctiva: a clinicopathologic study of five cases. Cancer 38(4):1699–1709

Robinson JW, Brownstein S, Jordan DR, Hodge WG (2006) Conjunctival mucoepidermoid carcinoma in a patient with ocular cicatricial pemphigoid and a review of the literature. Surv Ophthalmol 51(5):513–519

Soong HK, Feil SH, Elner VM et al (1999) Conjunctival mucoepidermoid carcinoma in a young HIV-infected male. Am J Ophthalmol 128(5):640–643

Ullman S, Augsburger JJ, Brady LW (1995) Fractionated epibulbar I-125 plaque radiotherapy for recurrent mucoepidermoid carcinoma of the bulbar conjunctiva. Am J Ophthalmol 119(1): 102–103

Conjunctiva: Spindle Cell Carcinoma 16

Hans E. Grossniklaus

Synonyms

Spindle cell variant of squamous cell carcinoma

Definition

Spindle cell carcinoma of the conjunctiva is a rare, aggressive variant of squamous cell carcinoma. Histologic examination shows that tumor cells are spindle-shaped and mimic other spindle cell, rather than epithelial neoplasms.

Etiology

The etiology is unknown, although there may be a relationship with sun exposure similar to conjunctival squamous cell carcinoma.

Clinical Presentation

This lesion, although rare, may present as an indistinct mass or nodule at the limbus (Fig. 16.1). The rare cases reported are usually in middle-aged men. There may be some conjunctival injection associated with the lesion.

H.E. Grossniklaus, M.D.
Emory University School of Medicine,
Emory Eye Center,
Department of Ophthalmology,
Atlanta, GA, USA
e-mail: ophtheg@emory.edu

H.E. Grossniklaus (ed.), *Pocket Guide to Ocular Oncology and Pathology*,
DOI 10.1007/978-3-642-29782-3_16,

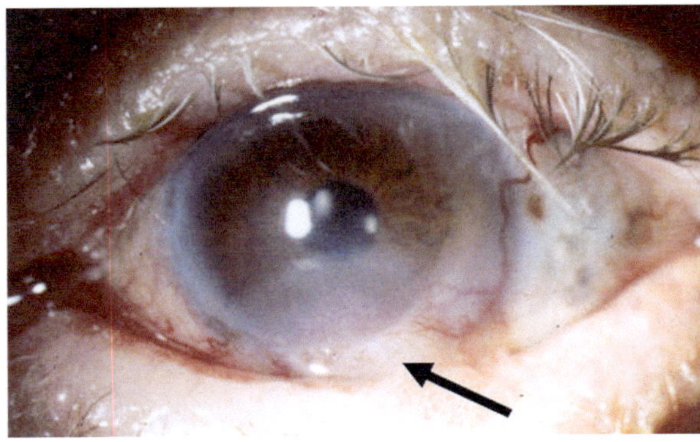

Fig. 16.1 Clinical appearance of inferior limbal spindle cell carcinoma of the conjunctiva (*arrow*) shows ill-defined, white mass

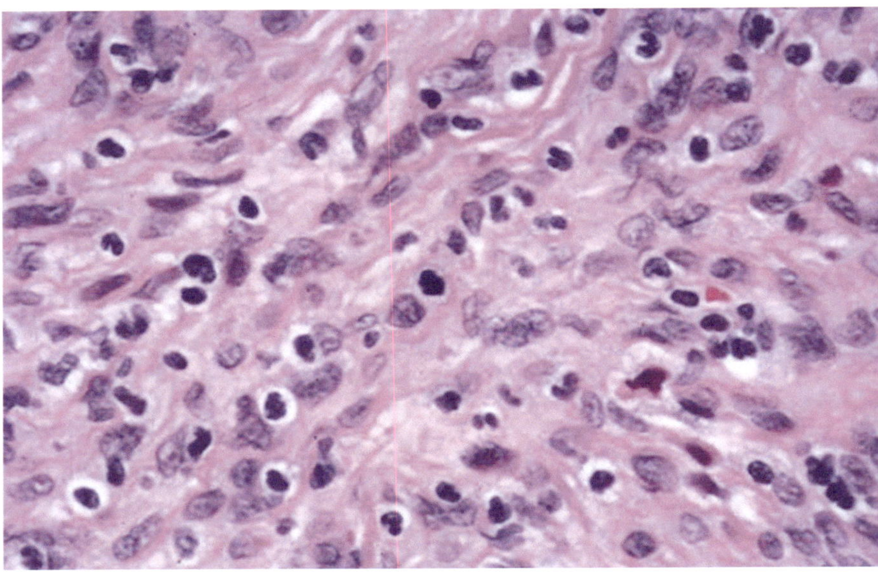

Fig. 16.2 The spindle cell carcinoma of the patient shown in Fig. 16.1 is composed of cells with vesiculated, elongated, fusiform to oval nuclei and variable amounts of cytoplasm. There are scattered lymphocytes in the tumor. (H&E, 100×)

Diagnosis

The diagnosis may be suspected clinically and confirmed by biopsy.

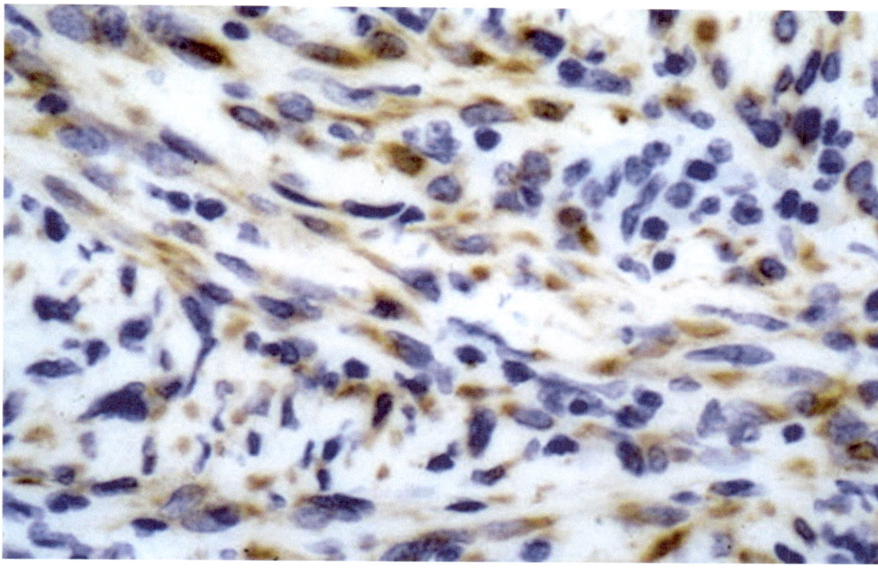

Fig. 16.3 Immunohistochemical stains are positive for cytokeratins in the spindle-shaped tumor cells. (peroxidase antiperoxidase, 100×)

Pathology

Histologic examination shows a spindle cell neoplasm (Fig. 16.2). The diagnosis is not obvious as it may represent a fibrous histiocytoma, spindle cell melanoma, or other spindle cell neoplasm. Positive immunohistochemical stains for cytokeratins (Fig. 16.3) confirm the diagnosis.

Differential Diagnosis

The differential diagnosis includes fibrous histiocytoma and spindle cell melanoma. These lesions will not stain for cytokeratins. Immunohistochemical stains are positive for vimentin and possible factor XIII alpha in fibrous histiocytoma and S100, HMB45, and/or Melan A in melanoma.

Prophylaxis

There is no known prophylaxis for spindle cell melanoma of the conjunctiva.

Therapy

The main therapy is complete excision of the lesion. If the lesion invades the sclera, a sclerectomy and partial- or full-thickness eye wall resection with a scleral patch graft may be performed. Another option for a deeply invasive lesion, as may be confirmed by ultrasound biomicroscopy (UBM), is plaque brachytherapy. If there is intraocular invasion that is otherwise untreatable, enucleation may be required.

Prognosis

The prognosis for spindle cell carcinoma of the conjunctiva is guarded, as it is an aggressive form of squamous cell carcinoma. Although it is possible to metastasize and cause death, this is unlikely. However, preservation of the eye is guarded due to the invasive nature of the tumor.

Epidemiology

Spindle cell carcinoma of the conjunctiva is rare and comprises approximately 0.1% of surgically excised conjunctival lesions. It may occur more commonly in men than women.

Cross-References

Conjunctival carcinoma-squamous cell, conjunctival carcinoma-mucoepidermoid, surgical techniques

Further Reading

Cohen BH, Green WR, Iliff NT et al (1980) Spindle cell carcinoma of the conjunctiva. Arch Ophthalmol 98:1809–1813

Grossniklaus HE, Green WR, Luckenbach M et al (1987) Conjunctival lesions in adults. A clinical and histopathologic review. Cornea 6:78–116

Huntington AC, Langloss JM, Hidayat AA (1990) Spindle cell carcinoma of the conjunctiva. An immunohistochemical and ultrastructural study of six cases. Ophthalmology 97:711–717

Schubert HD, Farris RL, Green WR (1995) Spindle cell carcinoma of the conjunctiva. Graefes Arch Clin Exp Ophthalmol 233:52–53

Seregard S, Kock E (1995) Squamous spindle cell carcinoma of the conjunctiva. Fatal outcome of a pterygium-like lesion. Acta Ophthalmol Scand 73:464–466

Shields JA, Eagle RC, Barr BP et al (2007) Invasive spindle cell carcinoma of the conjunctiva managed by full-thickness eye wall resection. Cornea 26:1014–1016

Slusker-Shtemfeld I, Syed NA, Sires BA (1997) Invasive spindle cell carcinoma of the conjunctiva. Arch Ophthalmol 115:288–289

Wise AC (1967) A limbal spindle-cell carcinoma. Surv Ophthalmol 12:244–246

Conjunctival Dysplasia

17

Jerome C. Ramos-Esteban, Arun D. Singh, Jill R. Wells, and Hans E. Grossniklaus

Synonyms

Conjunctival intraepithelial neoplasia

Definition

Conjunctival dysplastic lesions exhibit mild, moderate, or severe degrees of cellular atypia that may involve varying degrees of thickness of the epithelium, starting from the basal layer outwards.

J.C. Ramos-Esteban, M.D.
Department of Ophthalmic Oncology, Cole Eye Institute, Cleveland Clinic Foundation, 9500 Euclid Avenue, Cleveland, OH 44195, USA

A.D. Singh, M.D. (✉)
Department of Ophthalmic Oncology, Cole Eye Institute, Cleveland Clinic Foundation, 9500 Euclid Avenue, Desk i-329, Cleveland, OH 44195, USA
e-mail: singha@ccf.org

J.R. Wells, M.D.
Department of Ophthalmology, Emory University School of Medicine, Atlanta, GA, USA
e-mail: jwells4@emory.edu

H.E. Grossniklaus, M.D.
Emory University School of Medicine, Emory Eye Center, Department of Ophthalmology, Atlanta, GA, USA
e-mail: ophtheg@emory.edu

H.E. Grossniklaus (ed.), *Pocket Guide to Ocular Oncology and Pathology*,
DOI 10.1007/978-3-642-29782-3_17,

Etiology

Dysplasias are typically found in elderly white individuals with a history of chronic exposure to sunlight (UV radiation). Human papillomavirus has been demonstrated within some cases of dysplasia.

Clinical Presentation

Conjunctival dysplastic lesions occur within the interpalpebral fissure with a predilection for the limbus, although corneal and palpebral conjunctival involvement can also occur. Dysplasia may arise in the epithelium covering areas of solar elastosis, similar to actinic keratoses of the skin. The dysplasia is focal and well delineated associated with leukoplakic (keratinized) plaques (Fig. 17.1). When diffuse dysplasias occur in regions not exposed to the sun, the clinical appearance is more gelatinous and less well defined (Fig. 17.2).

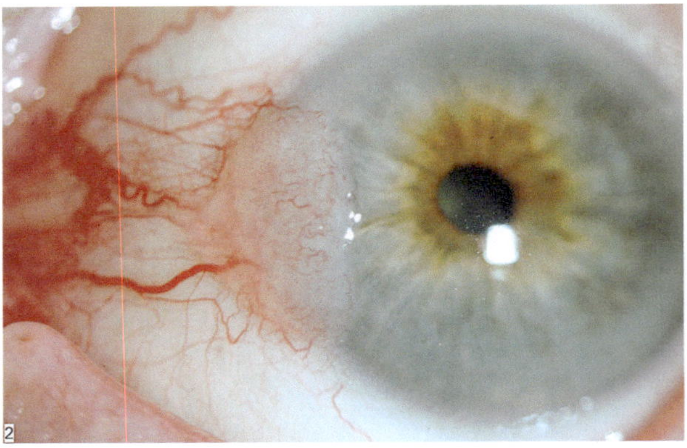

Fig. 17.1 A localized limbal gelatinous appearing ocular surface squamous neoplasia with intrinsic and feeder vessels

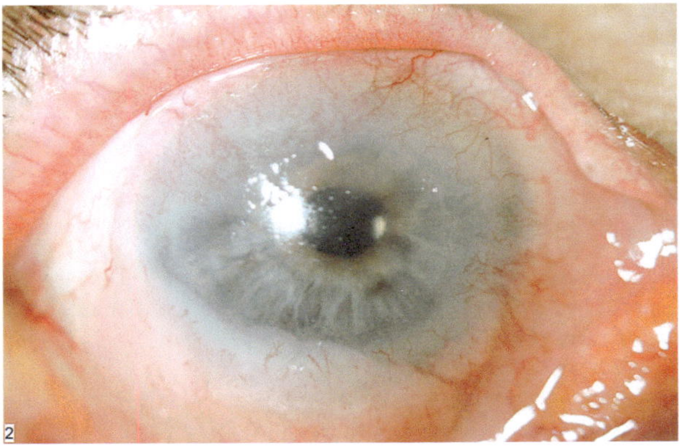

Fig. 17.2 Diffuse ocular surface squamous neoplasia involving all quadrants of the bulbar conjunctiva, all clock hours of the limbus, and large surface of the cornea

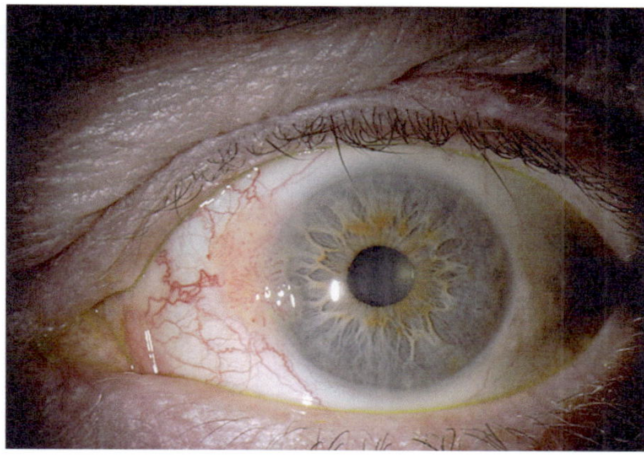

Fig. 17.3 Focal dysplasia in a papillomatous configuration is present near the limbus

Diagnostics

Clinical differentiation of this wide spectrum of lesions cannot be solely based on clinical evaluation. Histopathological evaluation of excised tissue is necessary to confirm the diagnosis. Dysplastic lesions are characterized by different levels of cellular atypia and depth of epithelial involvement. Carcinoma in situ is confined to the epithelium; in contrast, squamous cell carcinoma breaches the conjunctival basement membrane, and subepithelial invasion occurs.

Pathology

Dysplasia is graded as mild, moderate, or severe according to the degree of involvement of the epithelium. Mild dysplasia is defined as dysplasia confined to the lower third of the conjunctival epithelial thickness. Moderate dysplasia extends into the middle third and severe dysplasia into the upper third. The dysplasia may be focal (Figs. 17.3 and 17.4) or diffuse (Figs. 17.5 and 17.6). The surgical margins of excision should be evaluated and will usually be negative, except for the corneal margin, in focal dysplasia and positive in diffuse dysplasia.

Differential Diagnosis

Conjunctival papillomas, keratoacanthoma, benign hereditary intraepithelial dyskeratosis, conjunctival granuloma, pyogenic granuloma, carcinoma in situ, squamous cell carcinoma.

Prophylaxis

Unclear; avoidance of excessive sunlight exposure may be recommended.

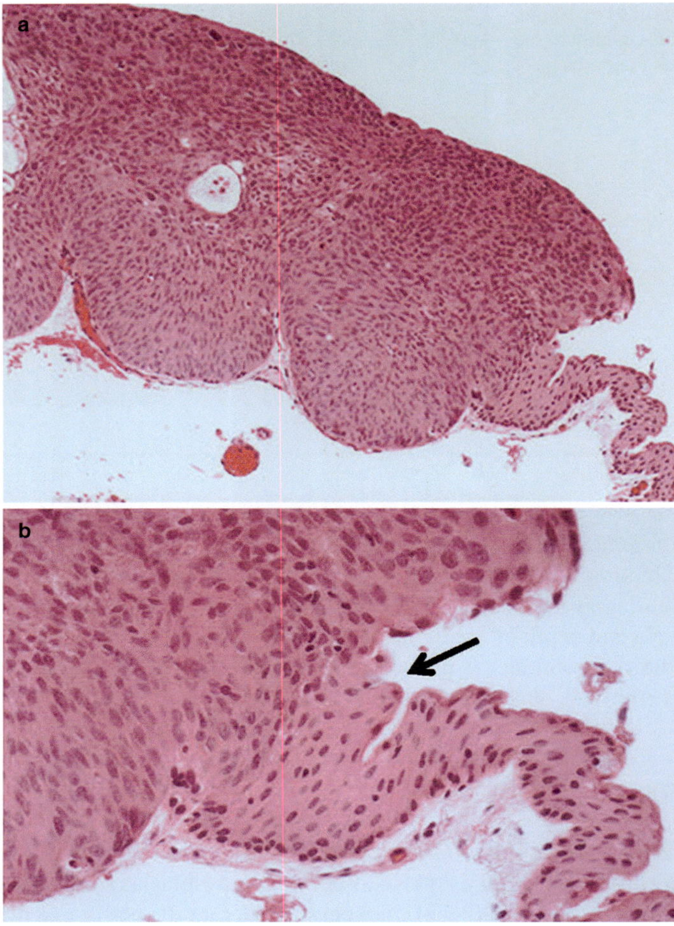

Fig. 17.4 Focal dysplasia (patient shown in Fig. 17.3). (**a**) The lesion is composed of a focally thickened epithelium containing keratinocytes that have lost their normal maturation sequence. (**b**) The junction between the dysplasia and normal conjunctiva is apparent (*arrow*). (**a** hematoxylin and eosin 25×, **b** hematoxylin and eosin 100×)

Therapy

Surgical excision with wide surgical margins (2–3 mm) is the recommended treatment. If corneal or scleral involvement is present, a corneal epitheliectomy and/or deep lamellar limbal keratectomy or sclerectomy must also be performed. Bowman's layer should not be violated. Additional cryotherapy to the surgical margins may also reduce the likelihood of recurrence. Alternative methods include brachytherapy with a recommended dose of 20–180 Gy to the tumor surface. Larger lesions which preclude surgical excision may be treated with topical chemotherapeutic agents such as mitomycin C, 5-fluorouracil, and interferon alpha-2b. Topical application of

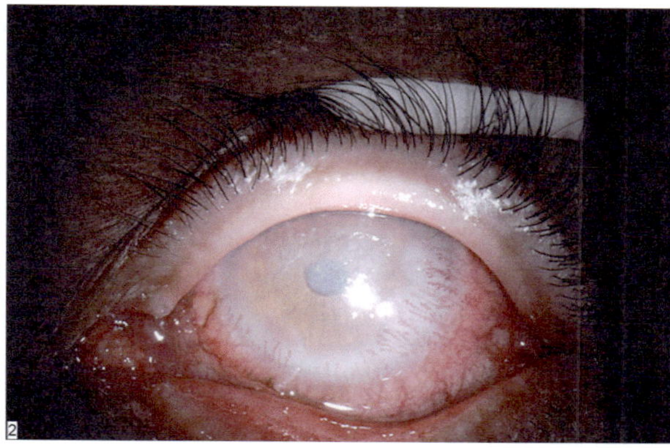

Fig. 17.5 Diffuse dysplasia encroaches onto cornea

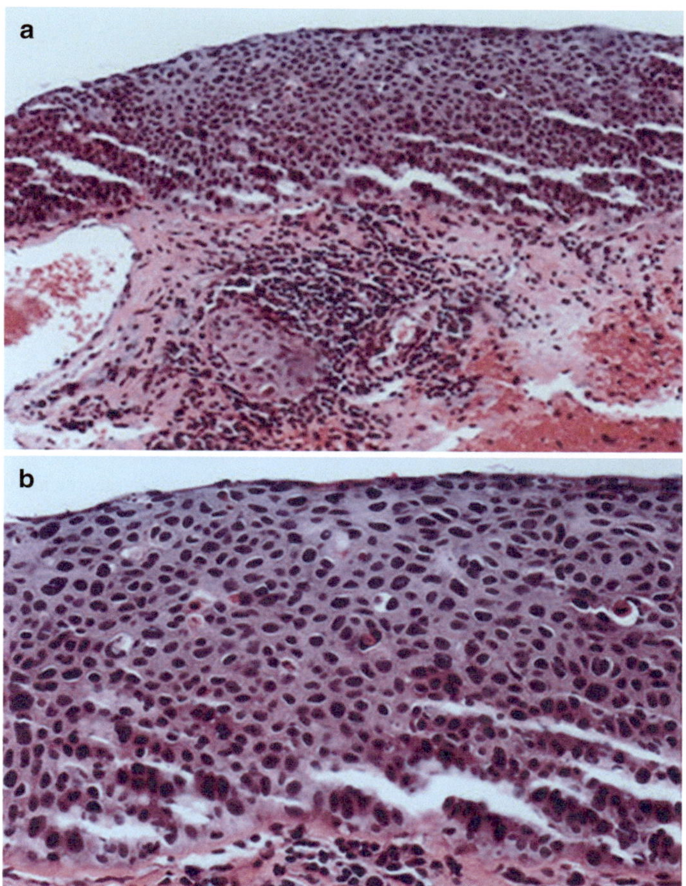

Fig. 17.6 Diffuse dysplasia (patient shown in Fig. 17.5). (**a**) The lesion is composed of diffusely thickened epithelium with loss of the normal maturation sequence of keratinocytes. (**b**) Keratinocytes have pleomorphic, hyperchromatic nuclei, and the process extends to the margin of excision. (**a**, hematoxylin and eosin 25×; **b**, hematoxylin and eosin 100×)

mitomycin C 0.04% four times a day given in 2-week cycles may cause regression of low-grade lesions. Interferon is given topically as ten million IU four times a day for several months until resolution. Ten million IU/1 cc of interferon alpha-2b may be injected into the lesion and/or around the lesion in refractory cases. These injections may be given every other week and repeated four to six times until resolution. Mitomycin C application may lead to ocular surface discomfort (hyperemia, burning sensation, and corneal epithelial toxicity). Addition of a topical corticosteroid may improve patient compliance.

Prognosis

The prognosis for conjunctival dysplasia is excellent. Local recurrences after surgical excision are dependent on the involvement of the surgical margins (5% when margins are free and 50% when margins are involved).

Epidemiology

This lesion is more prevalent in countries located near the equator.

Cross-References

Conjunctival squamous cell carcinoma, surgical techniques

Further Reading

Erie JC, Campbell RJ, Liesegang J (1986) Conjunctival and corneal intraepithelial and invasive neoplasia. Ophthalmology 93:176–183

Frucht-Pery J, Sugar J, Baum J et al (1997) Mitomycin C treatment for conjunctival-corneal intraepithelial neoplasia: a multicenter experience. Ophthalmology 104:2085–2093

Lee GA, Hirst LW (1995) Ocular surface squamous neoplasia. Surv Ophthalmol 39:429–450

Pe'er J (2005) Ocular surface squamous neoplasia. Ophthalmol Clin North Am 18:1–13

Pe'er J, Frucht-Pery J (2007) Ocular surface squamous neoplasia. In: Singh AD, Damato BE, Pe'er J, Murphree AL, Perry JD (eds) Clinical ophthalmic oncology. Saunders Elsevier, Philadelphia, pp 136–140

Conjunctival Choristomas

18

Martina C. Herwig, Karin U. Loeffler,
and G. Baker Hubbard III

Synonyms

Dermoid, Dermolipoma, Episcleral osseous choristoma, Lacrimal gland Choristoma, Complex choristoma

Definition

These tumors are composed of displaced tissue elements not normally found in the conjunctiva and hence fulfill the definition of choristomas. They are generally present at birth or become apparent shortly after birth.

Dermoid – yellowish white solid mass, usually found near the limbus, composed of dense fibrous tissue.

M.C. Herwig, M.D.
Department of Ophthalmology, Emory University School of Medicine,
Atlanta, GA, USA

Department of Ophthalmology, University of Bonn,
Bonn, Germany
e-mail: martina.herwig@ukb.uni-bonn.de

K.U. Loeffler, M.D.
Department of Ophthalmology, University Eye Clinic,
Bonn, Germany
e-mail: karinloeffler@uni-bonn.de

G.B. Hubbard III, M.D. (✉)
Department of Ophthalmology, Emory University School of Medicine,
Atlanta, GA, USA

The Emory Eye Center, Atlanta, GA, USA
e-mail: ghubba2@emory.edu

H.E. Grossniklaus (ed.), *Pocket Guide to Ocular Oncology and Pathology*,
DOI 10.1007/978-3-642-29782-3_18,

Dermolipoma – a soft, pale yellow mass visible just below the palpebral lobe of the lacrimal gland. It is composed of collagenous connective tissue and adipose tissue.

Episcleral osseous choristoma – an epibulbar mass consisting of mature bone surrounded by fibrous connective tissue.

Lacrimal gland choristoma – a pink stromal mass typically in the superotemporal quadrant of the conjunctiva consisting of lacrimal gland tissue.

Complex choristoma – distinguished from simple choristomas in that they are composed of a variety of tissue types.

Clinical Presentation

Dermoid – This pale solid mass is usually found near the inferotemporal corneoscleral limbus. It may have fine white cilia that can be seen with slit lamp biomicroscopy. Rarely it may extend to the central cornea. Some cases may be extensive and involve the cornea, anterior chamber, and iris stroma. Conjunctival dermoids may be isolated or may be associated with Goldenhar's syndrome (preauricular skin appendages, hearing loss, eyelid coloboma, dermolipoma, microphthalmia, and cervical vertebrae anomalies).

Dermolipoma – This choristoma is probably present at birth but usually remains asymptomatic for years, and it may not be detected until adulthood. It presents as a soft, yellow protrusion from the superior conjunctival fornix, and it may be confused with prolapsed orbital fat (Figs. 18.1 and 18.2). It is best visualized with the eye in inferonasal gaze. Occasionally, it can extend anteriorly to reach the limbus. Unlike herniated orbital fat, dermolipoma can contain fine white hairs on its surface, and it cannot be reduced with digital pressure into the orbit.

Episcleral osseous choristoma – This lesion usually presents as a solitary white or yellowish firm nodule in the upper temporal quadrant (Fig. 18.3). Size and shape vary from a small pea to an almond. The nodule is usually movable over the normal sclera, but it may be firmly adherent. Sometimes it involves the rectus muscle sheaths. These lesions are probably congenital and are usually detected in early infancy and childhood, but they can occasionally manifest in adulthood. There is no association with other malformations or systemic diseases.

Lacrimal gland choristoma – This congenital lesion is usually discovered in young children as an asymptomatic pink stromal mass, typically in the superotemporal portion of the conjunctiva.

Complex choristoma – This choristoma is quite variable in its clinical presentation depending on the predominant tissue type found in the lesion. It may cover much of the bulbar surface, or it may grow in a circumferential pattern around the limbus. Rarely these lesions enlarge over time. Complex choristomas may be found in association with the linear nevus sebaceous syndrome (linear sebaceous nevus of Jadassohn, skeletal deformities, heart defects, seizures, and intellectual disability).

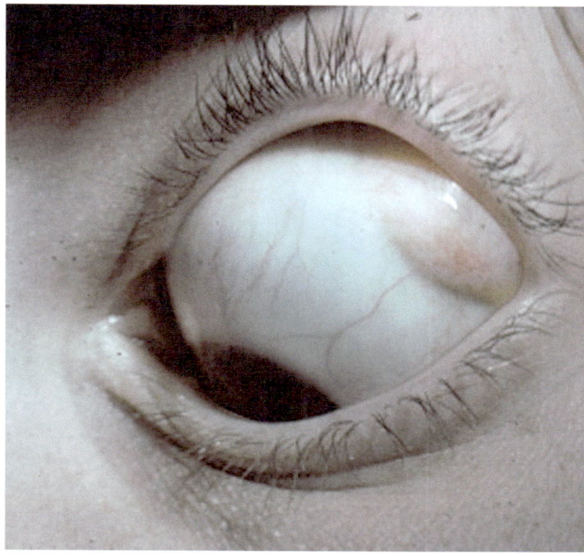

Fig. 18.1 Dermolipoma. A soft, yellow-white conjunctival mass is present superotemporally

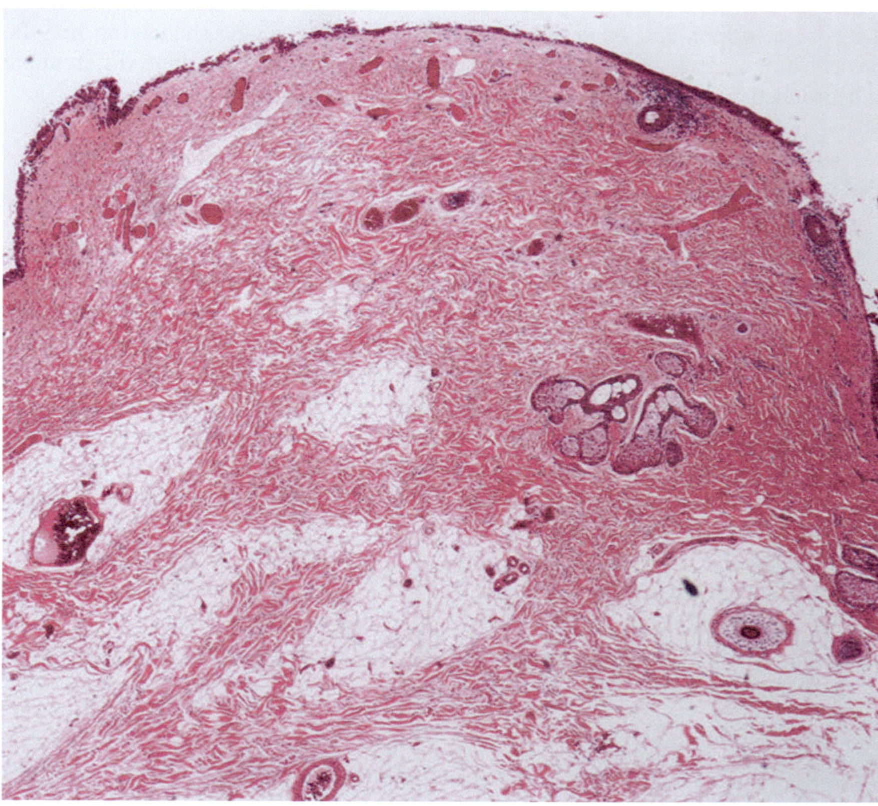

Fig. 18.2 Dermolipoma. The mass contains dermis, dermal appendages, adipose tissue, and surrounding dermis-like collagen (hematoxylin and eosin, 10×)

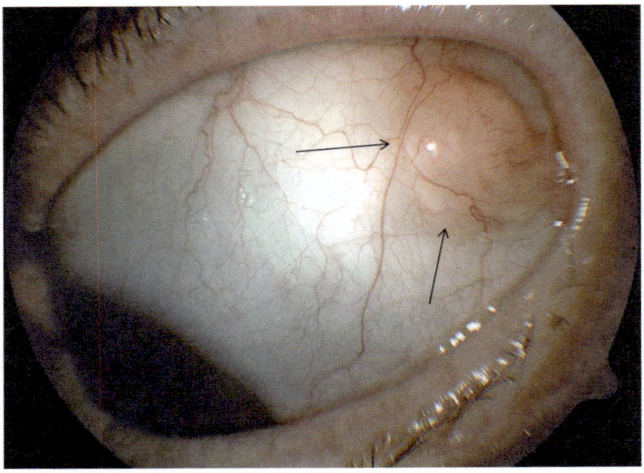

Fig. 18.3 Epibulbar osseous choristoma. Yellowish well-circumscribed subconjunctival nodule (*arrows*) of firm consistency located in the upper temporal quadrant of the left eye

Diagnostics

Ultrasound biomicroscopy may be utilized to determine the extent of the lesion into the cornea, sclera, and other structures. Pronounced acoustic shadowing may be present in episcleral osseous choristomas. CT and MR imaging help differentiate subconjunctival fat prolapse from dermolipoma.

Pathology

Dermoid – Histopathology shows dense fibrous connective tissue with variable hair follicles and sebaceous glands. The surface has conjunctival epithelium.

Dermolipoma – This lesion has conjunctival epithelium on the surface with variable quantities of collagenous connective tissue and adipose tissue below the epithelium (Fig. 18.2). Pilosebaceous units and lacrimal gland tissue may be present.

Episcleral osseous choristoma – Histopathology reveals mature compact bone surrounded by fibrous connective tissue (Fig. 18.4). The osteocytes appear essentially normal, and concentric lamellae of bone surround the Haversian canals. A periosteum is occasionally present. Hematopoietic marrow is rarely observed.

Lacrimal gland choristoma – This lesion is composed of normal lacrimal tissue with acini composed of two layers of cells placed on a thin hyaline basement membrane (Fig. 18.5).

Complex choristoma – These lesions may be composed of lacrimal tissue, cartilage, dermal appendages, bone, or other elements.

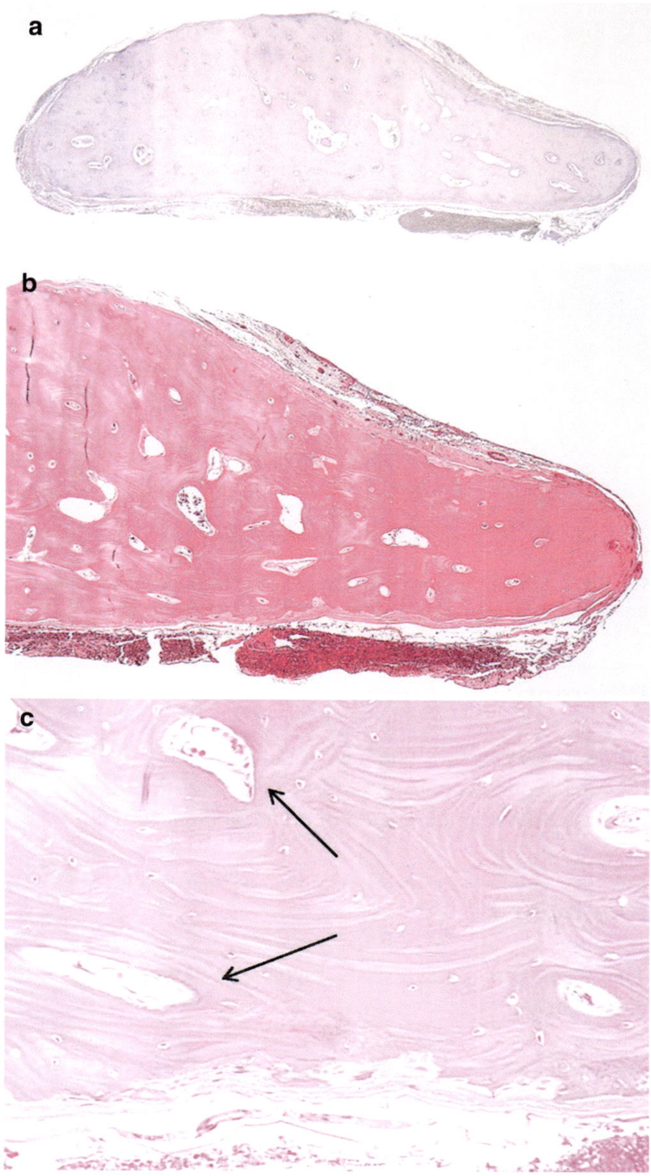

Fig. 18.4 Epibulbar osseous choristoma. Histopathologic examination shows mature bone with Haversian canals (*arrows*) surrounded by fibrous connective tissue (**a**: periodic acid Schiff, 4×; **b** hematoxylin and eosin, 25× and **c**: hematoxylin and eosin, 40×)

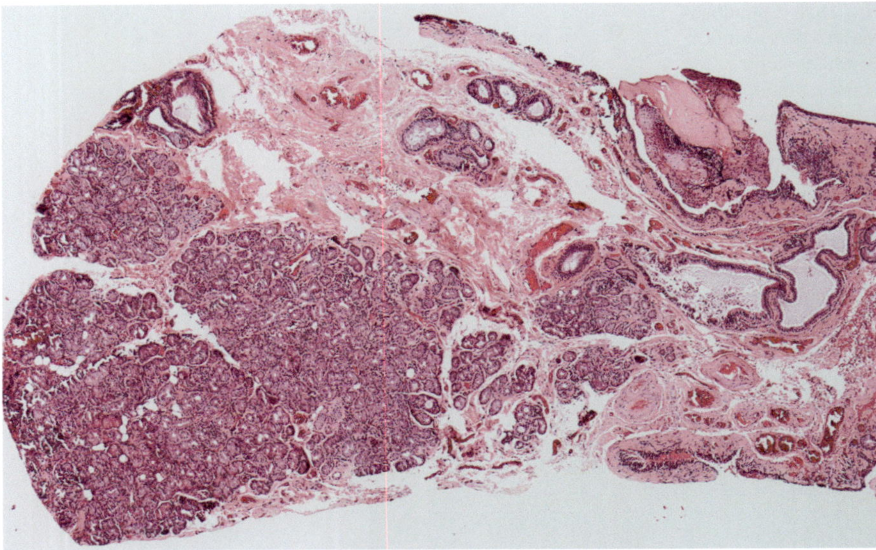

Fig. 18.5 Ectopic lacrimal gland. A lobule of lacrimal gland is present in the substantia propria of this bulbar conjunctival biopsy (hematoxylin and eosin, 25×)

Differential Diagnosis

Inflammatory lesions (such as granuloma, pyogenic granuloma), scars, and foreign bodies have to be considered in the differential diagnosis. These lesions may also mimic extraocular extension of an intraocular tumor.

Prophylaxis

There are no known risk factors or known ways to prevent conjunctival choristomas.

Therapy

The best management option is observation unless the lesion causes vision loss or an unacceptable cosmetic appearance in which case the lesion may be excised. Excision of larger lesions may be associated with significant scarring and may require mucous membrane grafting or lamellar or penetrating keratoplasty/patch graft.

Prognosis

These lesions do not have malignant potential and do not metastasize. Prognosis for vision is related to the size and extent of the lesion.

Epidemiology

These are generally rare lesions and the exact incidence is unknown.

Cross-References

Choristomas

Further Reading

Boniuk M, Zimmerman LE (1962) Epibulbar osteoma (episcleral osseous choristoma). Am J Ophthalmol 53:290–296

Duncan JL, Golabi M, Fredrick DR, Hoyt CS, Hwang DG, Kramer SG, Howes EL Jr, Cunningham ET Jr (1998) Complex limbal choristomas in linear nevus sebaceous syndrome. Ophthalmology 105:1459–1465

Gayre GS, Proia AD, Dutton JJ (2002) Epibulbar osseous choristoma: case report and review of the literature. Ophthalmic Surg Lasers 33:410–415

Hoops JP, Ludwig K, Boergen KP, Kampik A (2001) Preoperative evaluation of limbal dermoids using high-resolution biomicroscopy. Graefes Arch Clin Exp Ophthalmol 239:459–461

Shields CL, Shields JA (2004) Tumors of the conjunctiva and cornea. Surv Ophthalmol 49:3–24

Spencer WH (1996) Sclera. In: Spender WH (ed) Ophthalmic pathology: an atlas and textbook, 4th edn. WB Saunders Company, Philadelphia, pp 364–366

Conjunctival Fibrous Histiocytoma and Myxoma

19

Hans E. Grossniklaus

Synonyms

Benign and malignant fibrous histiocytoma (for fibrous histiocytoma)

Definition

Conjunctival fibrous histiocytoma is a mesenchymal spindle cell proliferation that usually occurs at the limbus. Conjunctival myxoma is a loosely cohesive spindle cell proliferation that may occur in the bulbar or palpebral conjunctiva.

Etiology

The etiology of fibrous histiocytoma is unknown. Myxoma may be associated with a mutation in the *PRKAR1A* gene on chromosome 17q2, which may be associated with Carney complex. Carney complex includes multiple myxomas, lentigenes, and endocrine abnormalities.

H.E. Grossniklaus, M.D.
Emory University School of Medicine,
Emory Eye Center,
Department of Ophthalmology,
Atlanta, GA, USA
e-mail: ophtheg@emory.edu

H.E. Grossniklaus (ed.), *Pocket Guide to Ocular Oncology and Pathology*,
DOI 10.1007/978-3-642-29782-3_19, © Springer-Verlag Berlin Heidelberg 2013

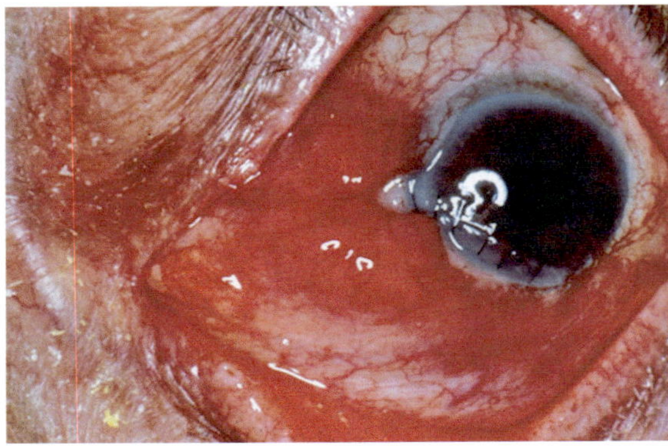

Fig. 19.1 A fleshy, red fibrous histiocytoma is present at the limbus

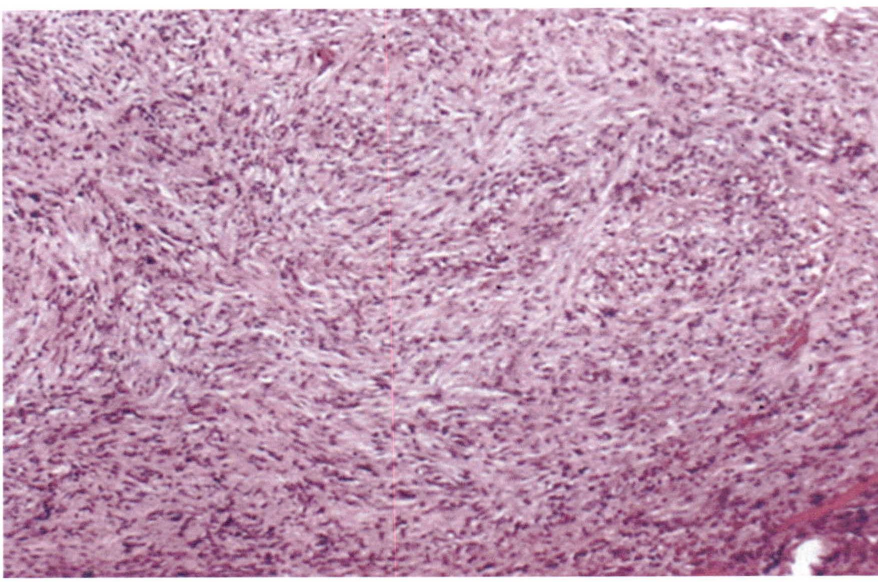

Fig. 19.2 The fibrous histiocytoma is cellular and composed of spindle-shaped cells arranged in a whorling or "storiform" pattern (hematoxylin and eosin, 100×)

Clinical Presentation

Fibrous histiocytoma may be an ill-defined, pink to red nodule, usually present at the limbus (Fig. 19.1). Myxoma is a white to colorless, soft mass that may appear in the bulbar (Fig. 19.2) or palpebral conjunctiva.

Diagnosis

The diagnosis for both fibrous histiocytoma and myxoma is made by histologic examination of an excisional biopsy.

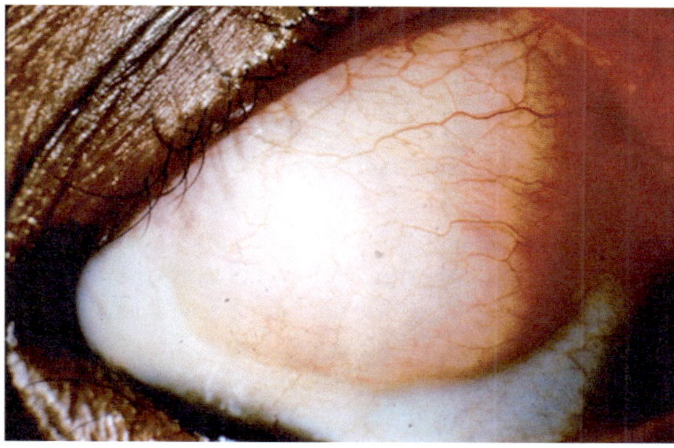

Fig. 19.3 A bulbar conjunctival myxoma appears as a soft, white mass

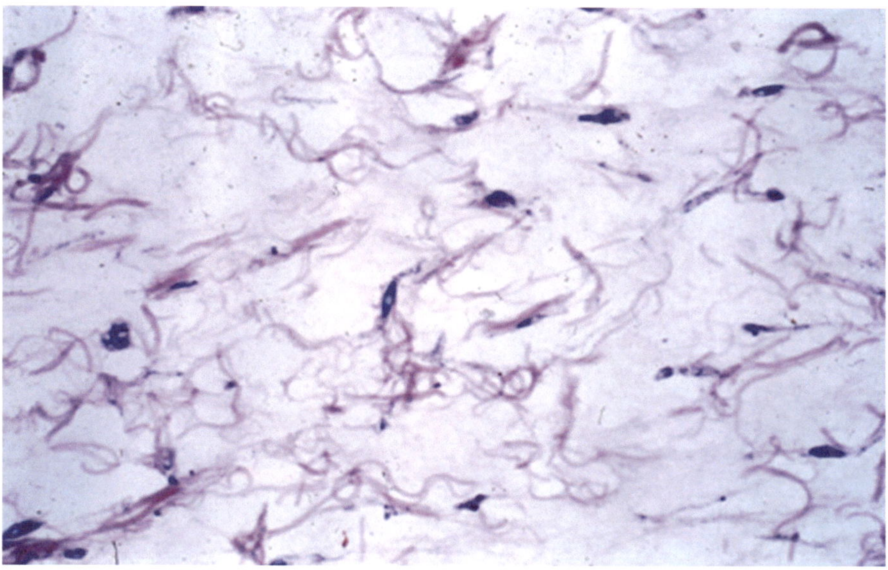

Fig. 19.4 The myxoma is composed of bland spindle-shaped cells in a loosely cohesive myxomatous matrix (hematoxylin and eosin, 100×)

Pathology

A fibrous histiocytoma forms whorling or "storiform" patterns of spindle-shaped cells (Fig. 19.3). The degree of cellularity, nuclear pleomorphism, and mitotic activity is used to determine if the fibrous histiocytoma is benign or malignant. Immunohistochemical stains are generally only positive for vimentin, and possibly factor XIIIa, in fibrous histiocytoma. Myxoma is composed of spindle-shaped cells with bland nuclei, some containing intranuclear pseudoinclusions, present in a loosely coherent matrix (Fig. 19.4). Stains for acid mucopolysaccharide, including alcian blue and colloid iron, will be positive in the matrix. Immunohistochemical stains are negative except for vimentin.

Differential Diagnosis

The differential diagnosis for fibrous histiocytoma includes giant cell angiofibroma, which on histologic examinations contains pseudovascular "angiectoid" spaces and giant cells, and solitary fibrous tumor, which will display a histologic "patternless pattern." The recently described entity, conjunctival stromal tumor, or "COST," shares histologic similarities with myxoma, although the cells in the lesion are CD34+ on immunostaining.

Prophylaxis

There is no prophylaxis for conjunctival fibrous histiocytoma or myxoma.

Therapy

The therapy for these lesions is surgical excision. If the lesion is classified as a malignant fibrous histiocytoma, incomplete excision will result in recurrence. Reexcision or plaque brachytherapy is utilized to treat recurrent malignant fibrous histiocytoma. Incomplete excision of myxoma may result in a local recurrence, which may be reexcised if desired.

Prognosis

The prognosis for fibrous histiocytoma is good, although incompletely excised malignant fibrous histiocytoma will recur and may invade the sclera. The prognosis for myxoma is good, although patients with conjunctival myxoma should be evaluated for Carney complex, including the possibility of atrial myxoma.

Epidemiology

Conjunctival fibrous histiocytoma appears to affect men more than women and usually occurs in 30- and 40-year-old patients. Myxoma affects men and women equally and occurs in adults.

Cross-References

Conjunctival vascular proliferations, conjunctival histiocytic proliferations, conjunctival lymphoma, surgical techniques

Further Reading

Allaire GS, Corriveau C, Teboul N (1999) Malignant fibrous histiocytoma of the conjunctiva. Arch Ophthalmol 117:685–687

Chen CL, Tai MC, Chen JT, Chen CH, Jin JS, Lu DW (2008) A rare case of conjunctival myxoma and review of the literature. Ophthalmologica 222:136–139

Demirci H, Shields CL, Eagle RC, Shields JA (2006) Report of conjunctival myxoma case and review of literature. Arch Ophthalmol 124:735–738

Herwig MC, Wells JR, Grossniklaus HE (2012) Conjunctival stromal tumor. Ophthalmology PMID 22200094: 682–687

Kim HJ, Shields CL, Eagle RC, Shields JA (2006) Fibrous histiocytoma of the conjunctiva. Am J Ophthalmol 142:1036–1042

Song A, Syed N, Kirby PA, Carter KD (2005) Giant cell angiofibroma of the ocular adnexae. Arch Ophthalmol 123:1438–1443

Conjunctival Vascular Proliferations 20

Hans E. Grossniklaus

Synonyms

There are a number of distinct conjunctival vascular proliferations, including pyogenic granuloma, lymphangiectasis, capillary hemangioma, cavernous hemangioma, and Kaposi sarcoma. These are all specific types of vascular proliferations.

Definition

Conjunctival vascular proliferations may be reactive/inflammatory (pyogenic granuloma), acquired (lymphangiectasis), hamartomatous (capillary/cavernous hemangioma), or neoplastic (Kaposi sarcoma). These proliferations contain vascular or pseudovascular channels lined by endothelium.

Etiology

Pyogenic granuloma occurs secondary to surgical or nonsurgical trauma and is essentially granulation tissue proliferation. Lymphangiectasis consists of dilated lymphatic channels secondary to congestion. Capillary and cavernous hemangioma may be hamartomatous vascular proliferations, although in some instance they may be acquired. Kaposi sarcoma is seen in the presence of HIV infection and is due to herpes hominis virus 8 (HHV8).

H.E. Grossniklaus, M.D.
Emory University School of Medicine,
Emory Eye Center,
Department of Ophthalmology,
Atlanta, GA, USA
e-mail: ophtheg@emory.edu

H.E. Grossniklaus (ed.), *Pocket Guide to Ocular Oncology and Pathology*,
DOI 10.1007/978-3-642-29782-3_20,

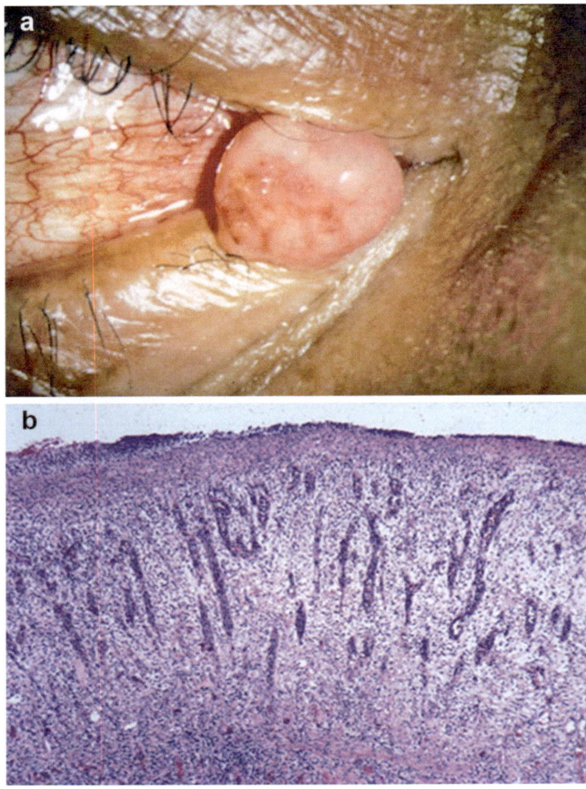

Fig. 20.1 Pyogenic granuloma. (**a**) A fleshy conjunctival growth is present at the site of a previous conjunctival incision. (**b**) The excised lesion displays a fanlike proliferation of reactive vascular channels in a loosely cohesive matrix (hematoxylin and eosin, 25×)

Clinical Presentation

The majority of vascular lesions of the conjunctiva are diagnosed in adults, typically aged 30–50 years. They are equally present in men and women. Pyogenic granuloma is a fleshy growth that appears at the site of surgery or trauma usually growing over a period of weeks (Fig. 20.1). Lymphangiectasias are fusiform, vesicular, or sausage-shaped cystic lesions that contain clear to yellow fluid (Fig. 20.2). A capillary hemangioma presents as a focal red to pink lesion that appears vascularized (Fig. 20.3). Capillary hemangiomas are more common in children than adults. A cavernous hemangioma is a focal blue to red vascular mass (Fig. 20.4). Cavernous hemangiomas are more common in adults than children. Kaposi sarcoma may be present in HIV + patients and clinically appears as a hemorrhagic mass (Fig. 20.5).

Diagnosis

Although the diagnosis may be clinically suspected in some instances, the definitive diagnosis is made by pathologic examination of the excised lesion.

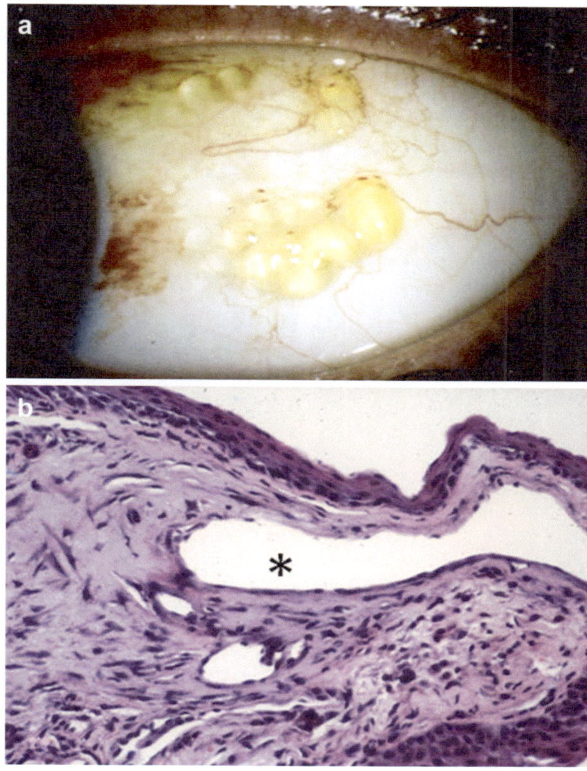

Fig. 20.2 Lymphangiectasis. (**a**) A lymphangiectasis appears as dilated, sausage-shaped channels filled with yellow fluid. (**b**) The excised lesion shows a dilated endothelial-lined vascular channel (*) in the substantia propria of the conjunctiva (hematoxylin and eosin, 100×)

Pathology

Pyogenic granuloma is histologically composed of a fanlike proliferation of vascular channels in a loosely cohesive matrix that contains inflammatory cells (Fig. 20.1). A lymphangioma is histologically composed of a dilated endothelial-lined vascular channel (Fig. 20.2). Conjunctival capillary hemangioma is histologically composed of tightly packed endothelial-lined capillary channels (Fig. 20.3). The histology of a cavernous hemangioma shows a collection of distended venous channels filled with erythrocytes (Fig. 20.4). Histologically, Kaposi sarcoma is a spindle-cell tumor that contains slit-like spaces, some of which containing erythrocytes (Fig. 20.5).

Differential Diagnosis

There is overlap among some of the vascular lesions of the conjunctiva, for instance, pyogenic granuloma/capillary hemangioma. Other uncommon vascular lesions of the conjunctiva include varix (a dilated vein that may be filled with a thrombus),

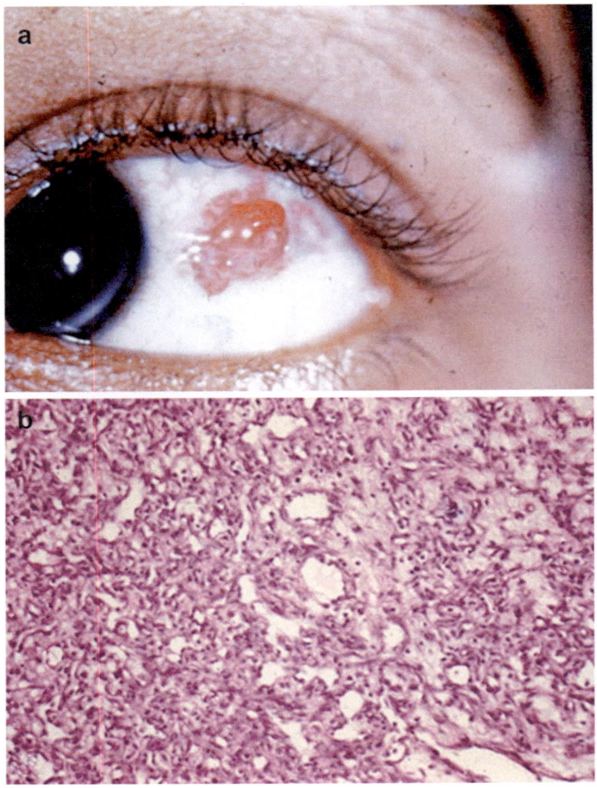

Fig. 20.3 Capillary hemangioma. (**a**) This lesion appears as a focal, red to pink, vascular mass. (**b**) The lesion is composed of compact endothelial-lined vascular channels (hematoxylin and eosin, 100×)

glomus tumor (glomangioma), hemangiopericytoma, bacillary angiomatosis, and conjunctival extension of orbital lymphangioma.

Prophylaxis

The prophylaxis for pyogenic granuloma is burying suture knots in conjunctival wounds and possibly topical corticosteroids. Control of HIV disease with antiretrovirals may be protective regarding development of Kaposi sarcoma.

Therapy

The therapy is excisional biopsy with cautery for hemangiomas and control of HIV disease for Kaposi sarcoma. Kaposi sarcoma may be excised, and any residual/recurrent tumor may be treated with 800–2,000 cGy low-dose external beam radiation therapy. Pyogenic granuloma may be surgically excised and treated with topical corticosteroids. Lymphangiectasis may be observed or surgically excised.

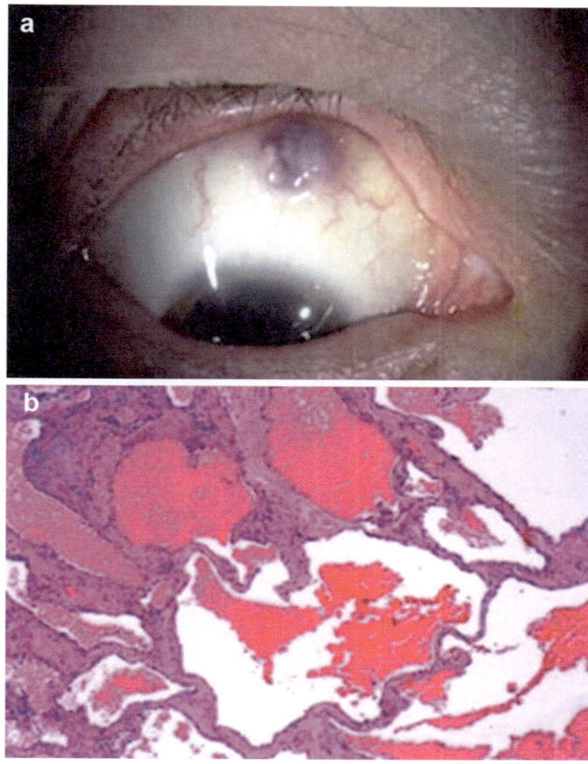

Fig. 20.4 Cavernous hemangioma. (**a**) This lesion is a focal, *blue* to *red* vascular mass. (**b**) The excised lesions are composed of dilated venous channels filled with erythrocytes (hematoxylin and eosin, 100×)

Prognosis

The prognosis for all of these entities is good for complete cure. Kaposi sarcoma may recur in HIV + patients not undergoing antiretroviral treatment.

Cross-References

Conjunctival fibrous histiocytoma/myxoma, conjunctival histiocytic proliferations, conjunctival peripheral nerve sheath tumor, surgical techniques

Epidemiology

These tumors occur sporadically in all ages of patients, with males equally affected as females.

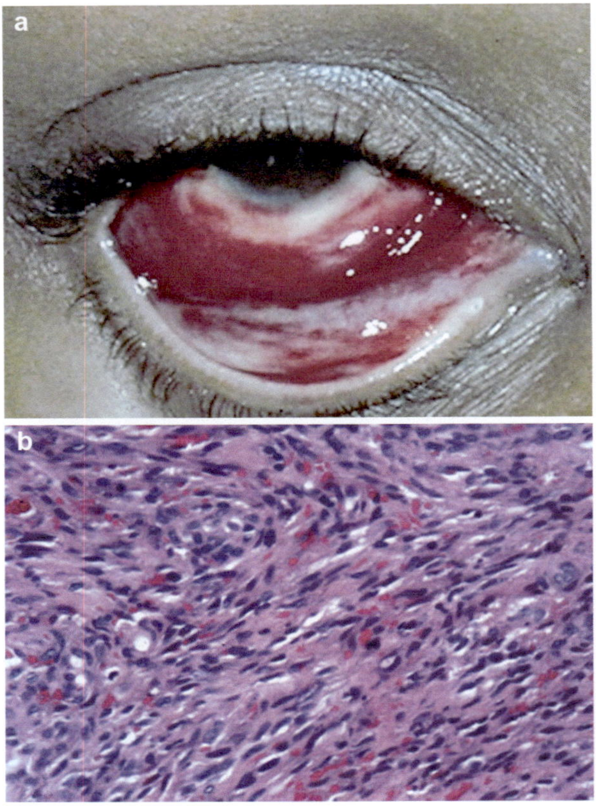

Fig. 20.5 Kaposi sarcoma. (**a**) This lesion appears as a hemorrhagic mass. It may be multifocal. (**b**) The excised lesion is composed of spindle-shaped cells with fusiform nuclei and slit-like spaces containing occasional erythrocytes (hematoxylin and eosin, 100×)

Further Reading

Ferry AP (1989) Pyogenic granulomas of the eye and ocular adnexa: a study of 100 cases. Trans Am Ophthalmol Soc 87:327–347

Fryer RH, Reinke KR (2000) Pyogenic granuloma: a complication of transconjunctival incisions. Plast Reconstr Surg 105:1565–1566

Jones IS (1961) Lympangiomas of the ocular adnexa. An analysis of sixty-two cases. Am J Ophthalmol 51:481–509

Shields JA, De Potter P, Shields CL, Komarnicky LT (1992) Kaposi sarcoma of the eyelids: response to radiotherapy. Arch Ophthalmol 110:1689

Shields JA, Mashayekhi A, Klingman BE, Kunz WB, Criss J, Eagle RC Jr, Shields CL (2011) Vascular tumors of the conjunctiva in 140 cases. Ophthalmology 118:1747–1753

Conjunctival Histiocytic Proliferations 21

Hans E. Grossniklaus

Synonyms

Although rare, there are several histiocytic proliferations that may occur in the conjunctiva. They include sinus histiocytosis with massive lymphadenopathy (Rosai–Dorfman disease), Langerhans cell histiocytosis (eosinophilic granuloma), and reticulohistiocytoma.

Definition

A local histiocytic proliferation that may be self-limited or part of a more generalized histiocytic proliferation.

Etiology

There is no known cause for these histiocytic proliferations that may result in localized masses.

Clinical Presentation

The proliferation usually results in a pink to yellow mass of the bulbar conjunctiva, including at the limbus (Fig. 21.1).

H.E. Grossniklaus, M.D.
Emory University School of Medicine, Emory Eye Center,
Department of Ophthalmology,
Atlanta, GA, USA
e-mail: ophtheg@emory.edu

H.E. Grossniklaus (ed.), *Pocket Guide to Ocular Oncology and Pathology*,
DOI 10.1007/978-3-642-29782-3_21,

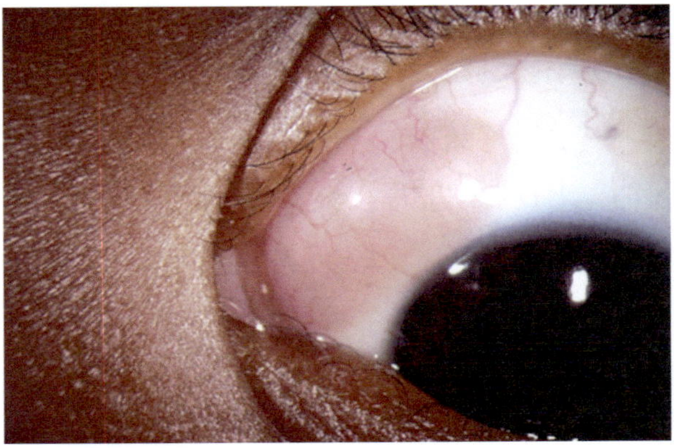

Fig. 21.1 Conjunctival sinus histiocytosis. The lesion in this patient is a lightly pink well-circumscribed mass

Diagnosis

The diagnosis is made by excisional biopsy. The lesion is composed of a proliferation of histiocytes that exhibit immunohistochemical positivity for S100 in cases of sinus histiocytosis and CD1a positivity in cases of Langerhans cell histiocytosis. Imaging of the head and neck, including an MRI and/or CT, plus systemic evaluation is indicated to determine the extent of the proliferation. Sinus histiocytosis may involve the paranasal sinuses. Langerhans cell histiocytosis may be localized (eosinophilic granuloma), multifocal with lytic lesions of the skull, orbital involvement, and diabetes insipidus (Hand–Schuller–Christian disease) or systemic (Letterer–Siwe disease).

Pathology

Conjunctival sinus histiocytosis with massive lymphadenopathy contains a histiocytic infiltrate surrounded by lymphocytes (Fig. 21.2). Some of the histiocytes will exhibit phagocytosis of lymphocytes (emperipolesis). Immunohistochemical stains are characteristically positive for S100 in these histiocytes. Conjunctival Langerhans cell histiocytosis will contain histiocytes and variable numbers of eosinophils (Fig. 21.3). Immunohistochemical stains will be positive for CD1a in the histiocytes. Ultrastructural examination will show intracytoplasmic pentalaminar inclusions (Birbeck granules) in the histiocytes.

Differential Diagnosis

The differential diagnosis includes granulomatous inflammation, xanthogranuloma, large cell lymphoma, and histiocytic sarcoma. These entities are excluded by histologic examination.

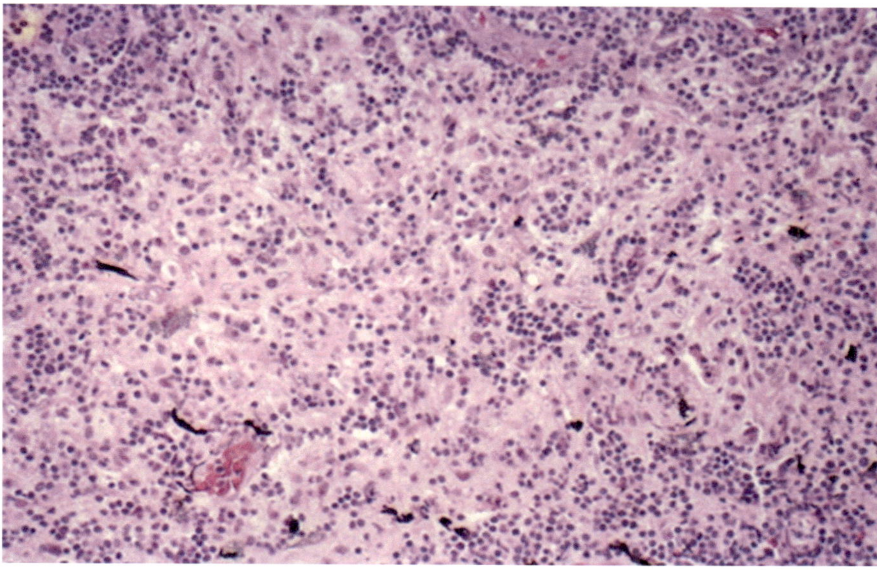

Fig. 21.2 Conjunctival sinus histiocytosis. The lesion is composed of a central area of histiocytes surrounded by small, round lymphocytes (hematoxylin and eosin, 100×)

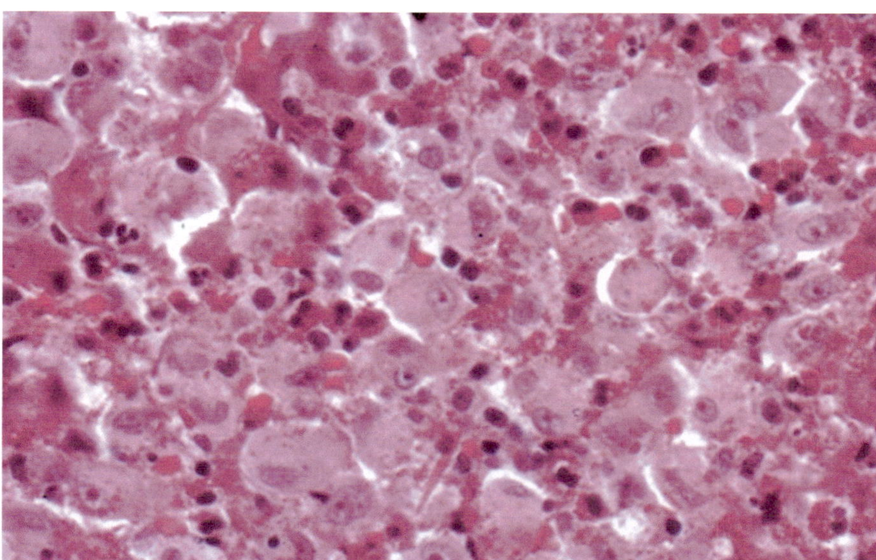

Fig. 21.3 Conjunctival Langerhans cell histiocytosis. In this case, there are many histiocytes surrounded by eosinophils (hematoxylin and eosin, 100×)

Prophylaxis

There is no prophylaxis for this condition.

Therapy

The therapy is excision if possible. Localized lesions are usually self-limited and may respond to topical corticosteroids. Extensive local involvement, for instance, of the orbit, or systemic involvement may require radiation therapy and/or chemotherapy in some instances. Consultation with a hematologist/oncologist is recommended.

Prognosis

The prognosis is good for localized lesions.

Epidemiology

These lesions tend to occur in children and young adults.

Cross-References

Conjunctival fibrous histiocytoma/myxoma, conjunctival vascular proliferations, conjunctival peripheral nerve sheath tumors

Further Reading

Allaire GS, Hidayat AA, Zimmerman LE, Minardi L (1990) Reticulohistiocytoma of the limbus and cornea. Ophthalmology 97:1018–1022

Fernandez FJ, Melcon B, Alvarez R, Honrubia FM (1998) Subconjunctival mass in Rosai-Dorfman disease. Eur J Ophthalmol 8:263–264

Ireland KC, Hutchinson AK, Grossniklaus HE (1999) Sinus histiocytosis presenting as bilateral epibulbar masses. Am J Ophthalmol 127:360–361

Kiratli H, Kocabeyo lu S, Sa lam A, Söylemezo lu F (2007) Langerhans cell histiocytosis of the caruncle. Clin Experiment Ophthalmol 35:661–663

Conjunctival Lymphoma 22

Ying Qian, Arun D. Singh, and Qing Zhang

Synonyms

Lymphoid proliferation of conjunctiva

Definition

Lymphoid proliferations of the conjunctiva represent a spectrum of disease, from benign lymphoid hyperplasia to malignant lymphoma. These tumors arise from the resident population of lymphoid tissue within the conjunctiva or may represent secondary ocular involvement of systemic lymphoma. Conjunctival lymphoma is best categorized as ocular adnexal lymphoma (OAL). A MALT lymphoma is a type of non-Hodgkin lymphoma involving the mucosa-associated lymphoid tissue (MALT), frequently of the stomach, but virtually of any mucosal site, including ocular adnexa. It is a cancer originating from B cells in the marginal zone of the MALT and is also termed extranodal marginal zone B cell lymphoma.

Y. Qian, M.D.
Department of Ophthalmology, Cole Eye Institute, Cleveland Clinic Foundation, Cleveland, OH, USA
e-mail: qiany2@ccf.org

A.D. Singh, M.D. (✉)
Department of Ophthalmology, Cole Eye Institute, Cleveland Clinic Foundation, 9500 Euclid Ave, Desk i-329, Cleveland, OH 44195, USA
e-mail: singha@ccf.org

Q. Zhang, M.D.
Department of Ophthalmology, Emory University School of Medicine, Atlanta, GA, USA
e-mail: qzhang7@emory.edu

H.E. Grossniklaus (ed.), *Pocket Guide to Ocular Oncology and Pathology*,
DOI 10.1007/978-3-642-29782-3_22, © Springer-Verlag Berlin Heidelberg 2013

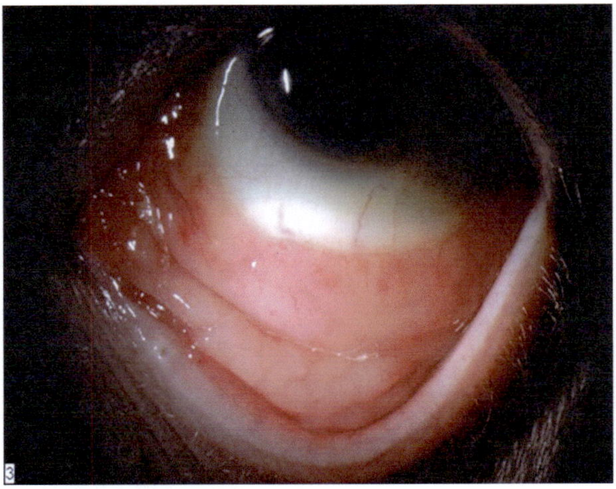

Fig. 22.1 Lymphoma of the conjunctiva appears as a diffuse "salmon patch" infiltrate

Etiology

Although there are several reports implicating infection by *C. psittaci* and other infective agents, the etiology of conjunctival lymphoma remains unclear.

Clinical Presentation

Conjunctival lymphomas generally present as slow-growing, smooth, elevated, and salmon pink masses in the subconjunctival space (Fig. 22.1) (a smooth, elevated, salmon pink masse in the subconjunctival space). They tend to be freely mobile, sharply demarcated, and nonulcerated. They usually do not cause symptoms and are not associated with feeder vessels. The most common locations are in the inferior fornix and bulbar conjunctiva. Most cases are unilateral. Burkitt's lymphoma and AIDS-associated lymphoma tend to grow rapidly.

Diagnostics

The distinction between benign lymphoid hyperplasia and malignant lymphoma is not clinically apparent, and all suspicious lesions warrant biopsy with immunohistochemical, flow cytometric, and gene arrangement analysis. Biopsy can be performed under local anesthesia. Lesions involving the bulbar conjunctiva are excised, and those involving the palpebral conjunctiva are incised. A portion of the surgical specimen is submitted in RPMI or other media for flow cytometry. Another portion is submitted in a fixative, either formalin, B5, or both. MALT lymphomas have a characteristic appearance (Fig. 22.2), which allows their differentiation

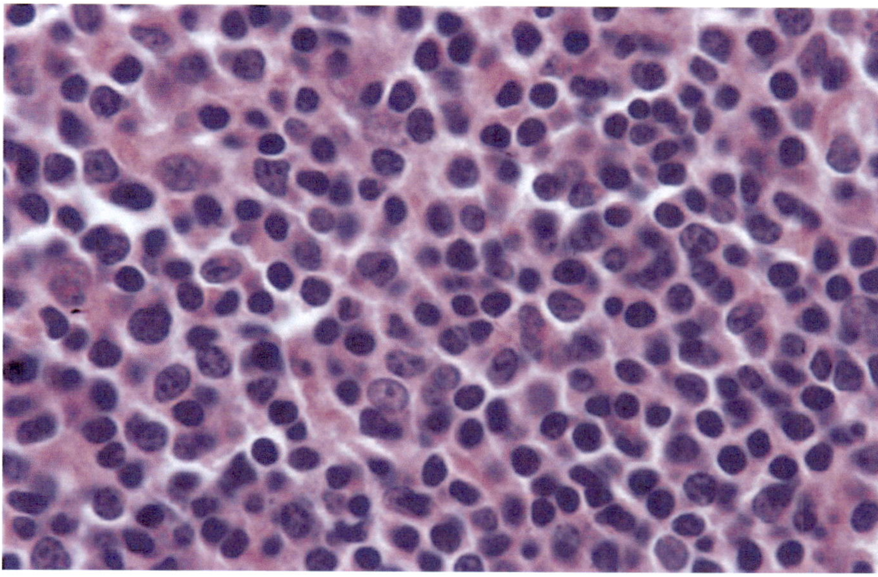

Fig. 22.2 Conjunctival lymphoma is composed of sheets of small, round lymphocytes and larger lymphocytes with open chromatin and prominent nucleoli (hematoxylin and eosin, 100×)

from reactive lymphoid hyperplasia and other small B cell lymphomas. They contain dense CD20+, CD79a+, CD10−, CD23−, BCL-2+, BCL-6−, cyclin-D1− malignant B cell lymphocytic infiltrates, with few interspersed CD3+ T lymphocytes. MALT lymphomas are almost always negative for CD5, distinguishing them from mantle cell lymphoma, small lymphocytic lymphoma, or chronic lymphocytic leukemia.

Pathology

Histopathologic features favoring reactive lymphoid hyperplasia include the presence of lymphoid follicles with germinal centers and an admixture of plasma cells and mature, small lymphocytes in the stroma. A diffuse sheet of monotonous, small, round lymphocytes is more characteristic of a low-grade lymphoma. If the sheets of lymphocytes have a high nuclear to cytoplasmic ratio with many mitotic figures, the diagnosis favors high-grade lymphoma.

Differential Diagnosis

The clinical differential diagnosis includes inflammation, reactive lymphoid hyperplasia, and pseudotumor.

Prophylaxis

None.

Therapy

Investigation for systemic lymphoma is performed first and includes lymph node palpation, complete blood count, sedimentation rate, antirheumatoid factor, serum protein electrophoresis, antinuclear antibodies, chest X-ray, computed tomography of chest, abdomen, and pelvis, bone scan, bilateral bone marrow biopsy, and liver–spleen scan. Systemic chemotherapy is indicated for systemic involvement. If the disease is localized to the conjunctiva, the gold standard therapy is low-dose fractionated external beam radiation (25–30 Gy), depending on the histology of the lymphoma. Patients are followed long term for local and systemic recurrence, typically every 6 months for 5 years, then yearly. Recurrence does not necessarily imply malignancy. Newer modalities include local interferon alpha-2b. Plaque therapy can be used for local disease, although there can be local complications. Cryotherapy is less effective than radiation and is reserved for patients in whom radiation is contraindicated. Benign lymphoid lesions may be observed or treated with corticosteroids. Most recently, mucosa-associated lymphoid tissue was successfully treated with rituximab, an anti-CD20 monoclonal antibody.

Prognosis

Prognosis and response to treatment are overall excellent. Diffuse and extensive involvement in forniceal and midbulbar conjunctival location are associated with systemic disease. In a recent series of patients with biopsy-proven conjunctival lymphoma, 12% developed systemic lymphoma at 1 year, 38% at 5 years, and 79% at 10 years. In patients with all types of lymphoid lesions, however, the rate of systemic lymphoma was 15% at 5 years and 28% at 10 years.

Epidemiology

About 20–30% of ocular adnexal lymphoid lesions arise in the conjunctiva. Most patients present in the sixth to seventh decade of life. More than 20% of patients have bilateral disease. Immunocompromised patients are at risk for developing conjunctival lymphoma.

Further Reading

Augsburger JJ, Schneider S (2004) Tumors of conjunctiva and cornea. In: Yanoff M, Duker JS (eds) Ophthalmology, 2nd edn. Mosby, Missouri, pp 541–543
Cohen VM, Sweetenham J, Singh AD (2008) Ocular adnexal lymphoma. What is the evidence for an infectious aetiology? Br J Ophthalmol 92(4):446–448
Pe'er J (2007) Conjunctival stromal tumors. In: Singh AD et al (eds) Clinical ophthalmic oncology. Saunders Elsevier, Philadelphia, pp 154–155
Warner MA, Jakobiec FA (2005) Subepithelial neoplasms of the conjunctiva. In: Krachmer JH et al (eds) Cornea, 2nd edn. Elsevier Mosby, Philadelphia, pp 593–595, 1780

Conjunctival Melanoma

23

Lynn Schoenfield and Arun D. Singh

Synonyms

There are no synonyms for conjunctival melanoma.

Definition

A conjunctival melanoma is an invasive malignant neoplasm arising from conjunctival melanocytes, often in the setting of primary acquired melanosis (PAM) with atypia also known as conjunctival melanocytic intraepithelial neoplasia (C-MIN) or, if severe enough, melanoma-in-situ.

Etiology

There is no clear evidence that UV radiation is a risk factor for melanoma. There is no association with cutaneous melanoma, dysplastic nevus syndrome, or oculodermal melanocytosis. The main precursors for conjunctival melanoma are PAM with atypia (C-MIN) and conjunctival nevi.

L. Schoenfield (✉)
Department of Pathology, Cleveland Clinic,
Cleveland, OH, USA
e-mail: schoenl@ccf.org

A.D. Singh, M.D.
Department of Ophthalmic Oncology,
Cole Eye Institute, Cleveland Clinic Foundation,
9500 Euclid Ave, Desk i-329, Cleveland, OH 44195, USA
e-mail: singha@ccf.org

H.E. Grossniklaus (ed.), *Pocket Guide to Ocular Oncology and Pathology*,
DOI 10.1007/978-3-642-29782-3_23, © Springer-Verlag Berlin Heidelberg 2013

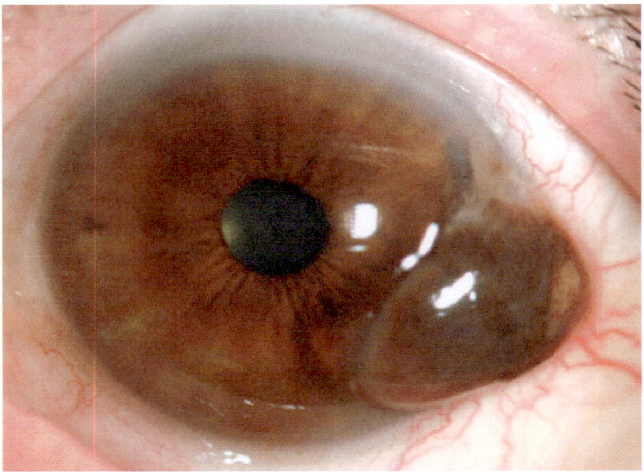

Fig. 23.1 Conjunctival melanoma arising at the limbus may appear as a discrete nodule

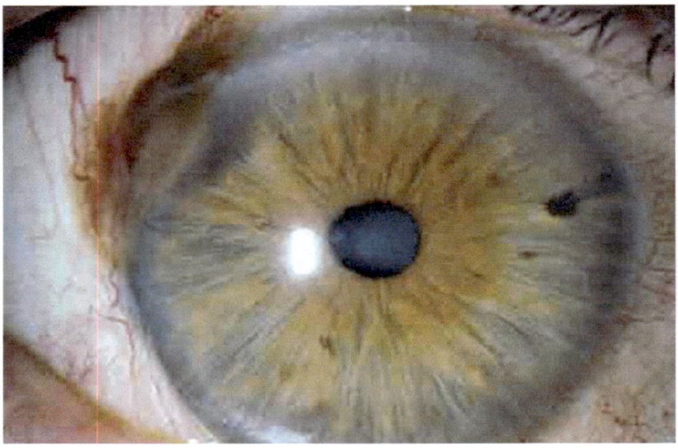

Fig. 23.2 This conjunctival melanoma arises within a bed of surrounding primary acquired melanosis (*PAM*)

Clinical Presentation

Conjunctival melanoma usually affects one eye and is found at the limbus in the interpalpebral region of the bulbar conjunctiva (Fig. 23.1). However, it may arise in any area of the conjunctiva (bulbar, palpebral, forniceal) or the caruncle or plica semilunaris. Conjunctival melanoma may be multifocal and in such cases associated with PAM with atypia , usually melanoma-in-situ (C-MIN of >4). (Fig. 23.2). The lesion is usually heavily vascularized, pigmented, and nodular. It may be amelanotic but in those cases, one can usually see flecks of pigmentation with high magnification using slit lamp biomicroscopy.

Diagnostics

Histopathologic examination is required for a definitive diagnosis. Other lesions, melanocytic or even non-melanocytic, may simulate melanoma and thus biopsy or excision is recommended in suspicious cases. Suspicious features include nodularity, growth, change in color, ulceration, and/or bleeding. Excisional biopsy is the best initial option to prevent spreading of tumor cells.

Pathology

Histopathologically, melanomas have diverse cellular morphology, ranging from pleomorphic, large, bizarre cells with prominent nucleoli to small, polygonal cells with mild anaplasia to spindle cells without identifiable melanin pigment (Fig. 23.3).

Invasion into the substantia propria by atypical melanocytes associated with melanoma-in-situ (or high C-MIN) constitutes invasive melanoma. Often one encounters C-MIN in one portion of the lesion (Fig. 23.4) and invasive melanoma in another portion (Fig. 23.5). Immunohistochemical stains for S100 protein,

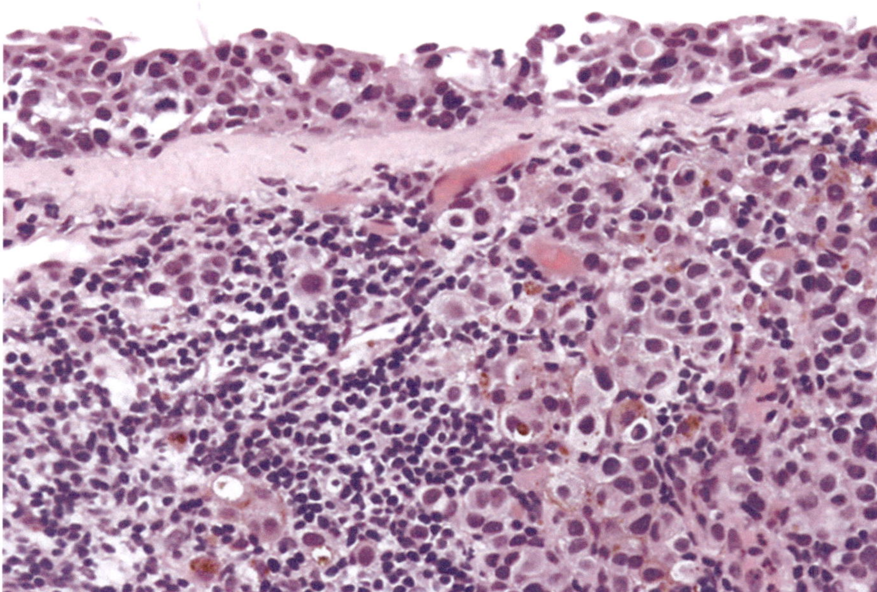

Fig. 23.3 Invasive malignant melanoma with overlying primary acquired melanosis from patient shown in Fig. 23.1 (hematoxylin and eosin, 40×)

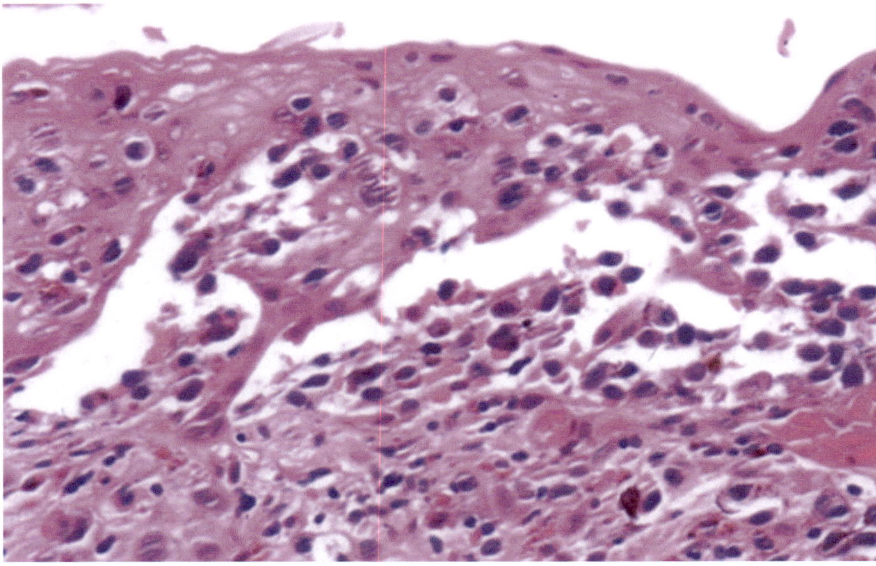

Fig. 23.4 Primary acquired melanosis with marked atypia is present at the junction between the epithelium and substantia propria. This corresponds with the patient shown in Fig. 23.2 (hematoxylin and eosin, 100×)

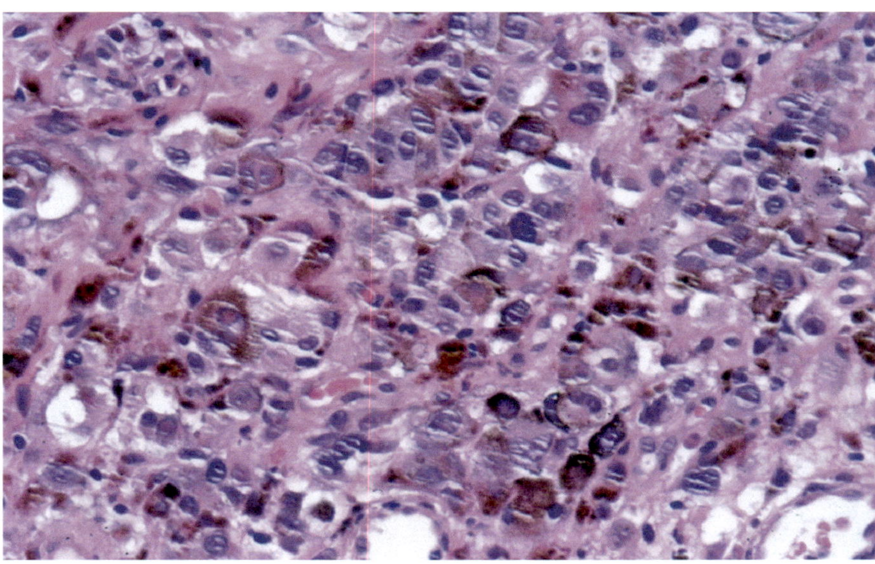

Fig. 23.5 Melanoma is found in other areas of the patient shown in Fig. 23.2. The melanoma cells have markedly pleomorphic nuclei which contain prominent nucleoli. Many tumor cells contain melanin pigment granules in their cytoplasm (hematoxylin and eosin, 100×)

HMB-45, and/or Melan-A may help to identify melanocytes in problematic cases. Features predicting an adverse prognosis include: pagetoid spread, lymphatic invasion, high numbers of mitotic figures, and deep stromal invasion. Generally, conjunctival melanomas less than 1.5 mm in thickness are associated with a good prognosis and greater than 1.5 mm in thickness with a less favorable prognosis. The pathology report should include whether tumor was present at the lateral and deep margins of resection and the tumor thickness. If site is known, this should also be included in the report, as melanomas involving the bulbar conjunctiva have a better prognosis than those of the caruncle, fornix or palpebral conjunctiva.

Differential Diagnosis

Several benign and malignant inflammatory and neoplastic processes can mimic conjunctival melanoma. The following are common lesions in the differential diagnosis: nevus, melanocytoma arising from conjunctiva or extension from uvea, primary acquired melanosis (PAM) without atypia, hematoma, foreign body, staphyloma, PAM with atypia, squamous cell carcinoma (SCC) especially pigmented squamous cell carcinoma, lymphoma, metastatic cutaneous melanoma (rare), and epibulbar extension of uveal melanoma.

Prophylaxis

Prophylaxis includes excision/cryotherapy of PAM lesions.

Therapy

Treatment requires surgical excision of the entire tumor with negative surgical margins of excision. A "no touch" technique is used to avoid dissemination of tumor cells. If deep limbal or scleral involvement is suspected, scleroconjunctivectomy should be considered. Alcohol debridement of the cornea is performed if there is extension onto the cornea. Generally, adjuvant therapy is also given, most commonly double freeze–thaw cryotherapy to the surgical margins and surgical bed. Brachytherapy using β-irradiation may be utilized in select recurrent tumors. It is important to also treat areas of PAM with atypia when present in order to prevent recurrence. Following excision, topical mitomycin C (0.02% QID off 1 week on 1 week for four cycles) may be used if there is any residual pigmentation. Exenteration, which was previously the preferred treatment, does not improve survival and is now reserved for palliative treatment for advanced stage local disease (without evidence of distant metastasis). Patients with conjunctival melanoma should be evaluated by an oncologist and examined for metastases, including regional lymph nodes. There may be some value in doing a sentinel node biopsy in patients with conjunctival melanoma greater than 1.5 mm in thickness.

Prognosis

Conjunctival melanoma-related mortality has ranged in various studies from 12% to 19% in 5 years and 23–30% in 10 years. Local recurrence (often amelanotic) has been reported in 56–65% of patients, and about half of these patients experience more than one recurrence. Surgical treatment without adjuvant therapy increases the recurrence rate, and patients with PAM with atypia are at higher risk for recurrence. Other risk factors are involved surgical margins and locations other than limbus and bulbar conjunctiva (especially the caruncle). Metastases may occur via lymphatic to regional lymph nodes (preauricular and submandibular). Systemic metastatic sites from hematogenous dissemination are frequently brain, liver, and lung. Tumor thickness correlates with prognosis and various studies give a critical thickness. Thin lesions (< 0.8 mm) without lymphatic space involvement rarely give rise to metastatic disease.

Epidemiology

The annual age-adjusted incidence is approximately 0.012/100,000 population. It is rare in black patients (white to black ratio of 13.6:1.0). This tumor makes up 2% of ocular malignancies and 5% of ocular melanomas. Recent studies have shown a higher incidence in males than females. Conjunctival melanoma is most likely to occur between the fourth to seventh decades of life.

Cross-References

PAM, conjunctival nevus, surgical techniques

Further Reading

Damato B and Coupland SE (2008) Conjunctival melanoma and melanosis: A reappraisal of terminology, classification and staging. Clinical and Experimental Ophthalmology; 36: 786–795

Font RL, Croxatto JO, Rao NA (2006) Tumors of the eye and ocular adnexa, AFIP atlas of tumor pathology, series 4, fascicle 5. American Registry of Pathology Press, Washington, DC, USA, pp 23, 47

Friedman NJ, Kaiser PK, Trattler WB (2005) Review of ophthalmology. Elsevier Saunders, Philadelphia, pp 206–207

Pe'er J, Folberg R (2007) Conjunctival melanoma. In: Singh AD, Damato BE, Pe'er J, Murphree AL, Perry JD (eds) Clinical ophthalmic oncology. Saunders Elsevier, Philadelphia, pp 146–149

Conjunctival Nevus

24

Deval Joshi, Sunir Joshi, Curtis E. Margo, Jerome C. Ramos-Esteban, and Arun D. Singh

Definition

A conjunctival nevus is a benign melanocytic lesion of the conjunctiva composed of nests of nevocellular nevus cells.

Etiology

The etiology of conjunctival nevi is unknown.

D. Joshi, M.D. (✉) • C.E. Margo, M.D., MPH
Department of Ophthalmology, University of Florida,
Gainesville, FL 33610, USA
e-mail: deval.joshi.md@gmail.com

S. Joshi, M.D.
Beraja Medical Institute,
Coral Gables, FL, USA
e-mail: sunirjoshi@gmail.com

J.C. Ramos-Esteban, M.D.
Department of Ophthalmic Oncology,
Cole Eye Institute, Cleveland Clinic Foundation,
9500 Euclid Avenue, Cleveland, OH 44195, USA
e-mail: ramosej@ccf.org

A.D. Singh, M.D.
Department of Ophthalmic Oncology,
Cole Eye Institute, Cleveland Clinic Foundation,
9500 Euclid Ave, Desk i-329, Cleveland, OH 44195, USA
e-mail: singha@ccf.org

H.E. Grossniklaus (ed.), *Pocket Guide to Ocular Oncology and Pathology*,
DOI 10.1007/978-3-642-29782-3_24, © Springer-Verlag Berlin Heidelberg 2013

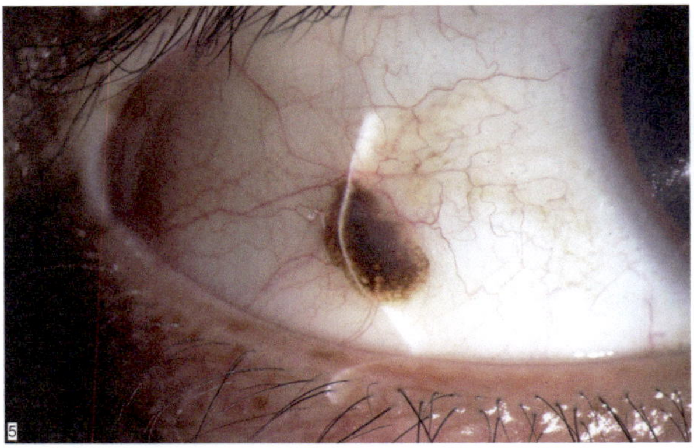

Fig. 24.1 Pigmented conjunctival nevus in the bulbar conjunctiva. Note the cysts within the lesion

Clinical Presentation

Conjunctival nevi are more prevalent in Caucasian patients than non-Caucasians. These melanocytic lesions are most commonly found in the interpalpebral bulbar conjunctiva near the limbus, although involvement of the caruncle and plica semilunaris can also occur. A conjunctival nevus located in the palpebral conjunctiva should raise suspicion for primary acquired melanosis or melanoma. These lesions may have variable sizes and degrees of pigmentation and elevation. The presence of multiple clear cystic structures within the lesion is characteristic for a compound nevus, as it contains epithelial inclusion cysts (Fig. 24.1). These cysts may greatly enlarge, causing the nevus to appear as a cyst (cystic nevus). Changes in the appearance of the nevus during adulthood should raise suspicion of malignant change and may warrant excisional biopsy.

Diagnostics

Conjunctival nevi are usually diagnosed clinically based on their characteristic, appearance, and distribution. Periodic observation with photographic documentation is recommended. Incisional biopsies are not recommended.

The criteria for surgical excision are discussed below.

Differential Diagnosis

Melanoma, primary acquired melanosis (PAM), secondary conjunctival pigmentation (racial melanosis), congenital melanosis oculi (congenital ocular melanocytosis), lymphoma, lymphangiectasia, epithelial inclusion cyst.

Prophylaxis

There is no known prophylaxis for conjunctival nevus.

Therapy

Most conjunctival nevi do not require excision and are observed with serial photographic documentation. Indications for surgical excision include: onset in adulthood; recent growth of the lesion; recent color change; location other than bulbar conjunctiva, plica semilunaris, or caruncle; prominent feeder vessels; and recurrence of an excised lesion. Cryotherapy may be applied to the margins of excision.

Prognosis

The overall risk of malignant transformation is less than 1%.

Epidemiology

Conjunctival nevi may be congenital or acquired. Conjunctival nevi are commonly encountered conjunctival lesions in clinical practice.

Pathology

There are numerous histologic and clinicopathologic variants of conjunctival nevi, as shown below. The most common variant is the compound nevus.

Histologic Variants

Junctional nevus—Nests of cells along the interface of the epithelium and the substantia propia. The cells contain abundant cytoplasm.

Compound nevus—Nests of nevus cells are present in the substantia propia in addition to the junctional area. There is maturation from the surface to the base of the lesion. The nevus contains epithelial inclusions or cysts (Fig. 24.2).

Subepithelial nevus—Nests of nevus cells confined entirely beneath the epithelium.

Balloon cell nevus—Nests of nevus cells with markedly vacuolated cytoplasm are present.

Melanocytoma—Plump polyhedral nevus cells contain heavily pigmented cytoplasm in this nevus. Bleaching of the slide is required for cytologic examination.

Clinicopathologic Variants

Blue nevus/cellular blue nevus—These nevi are subepithelial collections of cells with wavy, spindle-shaped nuclei enmeshed in a collagenous matrix. They may appear slate-gray or blue on slit lamp examination.

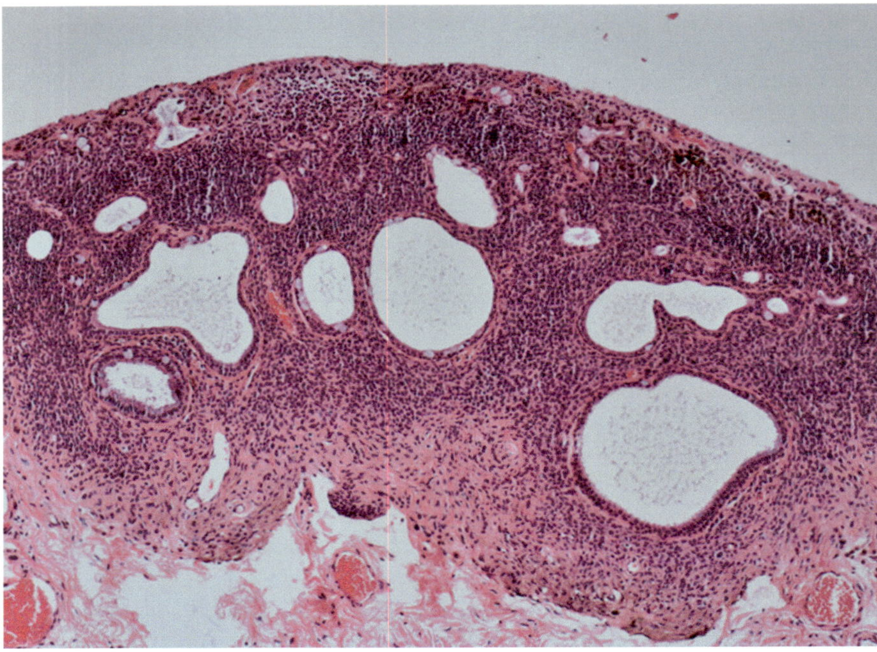

Fig. 24.2 Compound conjunctival nevus. This nevus is composed of junctival and subepithelial nevus cells with entrapped epithelial inclusion cysts (hematoxylin and eosin ×25)

Spitz nevus—This is a subset of common melanocytic nevus that has histological features that mimic melanoma. The majority of Spitz nevi have been reported in children. This distinguishing feature of Spitz nevus is its pleomorphic cells, which may be found individually or in clusters. These cells most often assume spindle shapes or look epithelioid. Spindle cells are often arranged in modified whorls that "rain down" vertically into the substantial propria (Fig. 24.3).

Congenital nevus—This refers to any birthmark or malformation of the conjunctiva present since birth. By convention, the term "congenital nevus" is often restricted to melanocytic malformations. Large congenital melanocytic malformations of the conjunctiva are often associated with contiguous skin involvement. The majority of larger lesions (>1 cm) of the skin tend to have the general architecture of compound nevus but with overlying epithelial hyperplasia and deeper penetration of melanocytes (Fig. 24.4).

Dysplastic nevus—In general, the term "dysplastic nevus" describes a melanocytic lesion occupying a conceptual position between nevus and melanoma. In reference to histological appearance, it describes either cytological atypia or architectural aberration, or both. Nuclei display a degree of pleomorphism and hyperchromatism that occupies a middle ground between benign and malignant. Unlike typical nevi, there may be asymmetry where the junctional activity extends beyond the subepithelial component (Fig. 24.5).

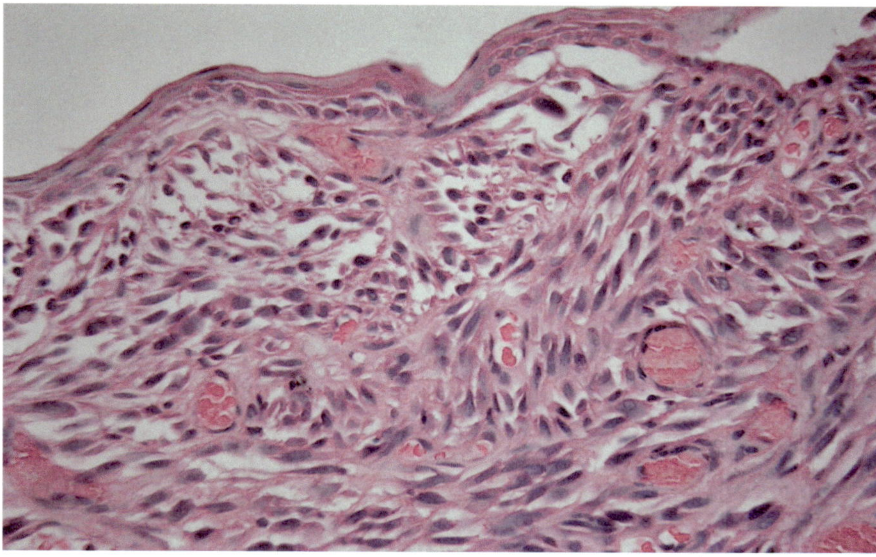

Fig. 24.3 Spitz nevus. Delicate melanocytes with no discernible pigment make up fascicles of spindle-shaped cells. Nuclear chromatin is bland, and no mitotic activity is present. Fascicles run both parallel and perpendicular to the surface epithelium (hematoxylin and eosin ×100)

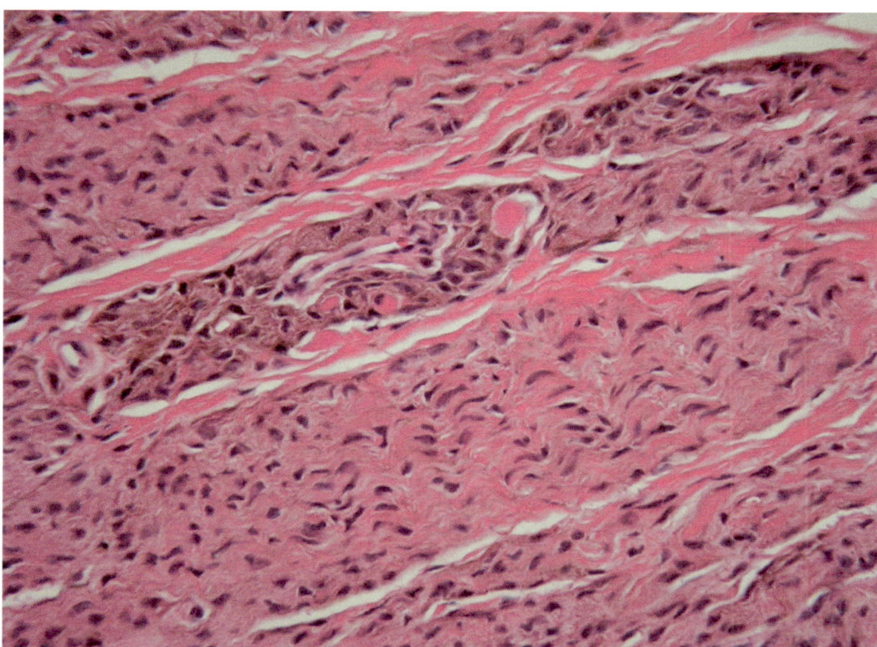

Fig. 24.4 Congenital conjunctival nevus with overlying epithelial hyperplasia and deeper penetration of melanocytes (hematoxylin and eosin ×100)

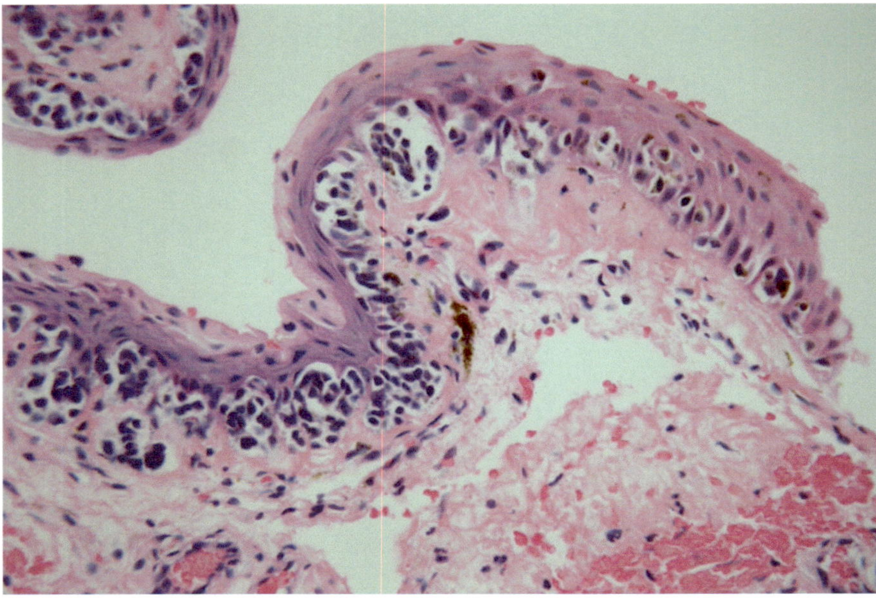

Fig. 24.5 Dysplastic nevus showing a proliferation of basilar melanocytes, in nests and individually, extending beyond the subepithelial component (hematoxylin and eosin ×100)

Cross-References

Conjunctival melanoma, primary acquired melanosis.

Further Reading

Pe'er J (2007) Benign conjunctival tumors. In: Singh AD, Damato BE, Pe'er J, Murphree AL, Perry JD (eds) Clinical ophthalmic oncology. Saunders Elsevier, Philadelphia, pp 129–135

Shields CL, Fasiudden AF, Mashayekhi A et al (2004) Conjunctival nevi: clinical features and natural course in 410 consecutive patients. Ach Ophthalmol 122:167–175

Conjunctiva Peripheral Nerve Sheath Tumors

25

Hans E. Grossniklaus

Synonyms

Peripheral nerve sheath tumors include neurolemmoma (schwannoma) and neurofibroma. There are several types of neurofibroma, including circumscribed, diffuse, and plexiform.

Definition

These tumors arise from the nerve sheath. In the conjunctiva, they likely arise from branches of cranial nerve V; therefore, "peripheral" nerve sheath tumor is a misnomer. These are generally benign and may be associated with neurofibromatosis, especially if the tumor is a plexiform neurofibroma.

Etiology

These tumors are usually isolated and of unknown etiology. However, patients with neurofibromatosis type 1 (17q11.2 mutation) or type 2 (22q11.2–13.1 mutation) may develop peripheral nerve sheath tumors.

H.E. Grossniklaus, M.D.
Emory University School of Medicine,
Emory Eye Center,
Department of Ophthalmology,
Atlanta, GA, USA
e-mail: ophtheg@emory.edu

H.E. Grossniklaus (ed.), *Pocket Guide to Ocular Oncology and Pathology*,
DOI 10.1007/978-3-642-29782-3_25,

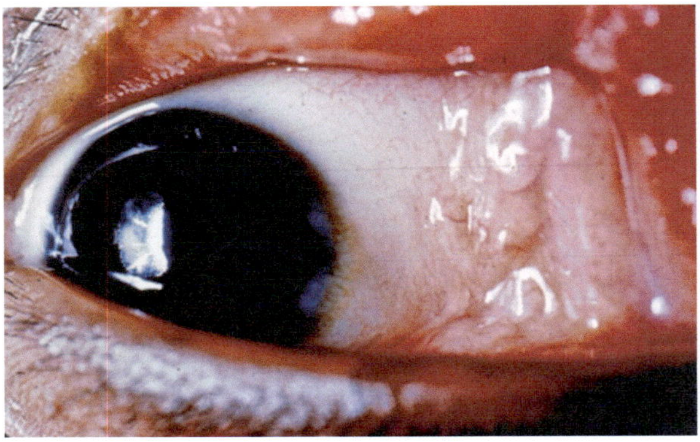

Fig. 25.1 Clinical appearance of conjunctival neurolemmoma (schwannoma) with an "S-shaped" appearance

Clinical Presentation

These tumors may appear on the bulbar and/or tarsal conjunctiva. They may appear as an isolated, discrete soft tissue mass or a more diffuse, irregular mass. In the case of neurolemmoma, it may have an "S-shaped" appearance (Fig. 25.1). They are soft to palpate and usually ballotable. They may have a white, pink, or yellowish appearance.

Diagnosis

The diagnosis is made by excisional biopsy. Persons with peripheral nerve sheath tumors should be evaluated for the presence of neurofibromatosis (see Chap. 19, 20, 75).

Pathology

Histologic evaluation of a neurolemmoma shows a subepithelial spindle cell tumor (Fig. 25.2). The cells in the tumor have bland, spindle-shaped nuclei arranged in bundles known as the "Antoni A" pattern (Fig. 25.3). Myxoid or "Antoni B" areas may be present in the tumor. Immunohistochemical stains are positive for S100 in the tumor (Fig. 25.4). Neurofibromas are composed of haphazard proliferations of endoneural and perineural fibroblasts and associated nerve fibers. They may be circumscribed, diffuse, or plexiform (enlarged nerve bundles), yielding to the clinical palpation "bag of worms" finding.

Differential Diagnosis

The differential diagnosis includes nonpigmented subepithelial conjunctival tumors, including fibrous histiocytoma, hemangiopericytoma, solitary fibrous tumor, and myxoma. These entities are excluded by pathologic examination of the excisional biopsy specimen.

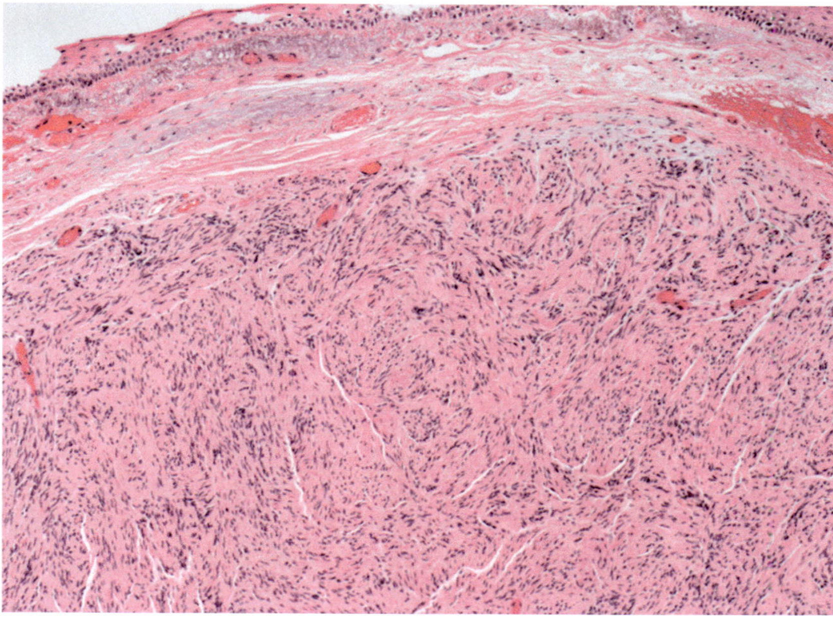

Fig. 25.2 The excised lesion is composed of a subepithelial mass of spindle-shaped cells (hematoxylin and eosin, ×25)

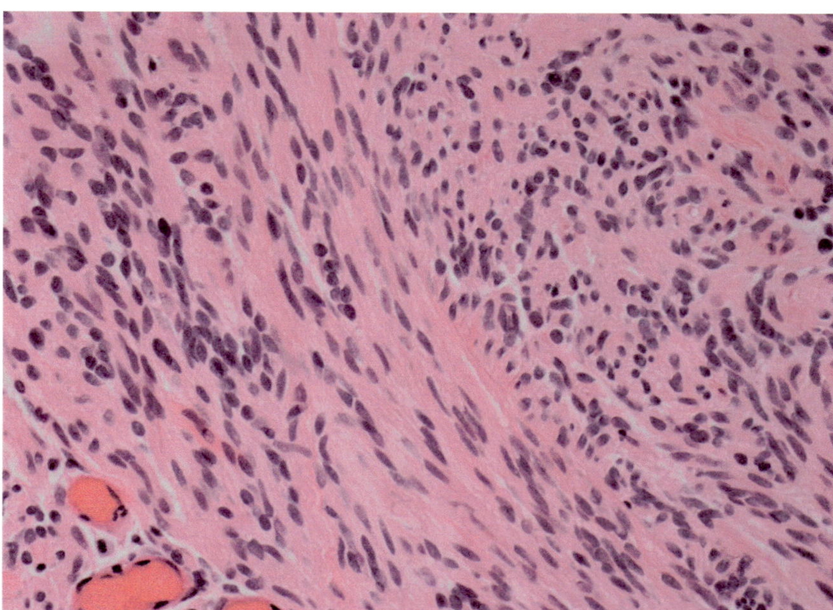

Fig. 25.3 The subepithelial mass contains bundles of cells with bland, spindle-shaped nuclei and abundant eosinophilic cytoplasm (hematoxylin and eosin, ×100)

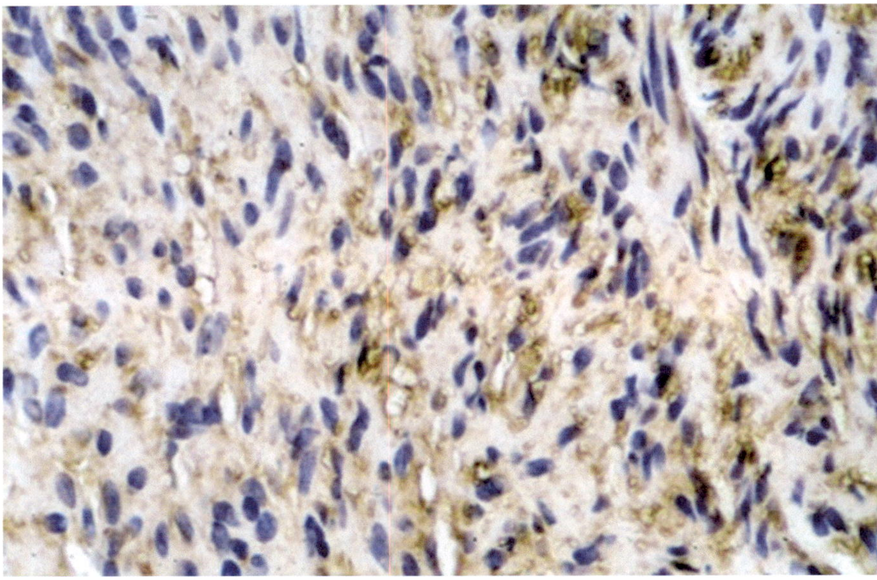

Fig. 25.4 Immunohistochemical stains for S100 are positive in the tumor (peroxidase-antiperoxidase, ×100)

Prophylaxis

There is no prophylaxis for conjunctival peripheral nerve sheath tumor.

Therapy

The therapy is complete surgical excision, as incompletely excised lesions may locally recur. Surgery may be accomplished by demarcating the tumor with a marking pen and dissecting with Westcott scissors and 12 forceps, with hemostasis maintained as needed with cautery.

Prognosis

The prognosis is excellent, as conjunctival peripheral nerve sheath tumor is virtually always a benign tumor.

Epidemiology

These tumors may occur in children or adults. They occur at an earlier age in patients with neurofibromatosis. They affect males and females equally.

Cross-References

Conjunctival fibrous histioctyoma/myxoma, conjunctival vascular proliferations, phakomatoses

Further Reading

Charles NC, Fox DM, Avendano JA, Marriquin LS, Appleman W (1997) Conjunctival neurolemmoma. Report of 3 cases. Arch Ophthalmol 115:547–549

Grossniklaus HE, Luckenbach M, Chan CC (1987) Conjunctival tumors in adults. A clinical and histopathologic review. Cornea 6:78–116

Kalina PH, Bartley GB, Campbell RJ, Buettner H (1991) Isolated neurofibromas of the conjunctiva. Am J Ophthalmol 111:694–698

Conjunctival Primary Acquired Melanosis

26

Jerome C. Ramos-Esteban, Arun D. Singh, Jill R. Wells, and Hans E. Grossniklaus

Synonyms

Lentigo maligna melanosis, precancerous melanosis, benign acquired melanosis (primary acquired melanosis, or PAM, without atypia), atypical melanocytic hyperplasia, melanoma-in-situ (PAM with atypia)

Definition

Primary acquired melanosis (PAM) is the term used to describe acquired intraepithelial/junctional proliferation of atypical melanocytes in the conjunctiva.

J.C. Ramos-Esteban, M.D. (✉)
Department of Ophthalmic Oncology,
Cole Eye Institute, Cleveland Clinic Foundation,
9500 Euclid Avenue, Cleveland, OH 44195, USA
e-mail: jre2020@aol.com

A.D. Singh, M.D.
Department of Ophthalmic Oncology,
Cole Eye Institute, Cleveland Clinic Foundation,
9500 Euclid Ave, Desk i-329, Cleveland, OH 44195, USA
e-mail: singha@ccf.org

J.R. Wells, M.D.
Departments of Ophthalmology, Emory University School of Medicine,
Atlanta, GA, USA
e-mail: jwells4@emory.edu

H.E. Grossniklaus, M.D.
Emory University School of Medicine,
Emory Eye Center,
Department of Ophthalmology,
Atlanta, GA, USA
e-mail: ophtheg@emory.edu

H.E. Grossniklaus (ed.), *Pocket Guide to Ocular Oncology and Pathology*,
DOI 10.1007/978-3-642-29782-3_26, © Springer-Verlag Berlin Heidelberg 2013

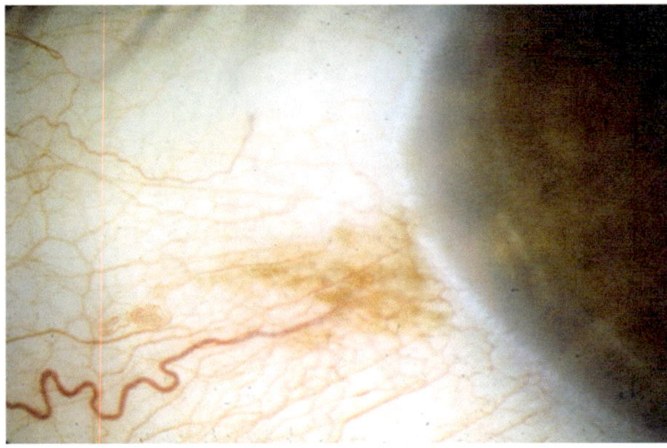

Fig. 26.1 Focal-acquired area of golden-brown pigmentation in the bulbar conjunctiva is suspicious for PAM

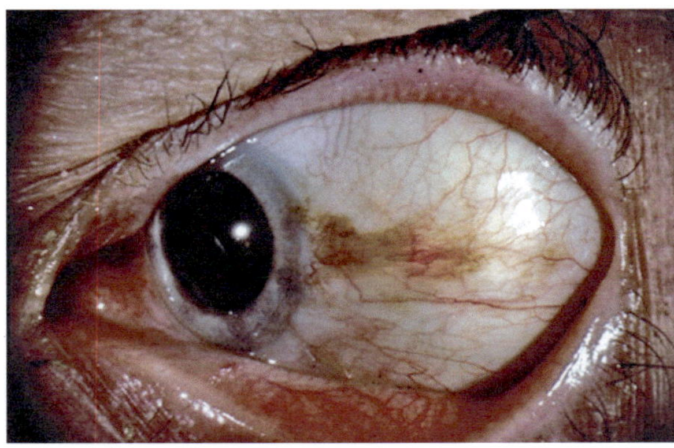

Fig. 26.2 This patient has more diffuse, patchy areas of acquired bulbar conjunctival pigmentation which is also highly suspicious for PAM

Etiology

Risk factors for the development of PAM may include sunlight exposure, cigarette smoking, and hypertension.

Clinical Presentation

PAM appears clinically as a flat and variably brown conjunctival lesion. It may be small and isolated (Fig. 26.1), patchy, golden brown, and diffuse (Fig. 26.2). PAM lesions occur primarily in middle-aged, fair-skinned individuals. PAM lesions do not have a uniform size and may exhibit different degrees of pigmentation. PAM lesions are commonly located in the limbal and perilimbal area and may extend into the corneal epithelium. Lesions may be isolated or grouped. Most are unilateral. Parts of the lesion may be amelanotic (sine pigmento), and therefore, the clinical borders may be misleading. There are no clinical criteria to determine if a lesion has atypia.

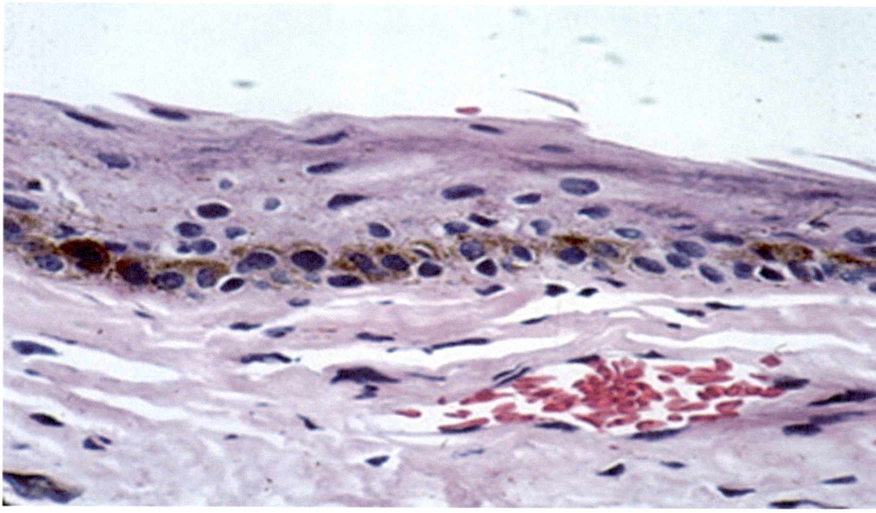

Fig. 26.3 PAM without atypia. This biopsy was obtained from the patient shown in Fig. 26.1 and consists of junctional melanocytes and pigmented basilar keratinocytes of the epithelium. There are no atypical features (hematoxylin and eosin, ×100)

Diagnostics

Periodic observation with photographic documentation is recommended. The eyelids must be everted to determine the extent of the lesion. If there are any clinical changes or the lesion has any nodularity/thickness, a biopsy should be performed. Map biopsies may be obtained to determine the extent of PAM.

Pathology

Histopathologically, PAM is divided into PAM without atypia (Fig. 26.3) and PAM with atypia (Fig. 26.4). PAM without atypia is histologically similar to a junctional nevus. The detection of any atypical growth pattern or cytologic features of the proliferating melanocytes is designated as PAM with atypia. Atypical growth patterns include basilar palisading, junctional nests, intraepithelial nests, pagetoid spread into the epithelium, or full-thickness epithelial replacement. Atypical cytology includes polyhedral, spindle, small epithelioid, and large epithelioid melanocytes. PAM with atypia may be classified with minimal atypia (basilar palisading growth pattern, spindle-shaped cells), moderate atypia (junctional nests, intraepithelial nests, and/or pagetoid spread with polyhedral or small epithelioid cells), or marked atypia (pagetoid spread, intraepithelial nests, and/or full-thickness epithelial replacement with large epithelioid cells). PAM without atypia or minimal atypia is highly unlikely to progress to melanoma. PAM with moderate atypia is likely to progress to melanoma. PAM with marked atypia is highly likely to progress to melanoma, and many consider this to be melanoma in situ.

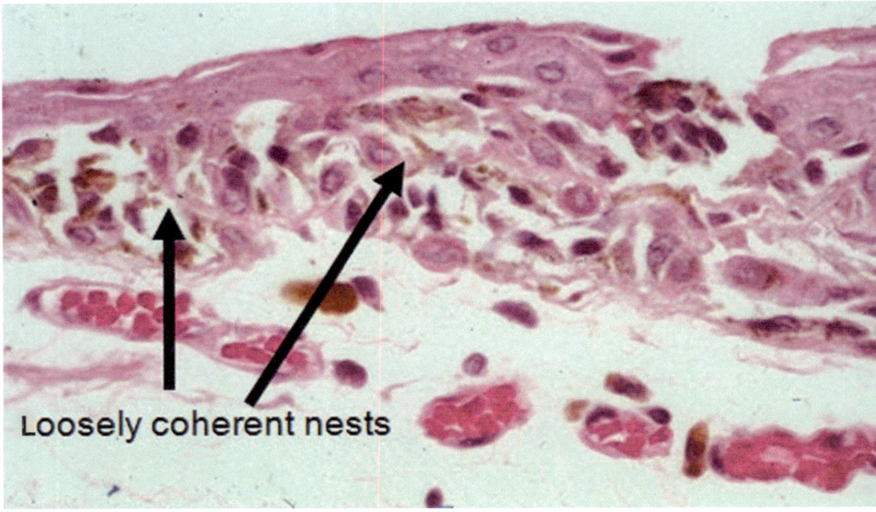

Fig. 26.4 PAM with atypia. This excisional biopsy was obtained from the patient shown in Fig. 26.2. Note the loosely cohesive junctional nests of melanocytes (*arrows*) (hematoxylin and eosin, ×100)

Differential Diagnosis

The differential diagnosis of PAM includes conjunctival nevus, ocular melanosis, conjunctival malignant melanoma, postinflammatory melanosis, complexion-associated conjunctival pigmentation (racial melanosis), congenital melanosis oculi (congenital ocular melanocytosis), and, in bilateral cases, Addison's disease.

Prophylaxis

There is no known prophylaxis for PAM.

Therapy

Management of PAM lesions includes observation, surgical excision, cryotherapy, and local chemotherapy with mitomycin C. All significant PAM lesions should be biopsied, depending on the size of the lesions, and an incisional or excisional technique may be used. If the lesion is less than 3 clock hours, it may be possible to excise with primary closure. If the lesion is greater than 3 clock hours, excision with a conjunctival autograft or amniotic membrane graft may be considered. Cryotherapy should be applied to the margins of excision.

In extensive lesions (greater than 1/3 of the conjunctiva), biopsy and serial double freeze-thaw cryotherapy are recommended. The cryotherapy may be applied to the undersurface of the conjunctiva that is exposed with Westcott scissors or the

CONJUNCTIVAL MELANOCYTIC PROLIFERATION

Name: ______________________ MRN No. ______________________

DOB:___ ___ ______ Path No.: ______________________

Eye: Left / Right

Specimen location:

1.
2.
3.
4.
5.
6.
7.
8.

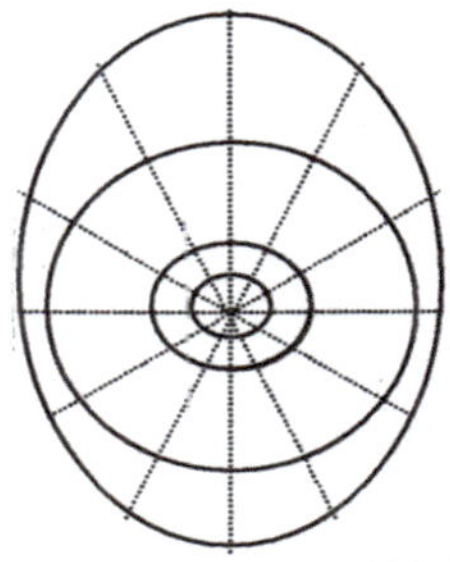

(Please check the box for each specimen)

Feature	**Description**	**Specimen**							
		1	2	3	4	5	6	7	8
Diagnosis	Nevus								
	Secondary melanosis								
	PAM without atypia								
	PAM with atypia								
	Melanoa								
PAM Degree of Atypia	Mild								
	Moderate								
	Severe								
	N/A								
Growth Pattern	Basilar pallisading								
	Junctional nests								
	Intraepithelial nests								
	Pagetoid								
	N/A								
PAM Cell Type	Dendritiform								
	Small epitheloid								
	Large epitheloid								
	Polyhedral								
	N/A								
Melanoma Growth Pattern	Discrete								
	Diffuse								
	N/A								
Melanoma Thickness	< 1.5 mm								
	> 1.5 mm								
	N/A								
Surgical Margin	Involved								
	Non-involved								

Comment: ______________________ Date: ___/___/___.

Fig. 26.5 Sample clinical/pathology submission form for suspected cases of conjunctival PAM/ melanoma

surface of the conjunctiva. Surgical specimens should undergo histopathological analysis to determine the presence of cellular atypia and free surgical margins. It is useful for the surgeon and pathologist to complete a form indicating the extent and pathology of PAM, including any areas where there are melanoma arising in the PAM. A sample submission form is shown (Fig. 26.5) based on the work of Damato and Coupland. Topical mitomycin C 0.02% may be used to treat extensive superficial lesions. Recurrent melanoma arising in PAM may be treated with reexcision, brachytherapy, or exenteration if extensive.

Prognosis

Local recurrence has been correlated with the presence of atypia (mild, moderate, or severe). It has been estimated that 60% of lesions with atypia can recur after excision and that 50% of those may recur as a malignant melanoma. The median interval between the biopsy of PAM and the biopsy of melanoma was 2.5 years in one series. Progression to melanoma 6 years after biopsy is very rare. Recurrence is more likely when there is incomplete resection of the lesion or when the cornea is involved. There is no mortality in PAM without transformation to melanoma, but it is important to remember the mortality of conjunctival melanoma is up to 25%.

Epidemiology

PAM lesions most often occur in middle-aged or elderly Caucasian individuals. Most cases of PAM are unilateral, although bilateral cases have been reported. The average age at the time of diagnosis ranges from 45 to 62 years. Men and women appear to be equally affected.

Cross-References

Conjunctival melanoma, conjunctival nevus, surgical techniques

Further Reading

Folberg R, McLean IW, Zimmerman LE (1985) Primary acquired melanosis of the conjunctiva. Hum Pathol 16:129–135

Glor P, Alexandrakis G (1995) Clinical characterization of primary acquired melanosis. Invest Ophthalmol Vis Sci 36:1721–1729

Jakobiec FA, Folberg R, Iwamoto T (1989) Clinicopathologic characteristics of premalignant and malignant melanocytic lesions of the conjunctiva. Ophthalmology 96:147–166

Pe'er J, Folberg R (2007) Primary acquired melanosis. In: Singh AD, Damato BE, Pe'er J, Murphree AL, Perry JD (eds) Clinical ophthalmic oncology. Saunders Elsevier, Philadelphia, pp 141–145

Singh AD (2007) Clinical ophthalmic oncology. WB Saunders Company, Philadelphia, pp 141–145

Damato B, Coupland SE (2008) Clinical mapping of conjunctival melanomas. Br J Ophthalmol 92:1542–9

Conjunctival Sebaceous Carcinoma

27

Sunir Joshi and Curtis Margo

Synonyms

Sebaceous gland carcinoma

Definition

The term is usually used in the context of secondary spread of sebaceous carcinoma to the conjunctiva from a primary site in the eyelid (meibomian gland or gland of Zeis). It is a malignant neoplasm capable of aggressive local behavior and metastases to regional lymph nodes and distant organs.

Sebaceous carcinoma is one of the most lethal ocular adnexal tumors.

Etiology

Prior radiation to the eye/orbit in patients with hereditary retinoblastoma may be associated with sebaceous carcinoma. Acne, eczema, and cutaneous hemangioma are risk factors. A possible relationship between SGC and HPV has been observed. There may be an association between sebaceous carcinoma and immune dysfunction at a relatively young age.

C. Margo, M.D., MPH (✉)
Department of Ophthalmology,
University of South Florida,
Tampa, FL, USA
e-mail: cmargo@health.usf.edu

S. Joshi, M.D.
Beraja Medical Institute,
Coral Gables, FL, USA
e-mail: sunirjoshi@gmail.com

H.E. Grossniklaus (ed.), *Pocket Guide to Ocular Oncology and Pathology*,
DOI 10.1007/978-3-642-29782-3_27,

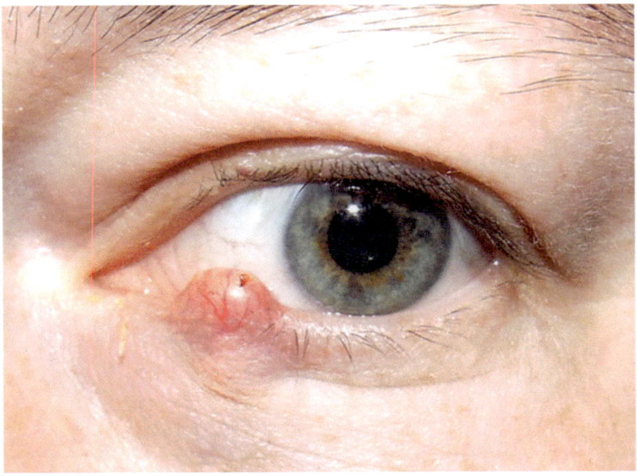

Fig. 27.1 Sebaceous carcinoma of the eyelid appearing as solitary, firm nodule fixed to the tarsus

Clinical Presentation

The majority of all periocular sebaceous carcinomas arise from the meibomian glands within the tarsus; 65% arise in the upper lid, 25% in the lower lid, and 5% involve both eyelids. Sebaceous carcinoma may arise primarily in the conjunctiva (primary intraepithelial sebaceous carcinoma). Sebaceous carcinoma most commonly appears as a solitary, firm, painless, and sessile round nodule fixed to the tarsus (Fig. 27.1). The tumor may demonstrate a yellow tint secondary to lipid. The second most common presentation is unilateral diffuse thickening of the eyelid (Fig. 27.2). Sebaceous carcinoma of the conjunctiva may also appear as chronic unilateral blepharoconjunctivitis in patients with "masquerade syndrome" (Fig. 27.3).

Diagnostics

A full-thickness excision or incisional biopsy of the eyelid is necessary in any eyelid suspicious for sebaceous carcinoma. After a diagnosis of sebaceous carcinoma is made, map biopsies are needed to determine the extent of disease. Fine needle aspiration biopsy (FNAB) and impression cytology are not recommended due to the limited amount of tissue obtained. Orbital imaging can be considered when there is diffuse involvement of the eyelids and conjunctiva to evaluate for posterior extension.

Pathology

Well-differentiated tumors consist of cells with typical foamy cytoplasm and centrally located hyperchromatic nuclei. Undifferentiated tumors consist of cells with high nuclear to cytoplasmic ratio and few discernible signs of sebaceous differentiation.

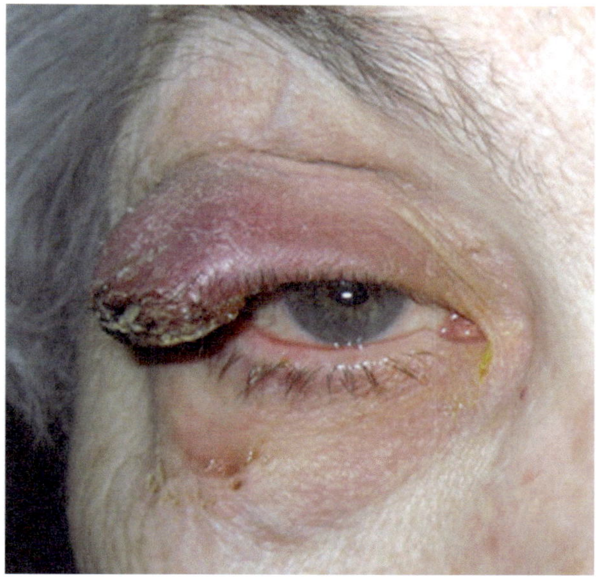

Fig. 27.2 Diffuse thickening of the eyelid in a patient with sebaceous carcinoma

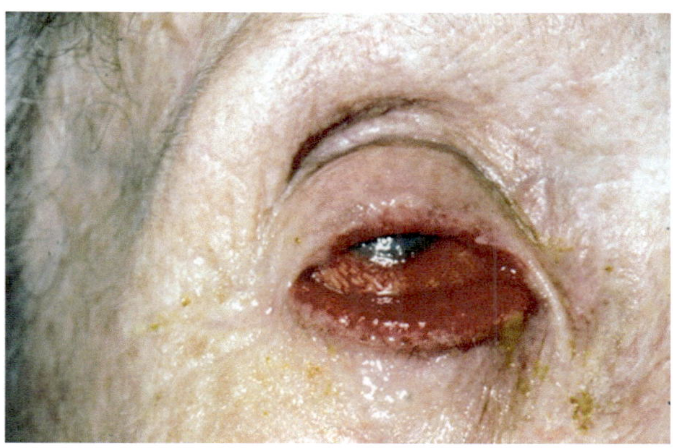

Fig. 27.3 Chronic unilateral blepharoconjunctivitis from intraepithelial sebaceous carcinoma causing "masquerade syndrome"

Two patterns are described: pagetoid, characterized by individual large cells in the suprabasilar layers (Fig. 27.4); and bowenoid, consisting of contiguous sheets of malignant cells (Fig. 27.5). Sebaceous carcinoma can also be classified into one of the following patterns: lobular (architecture similar to normal sebaceous gland with fewer differentiated cells peripherally and more differentiated lipid-producing cells located centrally), comedocarcinoma (a large necrotic central core surrounded by viable cells), papillary (papillary projections), and mixed (any combination of the above three). Positive oil red-O stains for lipid are helpful but not necessary. Immunohistochemistry stains may be positive for HMFG1, EMA, and BRST-1, but not cytokeratins.

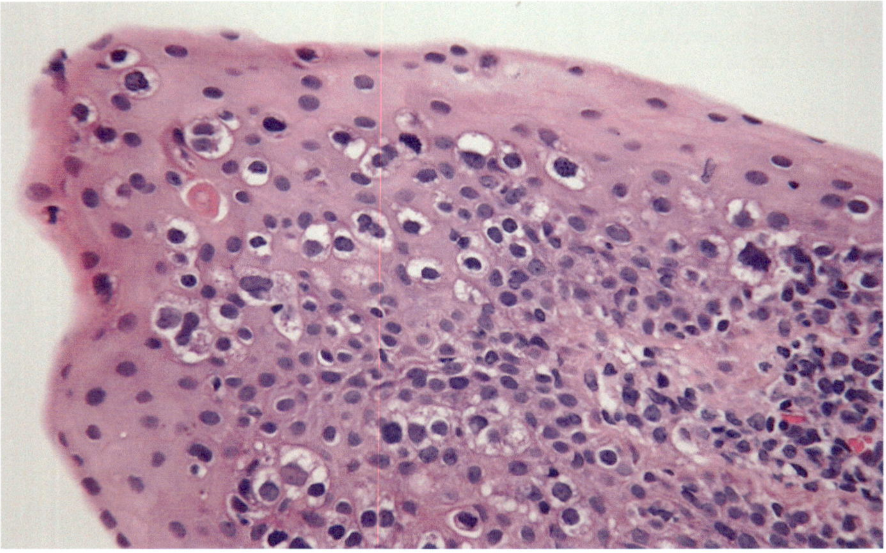

Fig. 27.4 Individual pagetoid cells with hyperchromatic nuclei are present in the suprabasilar epithelium close to the lid margin. These large cells have clear cytoplasm that stains negative for mucin and glycogen and positive for lipid (hematoxylin and eosin ×100)

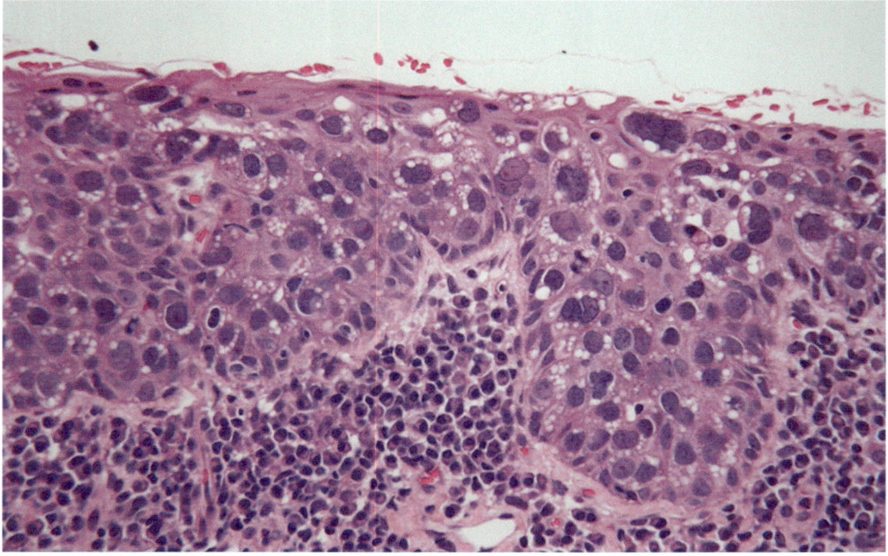

Fig. 27.5 Bowenoid spread shows the entire conjunctival epithelium replaced with large atypical cells with numerous clear cytoplasmic inclusions. There is a dense subepithelium inflammatory infiltrate

Differential Diagnosis

The clinical differential diagnosis includes: chalazion, blepharitis, conjunctivitis, meibomitis, superior limbic keratoconjunctivitis, cicatricial pemphigoid, conjunctival granuloma, basal cell carcinoma, squamous cell carcinoma, Merkel cell carcinoma, lymphoma, metastatic carcinoma, and amelanotic melanoma.

The pathologic differential diagnosis for well differeniated sebaceous carcinoma includes sebaceous adenoma and adenomatous hyperplasia. Poorly differentiated sebaceous carcinoma resembles other malignancies including metastatic carcinoma, melanoma, and poorly differentiated squamous cell and basal cell carcinomas.

Prophylaxis

There is no known prophylaxis for sebaceous carcinoma.

Therapy

Complete surgical excision is the preferred treatment for sebaceous carcinoma.

Either frozen section control or a Mohs technique is usually performed at the time of excision to evaluate the margins. Supplemental cryotherapy is indicated when the removal of wide margins is not possible. Topical chemotherapy with mitomycin C drops has been found to be effective in selected cases. Systemic chemotherapy is used to treat regional spread to lymph nodes and distant organs.

Prognosis

The 5-year local recurrence rate following wide excision ranges from 9% to 36%.

Older literature indicates that metastases occur in 30% of patients with sebaceous carcinoma, most commonly to regional lymph nodes. With early recognition, this rate may now be lowered. Advanced cases may spread hematogenously to liver, lung, bone, and brain. The 5-year tumor-related death rate in the past was 30%, but now, due to increased awareness, it is closer to 10%.

Risk factors associated with a worse prognosis include vascular, lymphatic, and orbital invasion; involvement of both upper and lower eyelids; poor differentiation; multicentric origin; duration of symptoms greater than 6 months; tumor diameter exceeding 10 mm; and pagetoid invasion.

Epidemiology

Sebaceous carcinoma accounts for 5% of all malignant eyelid tumors.

The annual incidence in the USA is 0.5 per million in the Caucasian population over age 20. This tumor is more common in Caucasians than African-Americans. A higher incidence has been observed in China, India, and other Asian countries than in the USA. The average age at the time of diagnosis is 57–72 years. There is a 70% predominance in women.

Cross-References

Conjunctival carcinoma-squamous cell, conjunctival dysplasia, map biopsies

Further Reading

Honavar SG, Shields CL, Maus M et al (2001) Primary intraepithelial sebaceous gland carcinoma of the palpebral conjunctiva. Arch Ophthalmol 119:764–767

Kass LG, Hornblass A (1989) Sebaceous carcinoma of the ocular adnexa. Surv Ophthalmol 33:477–490

Margo CE, Grossniklaus HE (1995) Intraepithelial sebaceous neoplasia without underlying invasive carcinoma. Surv Ophthalmol 39:239–301

Margo CE, Lessner A, Stern GA (1992) Intraepithelial sebaceous carcinoma of the conjunctiva and skin of the eyelid. Ophthalmology 99:227–231

Muqit MM, Roberts F, Lee WR et al (2004) Improved survival rates in sebaceous carcinoma of the eyelid. Eye 18:49–53

Shields CL, Naseripour M, Shields JA et al (2002) Topical mitomycin-C for pagetoid invasion of the conjunctiva by eyelid sebaceous gland carcinoma. Ophthalmology 109:2129–2133

Shields JA, Demirci H, Marr BP et al (2005) Sebaceous carcinoma of the ocular region: a review. Surv Ophthalmology 50:103–122

Sinard J (1999) Immunohistochemical distinction of ocular sebaceous carcinoma from basal cell and squamous cell carcinoma. Arch Ophthalmol 177:776–783

Singh AD (2007) Clinical ophthalmic oncology. WB Saunders Company, Philadelphia, pp 85–88

Sramek B, Lisle A, Loy T (2008) Immunohistochemistry in ocular carcinomas. J Cutan Pathol 35:641–646

Corneal Tumors

28

Sumitra Khandewal and Hans E. Grossniklaus

Synonyms

Corneal neoplasms; Corneal extension of conjunctival tumors

Definition

Although rare, there are many types of tumors that may potentially occur in the cornea. Epithelial tumors generally arise at the limbus and may involve the cornea secondarily, although they may also occur primarily in the cornea. Stromal tumors may also rarely occur. Corneal intraepithelial neoplasia (CIN) is a neoplastic intraepithelial proliferation that occurs on the cornea in the interpalpebral fissure. Squamous cell carcinoma is a malignant epithelial tumor with invasion beneath basement membrane of basilar epithelium. The mucoepidermoid carcinoma (Fig. 28.1) variant may invade into the cornea. Dermoid is a choristoma that included dermis-like connective tissue. Dermolipoma is the same as dermoid with associated

S. Khandewal, M.D. (✉)
Department of Ophthalmology,
Emory University School of Medicine,
Atlanta, GA, USA

Department of Ophthalmology,
Emory Eye Center, Atlanta, GA, USA
e-mail: ssubra9@emory.edu

H.E. Grossniklaus, M.D.
Emory University School of Medicine, Emory Eye Center,
Department of Ophthalmology,
Atlanta, GA, USA
e-mail: ophtheg@emory.edu

H.E. Grossniklaus (ed.), *Pocket Guide to Ocular Oncology and Pathology*,
DOI 10.1007/978-3-642-29782-3_28, © Springer-Verlag Berlin Heidelberg 2013

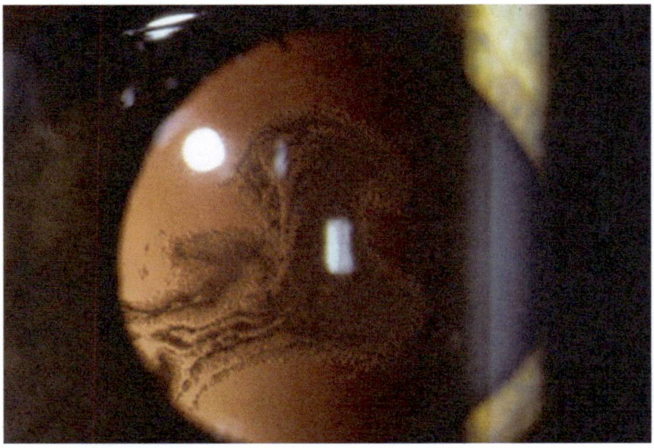

Fig. 28.1 A sheet of thickened corneal epithelium is seen by retroillumination in this patient with corneal epithelial dysplasia

adipose tissue. Melanoma of the conjunctiva may extend into the cornea or very rarely arise in the cornea. Conjunctival fibrous histiocytoma, xanthogranuloma, and papilloma may extend onto the cornea.

Etiology

CIN may be related to sun (UV light) exposure or corneal irritation. Squamous cell carcinoma is possibly related to UV light exposure or irritation. Dermoids and dermolipomas result from entrapment of epithelial elements at site of closure of a fetal fissure. Melanoma may arise at the limbus, often from primary acquired melanosis (PAM) with atypia, and extend onto the cornea, although melanoma may rarely arise in the cornea from displaced melanocytes. Papilloma may be associated with HPV 6 and 11 in children or HPV 16 and 18 in adults.

Clinical Presentation

CIN varies from a distinct limbal lesion to a gray, avascular semitransparent lesion with thickened sheets of epithelium that may be seen on retroillumination (Figs. 28.1 and 28.2). It may be slightly elevated, well-demarcated, and accompanied by feeder vessels at the limbus temporally or nasally. Squamous cell carcinoma is larger and more elevated than CIN and may have a variable leukoplakia (white plaque appearance). A dermoid is a well-circumscribed yellow-white solid mass that may contain fine white hairs. It may be isolated or occur in association with Goldenhar syndrome; it may be grade 1 (ocular surface), grade 2 (involving anterior intraocular structures), or grade 3 (involving posterior intraocular structures) (Figs. 28.3 and 28.4). A dermolipoma appears the same as dermoid, although it appears more yellow, may be pale yellow, flocculant fusiform mass. A melanoma may be a pigmented to fleshy lesion with variable growth patterns. Fibrous histiocytoma and

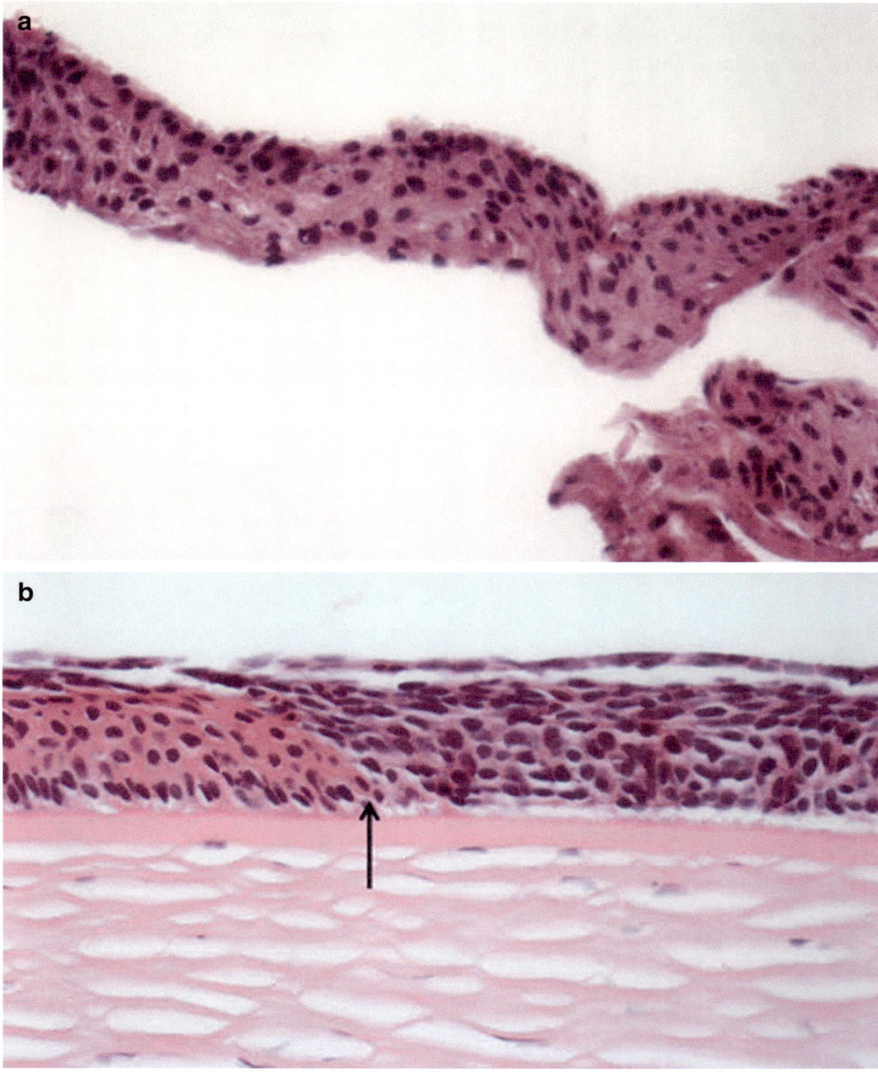

Fig. 28.2 (**a**) The epithelial lesion from the patient shown in Fig. 28.1 was removed and shows atypical keratinocytes with a loss of normal maturation. (**b**) A corneal specimen shows a demarcation (*arrow*) between normal epithelium to the left and severe dysplasia to the right (A&B, hematoxylin and eosin, ×100)

xanthogranuloma may appear yellow to white firm lesion with prominent superficial vascularity; they may be diffused with poorly defined margins and extensive infiltration. They usually involve the limbus but rarely may arise in the cornea. Papillomas are pink, fibrovascular fronds of tissue with translucent epithelium overlying fibrovascular cores containing corkscrew-shaped vessels.

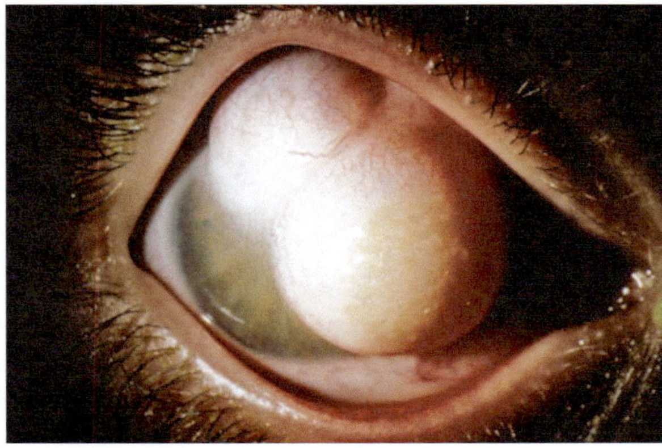

Fig. 28.3 A bilobed corneal white to yellow mass is seen in this patient with a corneal dermoid

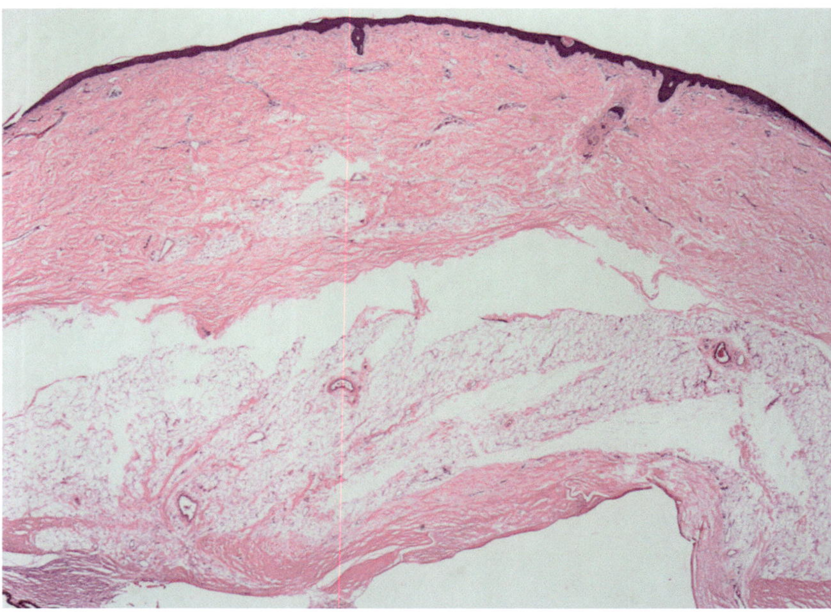

Fig. 28.4 This dermoid in the patient shown in Fig. 28.3 was grade 3, with associated intraocular malformation. The enucleation specimen shows dermis-like tissue in the corneal stroma and malformed anterior ocular structures (hematoxylin and eosin, ×10)

Diagnostics

In CIN, exfoliative/impression cytology, biopsy, and in vivo confocal microscopy show hyperreflective cells with bright nuclei and high resolution OCT; pathology shows acanthosis and varying degrees of replacement of epithelium with dysplastic keratinocytes from mild, basilar (grade 1) to moderate, up to mid level (grade 2), and severe near full thickness (grade 3) or full thickness carcinoma-in-situ. The diagnosis

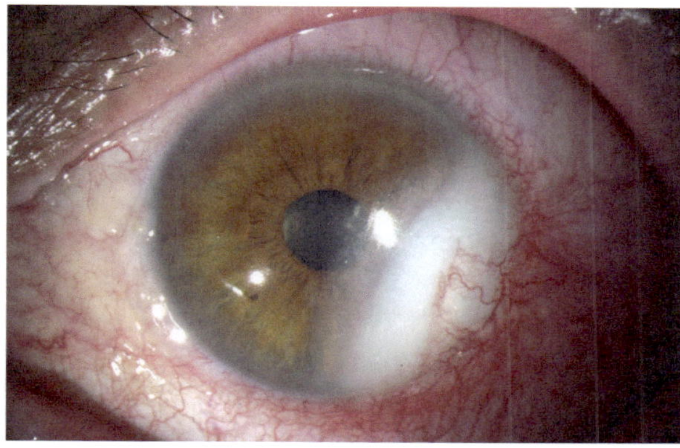

Fig. 28.5 This patient with a previously excised limbal mucoepidermoid carcinoma developed segmental corneal stromal haze due to corneal invasion of the tumor

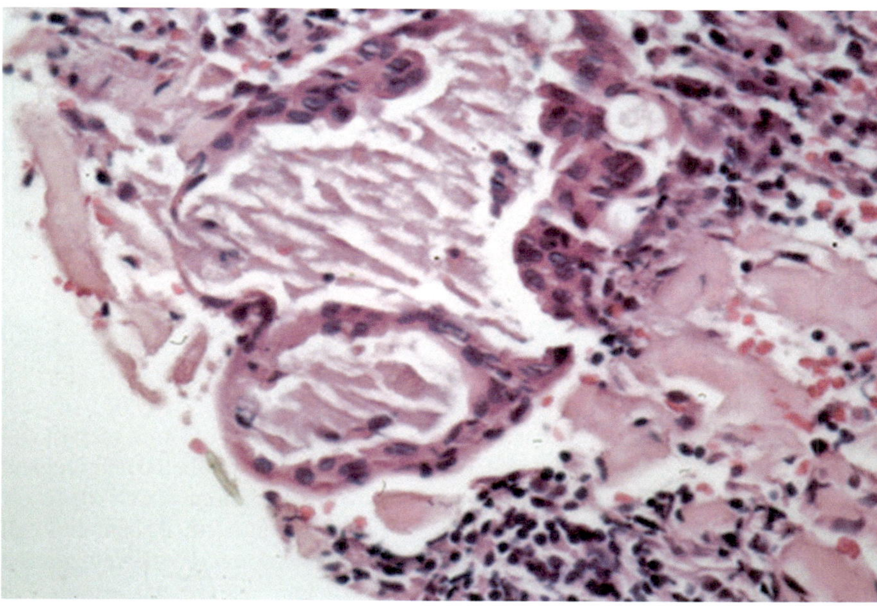

Fig. 28.6 A biopsy of the patient shown in Fig. 28.5 shows mucoepidermoid carcinoma in a sea of mucin within the corneal stroma (hematoxylin and eosin, ×100)

of squamous cell carcinoma is similar to CIN, although a biopsy containing the full thickness of the lesion is advised. Invasive variants of squamous cell carcinoma, such as mucoepidermoid carcinoma, may extend into the corneal stroma and are diagnosed by biopsy (Figs. 28.5 and 28.6). Dermoid and dermolipoma may be suspected by clinical appearance, although a biopsy may be diagnostic. Melanoma is diagnosed by incisional or excisional biopsy. Fibrous histiocytoma and xanthogranuloma are diagnosed by biopsy. A papilloma is diagnosed by its clinical appearance and excisional biopsy.

Pathology

The pathologic features are the same as those described for conjunctival lesions with the same diagnosis.

Differential Diagnosis

The differential diagnosis for CIN and squamous cell carcinoma includes pterygium, pannus, viral keratitis, epithelial/basement membrane dystrophy, fatty degeneration, and band keratopathy. The dermoid and dermolipoma differential diagnosis includes other causes of cloudy cornea at birth including sclerocornea, mucopolysaccharidosis, and Peter's anomaly. Melanoma may appear clinically similar to pigmented squamous cell carcinoma. Fibrous histiocytoma/xanthogranuloma may appear clinically similar to squamous cell carcinoma, melanoma, and lymphoma.

Prophylaxis

For CIN and squamous cell carcinoma, possible limitation of sun exposure and UV protection may be indicated. Sunglasses with UV protection may be helpful for CIN, squamous cell carcinoma, and melanoma, but this is not proven. There is no known prophylaxis for other corneal tumors.

Therapy

For CIN and squamous cell carcinoma, surgical excision with 2–3-mm margin and cryotherapy to the base/margin of limbal lesion are indicated. Epithelial debridement may be performed with ethyl alcohol, and adjuvant topical mitomycin C (MMC) or interferon alpha 2b (IFNa2b) may be utilized similar to conjunctival squamous cell carcinoma. For dermoid/dermolipoma grade 1, lamellar excision is indicated; grade 2 may require a penetrating keratoplasty, and grade 3 may require enucleation. For melanoma, complete surgical excision is indicated. If the melanoma arises in the limbus, an ethyl alcohol epitheliectomy and excision with no-touch technique with avoidance of violating Bowman's layer are recommended. If the melanoma is entirely in the cornea, it may require lamellar resection/penetrating keratoplasty. Fibrous histiocytoma and xanthogranulomas are surgically excised. Papillomas are excised with adjuvant MMC or interferon alpha 2b as needed.

Prognosis

The prognosis for CIN and squamous cell carcinoma is very good with complete removal. Mucoepidermoid and spindle cell variants that may occur at the limbus have more guarded prognosis as there may be corneal stromal invasion.

The visual prognosis for eyes with corneal dermoid/dermolipoma is guarded and depends on the grade of the lesion. Melanoma has a guarded prognosis, depending on depth of invasion (<1.5 mm favorable; >1.5 mm unfavorable). The prognosis for fibrous histiocytoma and xanthogranuloma is good.

Epidemiology

CIN and squamous cell carcinoma occur in older individuals, with men being more affected than women. Corneal dermoid/dermolipoma are congenital lesions that equally arise in boys and girls. Melanoma arises most often in adults with men and women equally affected. Fibrous histiocytoma most often arises in adults, whereas 70% of juvenile xanthogranulomas present within the first year of life. Papillomas typically arise in young adults.

Cross-References

Conjunctival squamous cell carcinoma, mucoepidermoid carcinoma, spindle cell carcinoma, melanoma, fibrous histiocytoma

Further Reading

Alomar TS, Nubile M, Lowe J, Dua HS (2011) Corneal intraepithelial neoplasia: in vivo confocal microscopic study with histopathologic correlation. Am J Ophthalmol 151:238–247

Ash JE (1950) Epibulbar tumors. Am J Ophthalmol 33:1203–1219

Conway RM, Holbach LM, Naumann GOH, Conway RM (2003) Benign fibrous histiocytoma of the corneoscleral limbus: unique clinicopathologic features. Arch Ophthalmol 121:1776–1779

Divine RD, Anderson RL (1983) Nitrous oxide cryotherapy for intraepithelial epithelioma of the conjunctiva. Arch Ophthalmol 101:782–786

Dua HS, Lagnado R, Raj D et al (2006) Alcohol delaminations of the corneal epithelium: an alternative in the management of recurrent corneal erosions. Ophthalmology 113(3):404–411

Hamam R, Bhat P, Foster CS (2009) Conjunctival/corneal intraepithelial neoplasia. Int Ophthalmol Clin 49(1):63–70

Hermel M, Donner A, Remky A (2010) New treatment option for adult-onset limbal xanthogranuloma. Cornea 29(1):113–116

Iliff WJ, Marback R, Green WR (1975) Invasive squamous cell carcinoma of the conjunctiva. Arch Ophthalmol 93:119–122

Kobayshi A, Shirao Y, Takata Y et al (2002) Adult-onset limbal juvenile xanthogranuloma. Arch Ophthalmol 120:96–97

Lim-I-Linn Z, Li L (2005) Juvenile xanthogranuloma of the corneoscleral limbus. Cornea 24(6):745–747

Lommatzsch PK, Lommatzsch RE, Kirsch I, Fuhrmann P (1990) Therapeutic outcomes of patients suffering from malignant melanoma of the conjunctiva. Br J Ophthalmol 74:615–619

Mansour AM, Wang F, Henkind P et al (1985) Ocular findings in the facioauriculovertebral sequences (Goldenhar-Gorlin syndrome). Am J Ophthalmol 100:555–559

Mansour AM, Barber JC, Reinecke RD, Wang FM (1989) Ocular choristomas. Surv Ophthalmol 33:5

Mohamed SR, Matthews N, Calcagni A (2002) Juvenile xanthogranuloma of the limbus in an adult. Arch Ophthalmol 120:976–977

Park CY, Kim EJ, Choi JS, Chick RS (2011) Isolated corneal papilloma-like lesion associated with human papilloma virus type 6. Cornea 30(5):600–603

Peksayar G, Soyturk MK, Demiryont M (1989) Long-term results of cryotherapy on malignant epithelial tumors of the conjunctiva. Am J Ophthalmol 15:337–340

Sheilds JA, Eagle RC, Sheilds CL, Depotter P, Schnall BM (1997) Epibulbar osseous choristoma: computed tomography and clinicopathologic correlation. Ophthal Pract 15:110–112

Shields CL, Shields JA (2004a) Tumors of the conjunctiva and cornea. Surv Ophthalmol 49:1

Shields CL, Shields JA (2004b) Tumors of the conjunctiva and cornea. Surv Ophthalmol 49:1

Shields CL, Lally MR, Singh AD et al (1999) Oral cimetidine for recalcitrant, diffuse conjunctival papillomatosis. Am J Ophthalmol 128:362–364

Shousha MA, Karp CL, Perez VL, Hoffmann R, Ventura R, Chang V, Dubovy SR, Wang J (2011) Diagnosis and management of conjunctival and corneal intraepithelial neoplasia using ultra high-resolution optical coherence tomography. Ophthalmology 118:1531–1537

Strempel I, Kroll P (1999) Conjuncitval malignant melanoma in children. Ophthalmologica 213:129–132

Tuomaala S, Aine E, Saari KM, Kevela T (2002a) Corneally displaced malignant conjunctival melanoma. Ophthalmology 109:914–9191

Tuomaala S, Aine E, Saari KM, Kevela T (2002b) Corneally displaced malignant conjunctival melanoma. Ophthalmology 109:914–9191

Part III

Retinal, RPE, and Ciliary Epithelial Tumors

Retinal Astrocytoma

29

Harpreet Singh Walia, Hans E. Grossniklaus,
Mehran Taban, and Arun D. Singh

Synonyms

Retinal astrocytic hamartoma, giant cell astrocytoma

Definition

The astrocytoma of the retina and optic disc is a benign tumor that typically occurs in patients with tuberous sclerosis, although it can also be seen in patients with neurofibromatosis, retinitis pigmentosa, or as an isolated finding.

H.S. Walia, M.D. (✉)
Department of Ophthalmology,
Emory University School of Medicine,
Atlanta, GA, USA
e-mail: hwalia@emory.edu

H.E. Grossniklaus, M.D.
Emory University School of Medicine, Emory Eye Center,
Department of Ophthalmology,
Atlanta, GA, USA
e-mail: ophtheg@emory.edu

M. Taban, M.D.
Taban-Department of Ophthalmology, Cleveland Clinic,
Cleveland, OH, USA
e-mail: tabanm@ccf.org

A.D. Singh, M.D.
Department of Ophthalmic Oncology, Cole Eye Institute,
Cleveland Clinic Foundation,
9500 Euclid Ave, Desk i-329, Cleveland, OH 44195, USA
e-mail: singha@ccf.org

H.E. Grossniklaus (ed.), *Pocket Guide to Ocular Oncology and Pathology*,
DOI 10.1007/978-3-642-29782-3_29, © Springer-Verlag Berlin Heidelberg 2013

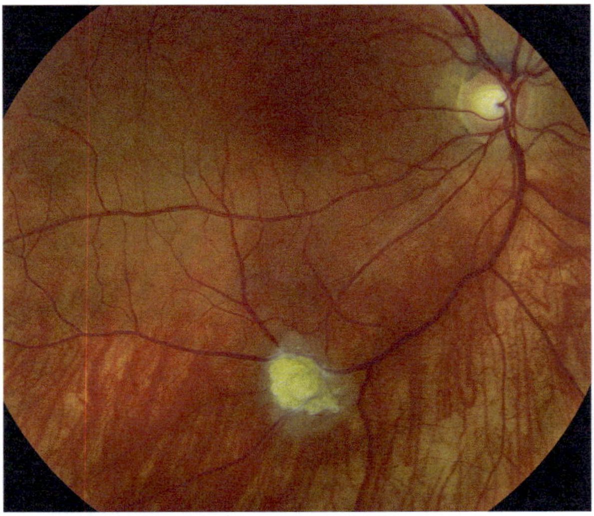

Fig. 29.1 Fundus appearance of an astrocytic hamartoma with central calcification

Etiology

Tuberous sclerosis arises due to mutations in the TSC1 or TSC2 genes. These genes encode for hamartin and tuberin respectively. Hamartin/tuberin suppress PI3K signaling and are involved with integration of growth factor and nutrient signals.

Clinical Presentation

These tumors are usually asymptomatic and are detected as part of screening for tuberous sclerosis. Occasionally, patients can develop painless blurred vision. They may be solitary or there may be several astrocytic hamartomas in one eye. The lesion is usually indolent, although giant cell astrocytoma may grow. Clinically, there are three recognized morphologic types of retinal astrocytic hamartomas: (1) subtle, flat, round, semitranslucent lesion (most common type); (2) large, elevated, nodular, and calcified mulberry lesion; and (3) mixed type of lesion possessing features of the other two (Fig. 29.1). Retinal astrocytoma may be the first clinical manifestation of tuberous sclerosis. Although the exact prevalence of retinal astrocytoma in tuberous sclerosis is not known, approximately 1/3 to 1/2 of patients with tuberous sclerosis have retinal or optic nerve hamartomas, and in half of these patients, the astrocytoma occurs bilaterally. "Acquired" retinal astrocytoma is a term applied to retinal astrocytomas that develop at any age and are not associated with tuberous sclerosis. These tumors may be a solitary intraocular counterpart of the astrocytoma that occurs in the brain. For the most part, clinical features, pathology, diagnostic approaches, management, and prognosis of the acquired form of retinal astrocytoma are the same as retinal astrocytic hamartoma associated with tuberous sclerosis.

Fig. 29.2 Optical coherent tomography reveals full-thickness replacement of the retinal anatomic layers with the tumor and shadowing corresponding to the intralesional calcification

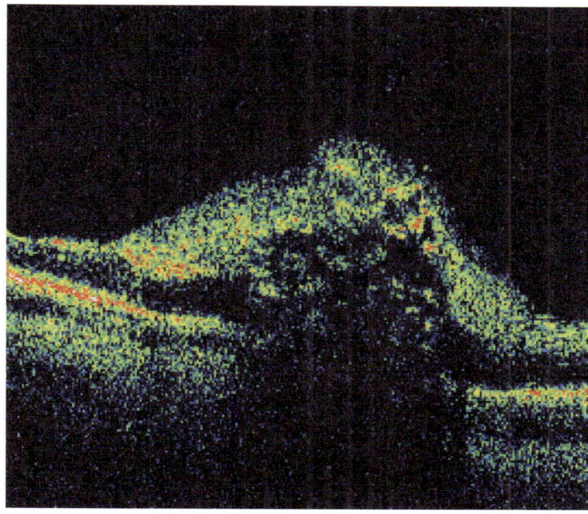

Diagnostics

In majority of cases, the diagnosis of retinal astrocytoma can be made with ophthalmoscopy and clinical evaluation looking for signs of tuberous sclerosis. However, ancillary studies can be useful. Fluorescein angiography shows prominent superficial network of fine vessels in the arterial phase with leakage in the venous phase, and late angiograms show intense diffuse homogenous staining of the mass. Optical coherent tomography reveals full-thickness replacement of the retinal anatomic layers with the tumor and shadowing corresponding to the intralesional calcification (Fig. 29.2). B-scan ultrasonography of calcified lesions shows characteristic features including acoustic solidity and shadowing (Fig. 29.3).

Pathology

Histologically, retinal astrocytic hamartomas are composed of a proliferation of well-differentiated spindle-shaped cells with bland, fusiform nuclei and fibrillar cytoplasm (Fig. 29.4). Giant cell astrocytomas of the retina have been described in which the tumor also displays giant round cells. This variant of the tumor may exhibit aggressive growth.

Differential Diagnosis

Despite many characteristic features of astrocytic hamartoma, certain entities can closely resemble astrocytic hamartoma. For example, similarity between optic disc drusen and optic disc astrocytoma has led to the term "giant drusen" for the calcified

Fig. 29.3 B-scan ultrasonography shows characteristic features of calcification including acoustic solidity and shadowing

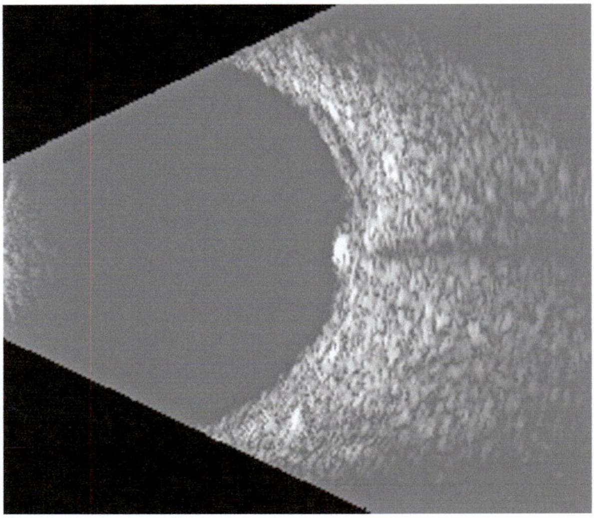

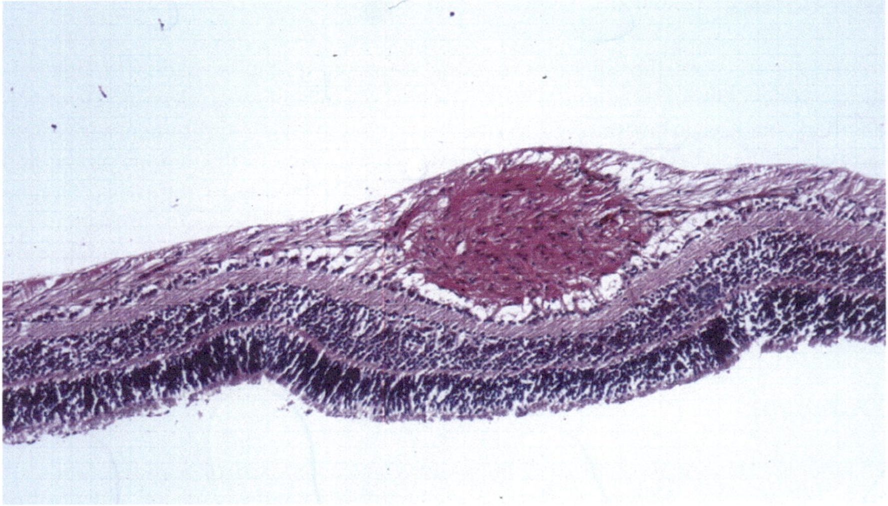

Fig. 29.4 A retinal astrocytic hamartoma in the inner retina is composed of a proliferation of bland spindle-shaped cells (hematoxylin and eosin, ×25)

astrocytic hamartoma seen with tuberous sclerosis. However, optic disc drusen are usually bilateral and lie within the disc, whereas astrocytic hamartoma is unilateral, protrudes above the optic disc, and characteristically obscures the disc and retinal blood vessels. Other considerations in the differential include retinoma, retinoblastoma, and retinal gliosis.

Prophylaxis

There are no known risk factors or prophylactic strategies for retinal astrocytoma.

Therapy

Lesions are usually followed by observation. Lesions that grow may be treated. Treatment options include photodynamic therapy (PDT), laser photocoagulation, intravitreal anti-VEGF agents (if there is concurrent neovascularization), and enucleation for large lesions.

Prognosis

In general, astrocytomas have excellent visual prognosis. They are not known to undergo malignant transformation. However, rarely they have been associated with vitreous seeding, vitreous or subretinal hemorrhage, and subretinal exudation or detachment. Giant cell astrocytomas may grow and eventually require enucleation.

Epidemiology

The incidence of tuberous sclerosis is approximately 1:14,000–25,000 individuals. Approximately 1/3 to 1/2 will have retinal astrocytoma. The incidence of retinal astrocytoma not associated with tuberous sclerosis is unknown, but it is rare.

Cross-References

Phakomatoses

Further Reading

Hallett L, Foster T, Liu Z, Blieden M, Valentim J (2011) Burden of disease and unmet needs in tuberous sclerosis complex with neurological manifestations: systematic review. Curr Med Res Opin 27:1571–1583

Jung CS, Hubbard GB 3rd, Grossniklaus HE (2009) Giant cell astrocytoma of the retina in a 1-month-old infant. J Pediatr Ophthalmol Strabismus 2:1–4

Mennel S, Hausmann N, Meyer CH, Peter S (2006) Photodynamic therapy for exudative hamartoma in tuberous sclerosis. Arch Ophthalmol 124(4):597–599

Mennel S, Meyer CH, Peter S, Schmidt JC, Kroll P (2007) Current treatment modalities for exudative retinal hamartomas secondary to tuberous sclerosis: review of the literature. Acta Ophthalmol Scand 85(2):127–132

Shields CL, Materin MA, Shields JA (2005a) Review of optical coherence tomography for intraocular tumors. Curr Opin Ophthalmol 16:141–154
Shields JA, Eagle RC, Shields CL et al (2005b) Aggressive retinal astrocytomas in 4 patients with tuberous sclerosis complex. Arch Ophthalmol 123:856–863
Williams R, Taylor D (1985) Tuberous sclerosis. Surv Ophthalmol 30:143–154
Zimmer-Galler IE, Robertson DM (1995) Long-term observation of retinal lesions in tuberous sclerosis. Am J Ophthalmol 119(3):318–324

Coats' Disease

30

Ron Margolis, Arun D. Singh, and G. Baker Hubbard III

Synonyms

Leber's miliary aneurysms

Definition

Coats' disease is an idiopathic condition characterized by retinal vascular telangiectasis and aneurysmal dilation with intraretinal and subretinal exudation that can progress to massive retinal detachment, with secondary cataract and glaucoma.

Etiology

Coats' disease is an idiopathic condition. There is some evidence that a mutation in the NDP gene on chromosome Xp11.2, which codes for the retinal protein norrin, may play a role in the disease.

R. Margolis, M.D. (✉)
Department of Ophthalmic Oncology,
Cole Eye Institute, Cleveland Clinic Foundation, Cleveland, OH, USA
e-mail: ron_margolis@yahoo.com

A.D. Singh, M.D.
Department of Ophthalmic Oncology, Cole Eye Institute, Cleveland Clinic Foundation,
9500 Euclid Ave, Desk i-329, Cleveland, OH 44195, USA
e-mail: singha@ccf.org

G.B. Hubbard III, M.D.
Department of Ophthalmology,
Emory University School of Medicine, Atlanta, GA, USA

The Emory Eye Center, Atlanta, GA, USA
e-mail: ghubba2@emory.edu

H.E. Grossniklaus (ed.), *Pocket Guide to Ocular Oncology and Pathology*,
DOI 10.1007/978-3-642-29782-3_30,

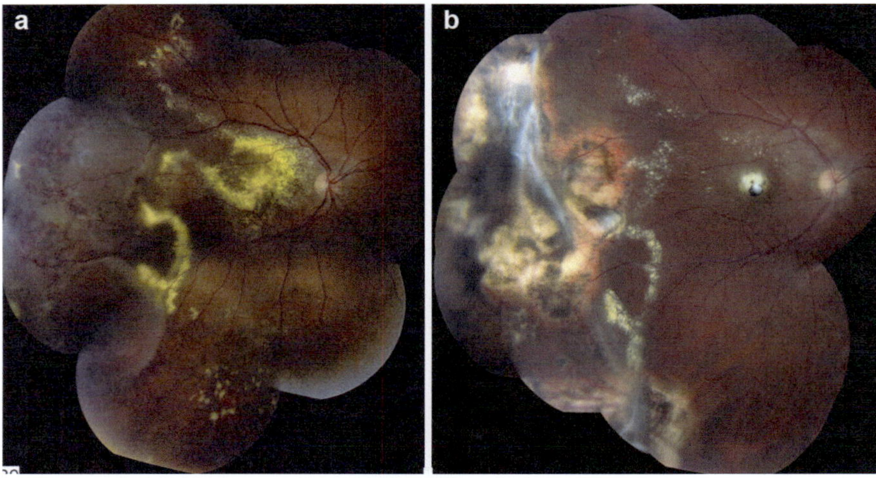

Fig. 30.1 (**a**) Retinal vascular telangiectasias and aneurysms in Coats' disease are associated with lipid exudation and exudative retina detachment. (**b**) The lipid exudates and detachment have largely resolved after laser and cryotherapy

Clinical Presentation

Most cases of Coats' disease present within the first decade of life with leukocoria, strabismus, or decreased vision. Fundus examination reveals yellow subretinal lipid exudates that can range from minimal to a total exudative retinal detachment. Lipid exudation results from leakage of retinal vascular abnormalities usually found in the peripheral retina. Characteristic findings include telangiectasia, tortuosity, aneurysm, capillary nonperfusion, and occasionally neovascularization (Fig. 30.1). Other posterior segment complications include retinal macrocysts and vasoproliferative tumor. Secondary anterior segment complications include cataract, neovascular glaucoma, and phthisis bulbi.

Diagnostics

Fluorescein angiography is essential to identify the extent of vascular anomalies and to direct treatment to all involved areas of the retina. Typical findings include telangiectatic vessels, aneurysms (light bulb lesions), and beading of vessel walls. These anomalies show early and persistent leakage. Diffuse areas of capillary nonperfusion are common and are typically surrounded by a characteristic pattern of anomalous vessels (Fig. 30.2).

Pathology

Most of our knowledge of the pathologic findings in Coats' disease results from study of end-stage eyes enucleated for pain and blindness. Gross examination of the

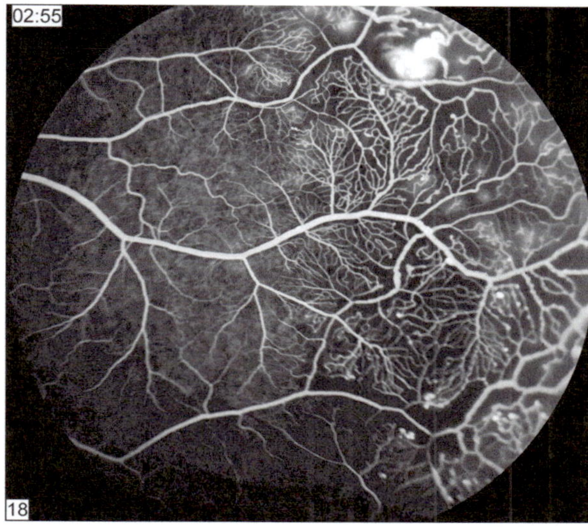

Fig. 30.2 Fluorescein angiography showing the typical retinal vascular changes of Coats' disease

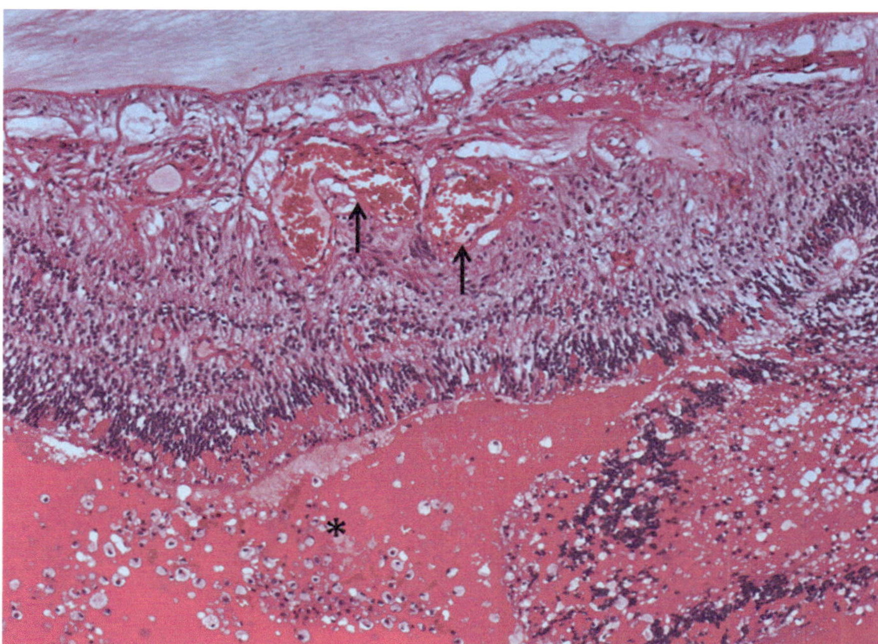

Fig. 30.3 The retina is detached by proteinaceous material and lipid-laden histiocytes (*). There are dilated telangiectatic vessels (*arrows*) in the inner retina (hematoxylin and eosin, ×25)

posterior segment typically reveals total retinal detachment with clumps of subretinal yellow material. Microscopic evaluation may reveal a fibrovascular membrane on the anterior surface of the iris with angle closure in cases with neovascular glaucoma. The neurosensory retina may be thickened with lipoproteinaceous material and lipid-laden macrophages. Cholesterol clefts are seen in the retina and in the eosinophilic subretinal fluid. The retina may be detached by proteinaceous material, and the peripheral retinal vessels are larger than normal caliber, corresponding to areas of telangiectasia seen clinically (Fig. 30.3). These vessels have markedly thickened basement membrane with periodic acid-Schiff (PAS)-positive material. Glial cells and RPE cells may wall off subretinal exudates to form nodules.

Differential Diagnosis

Coats' disease should be considered in the differential diagnosis of childhood leukocoria, which includes retinoblastoma, retinal detachment, persistent fetal vasculature syndrome, Norrie's disease, and familial exudative vitreoretinopathy. Most cases of Coats' disease can be accurately diagnosed by identifying the typical ophthalmoscopic features. Advanced disease, however, can be difficult to diagnose because the typical features are not always evident. B-scan ultrasonography is useful in ruling out retinoblastoma, as there is no retinal mass in Coats' disease. Several conditions including retinitis pigmentosa, pars planitis, and facioscapulohumeral muscular dystrophy are known to be associated with a Coats-like exudative retinopathy that should be distinguished from true Coats' disease.

Therapy

The goal of treatment is destruction of the vascular abnormalities in order to prevent further leakage and allow resorption of exudates. Mild cases can be treated with scatter laser photocoagulation using green or yellow wavelengths. Cryotherapy may be necessary for advanced cases as retinal detachment can preclude adequate uptake of laser energy. Cryotherapy is applied using a double freeze-thaw technique. Laser and cryotherapy may be used together, and typically several treatment sessions are required. Drainage of subretinal fluid combined with an anterior chamber or vitreous infusion may be necessary to obtain sufficient retinal freezing. Diathermy and transpupillary thermotherapy have also been used. Surgical repair of retinal detachment using vitrectomy with internal drainage of subretinal fluid and intraocular tamponade has been used in selected cases.

Prognosis

Even after all telangiectasias are ablated and active exudation and retinal detachment resolve, subretinal fibrosis in the macula and pigmentary alterations often limit visual recovery. In one large series, only 14% of 124 eyes achieved final visual acuity of 20/50 or better, and vision of hand motions or light perception was present in 40%. Enucleation was ultimately necessary in 16%. Risk factors for poor visual outcome were postequatorial, diffuse or superior location of the telangiectasis and exudation, failed resolution of subretinal fluid after laser photocoagulation or cryotherapy, and presence of retinal macrocyst.

Epidemiology

Coats' disease is an uncommon condition that is usually diagnosed in children in the first decade of life. It is a sporadic nonhereditary condition, and it is not associated with any systemic abnormality. There is no racial or ethnic predilection, but >75% of cases occur in males.

Cross-References

Retinoblastoma, retinal vascular tumors

Further Reading

Aaberg TM Jr (2007) Coats' disease. In: Singh AD, Damato BE, Pe'er J, Murphree AL, Perry JD (eds) Clinical ophthalmic oncology. Saunders-Elsevier, Philadelphia, pp 348–353

Black GC, Perveen R, Bonshek R et al (1999) Coats' disease of the retina (unilateral retinal telangiectasis) caused by somatic mutation in the NDP gene: a role for norrin in retinal angiogenesis. Hum Mol Genet 8:2031–2035

Jones JH, Kroll AJ, Lou PL, Ryan EA (2001) Coats' disease. Int Ophthalmol Clin 41:189–198

Rubin MP, Mukai S (2008) Coats' disease. Int Ophthalmol Clin 48:149–158

Shields JA, Shields CL (2001) Differentiation of Coats' disease and retinoblastoma. J Pediatr Ophthalmol Strabismus 38:262–266

Shields JA, Shields CL (2002) Review: coats disease: the 2001LuEsther T. Mertz lecture. Retina 22:80–91

Shields JA, Shields CL, Honavar SG, Demirci H, Cater J (2001a) Classification and management of coats disease: the 2000 proctor lecture. Am J Ophthalmol 131:572–583

Shields JA, Shields CL, Honavar SG, Demirci H (2001b) Clinical variations and complications of coats disease in 150 cases: the 2000 Sanford Gifford memorial lecture. Am J Ophthalmol 131:561–571

Retinal Hemangioblastoma

31

Joshua Robinson and Hans E. Grossniklaus

Synonyms

Retinal capillary hemangioblastoma, Retinal capillary hemangioma, Retinal angioma, von Hippel tumor

Definition

Hemangioblastomas are proliferative retinal angiomatous hamartomas of the retina and optic nerve head. They can be peripheral (referred to as the von Hippel tumor) or juxtapapillary and may primarily involve the inner retina (endophytic) or outer retina (exophytic). Most are endophytic and located peripherally, typically in the superotemporal quadrant. These tumors may occur sporadically or as part of von Hippel-Lindau (VHL) disease, which is an uncommon autosomal dominant disorder associated with multisystem tumor formation including hemangioblastoma of the central nervous system, renal cell carcinoma, and pheochromocytoma.

J. Robinson, M.D. (✉)
Department of Ophthalmology,
Emory University Eye Center,
Atlanta, GA, USA
e-mail: jrobi25@emory.edu

H.E. Grossniklaus, M.D.
Emory University School of Medicine,
Emory Eye Center,
Department of Ophthalmology,
Atlanta, GA, USA
e-mail: ophtheg@emory.edu

H.E. Grossniklaus (ed.), *Pocket Guide to Ocular Oncology and Pathology*,
DOI 10.1007/978-3-642-29782-3_31,

Etiology

Retinal hemangioblastomas arise from a loss-of-function mutation in the von Hippel-Lindau (VHL) gene on 3p25–26, which encodes a ubiquitously expressed protein (VHL protein) involved in the degradation of hypoxia-inducible factors (HIFs). Unregulated expression of HIFs leads to overexpression of vascular endothelial growth factor (VEGF) and platelet-derived growth factor (PDGF), which in turn lead to angiogenesis and tumor formation. In this regard, the VHL gene can be thought of as a tumor suppressor gene. Findings from age-incidence analyses of retinal hemangioblastoma have been consistent with a "two-hit" mutation model similar to that originally described by Knudsen regarding the tumorigenesis of retinoblastoma.

Clinical Presentation

There is no sex or racial predisposition for retinal capillary hemangioma. The tumor is usually diagnosed in the second or third decade of life. The lesions may be discovered on a routine evaluation or a screening exam because of a history of VHL. Patients may be asymptomatic or complain of progressive worsening vision secondary to retinal exudation.

Diagnostics

Diagnosis is usually made by the characteristic appearance ophthalmoscopically. The lesions are circumscribed with an orange-red color and have prominent feeder vessels that often emanate from the optic disc (Fig. 31.1). Fluorescein angiography is generally not necessary for diagnosis but can help distinguish feeder arterioles from draining venules.

Pathology/Histology

The histologic appearance of hemangioblastomas is similar whether the tumor arises as part of the systemic VHL syndrome or as a solitary retinal lesion. In general, they are composed of an extensive network of small-caliber vascular channels lined by endothelial cells. This vascular network is enmeshed in a stroma consisting of sheets of polyhedral cells with abundant eosinophilic cytoplasm, spindle-shaped cells, and vacuolated "foamy" cells (Figs. 31.2, 31.3 and 31.4). The spindle-shaped cells and extensive capillary network are generally considered to represent reactive proliferations, whereas the primary, or intrinsic, tumor cells are thought to consist of the polyhedral and foamy cells.

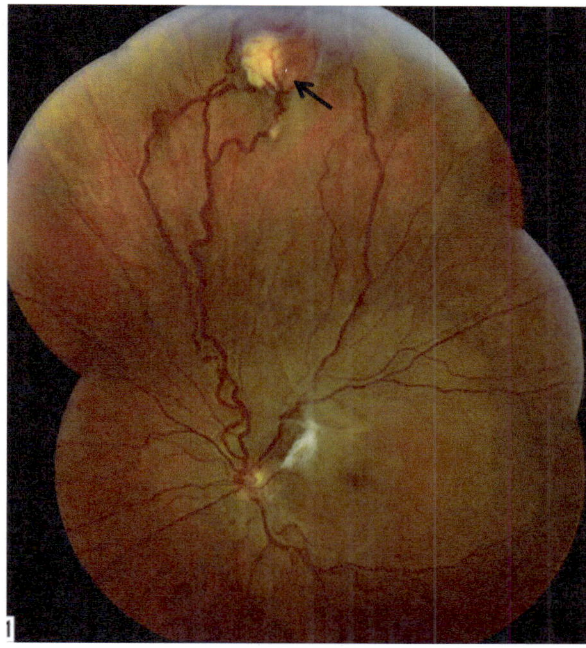

Fig. 31.1 Color fundus photograph of a peripheral retinal hemangioblastoma (von Hippel tumor) in the left eye of a 43-year-old female patient. The tumor (*arrow*) is a pink, fleshy, well-circumscribed mass with feeder vessels

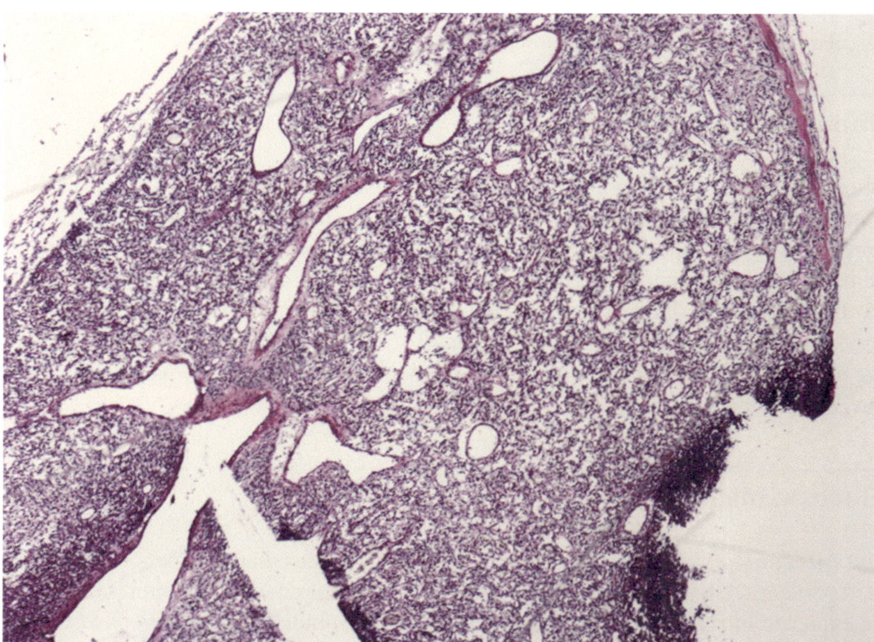

Fig. 31.2 Low-magnification image of a section of a retinal hemangioblastoma status postenucleation. The tumor is composed of stromal cells with foamy cytoplasm and scattered vascular channels, which appear tubular in this PAS-stained section (Periodic acid Schiff, ×25)

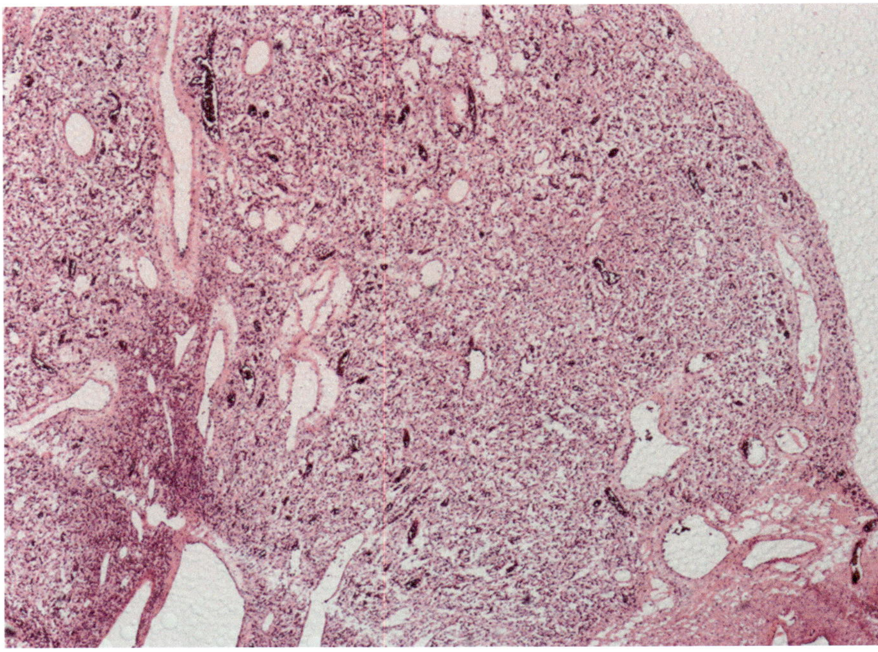

Fig. 31.3 The tumor is composed of stromal cells, some of which contain foamy cytoplasm and vascular channels (hematoxylin and eosin, ×25)

Immunohistochemistry

The immunohistochemical features of retinal hemangioblastoma are similar to hemangioblastoma of the central nervous system. Factor VIII-associated antigen and Ulex europaeus agglutinin (endothelial markers) stain the vascular endothelium, but do not stain the tumor stromal cells. Stromal polyhedral, foamy, and spindle cells stain positively for glial fibrillary acid protein and neuron-specific enolase. Other histiocyte markers including MAC-387, factor XIIIa, lysozyme, and alpha 1-antichymotrypsin are not positive in tumor sections, nor are the neural/neuroendocrine markers for chromogranin or neurofilament.

Electron Microscopy

Ultrastructural examination reveals endothelial-lined vascular channels with associated pericytes. Elongated cells with intracytoplasmic intermediate filaments, as would be expected in retinal glial cells, correspond to the spindle-shaped cells observed on light microscopy. The foamy stromal cells appear as plump, vacuolated cells with intracytoplasmic intermediate filaments. Adjacent vacuolated cells are adjoined by intercellular junctions, with discontinuous patches of basement membrane noted in

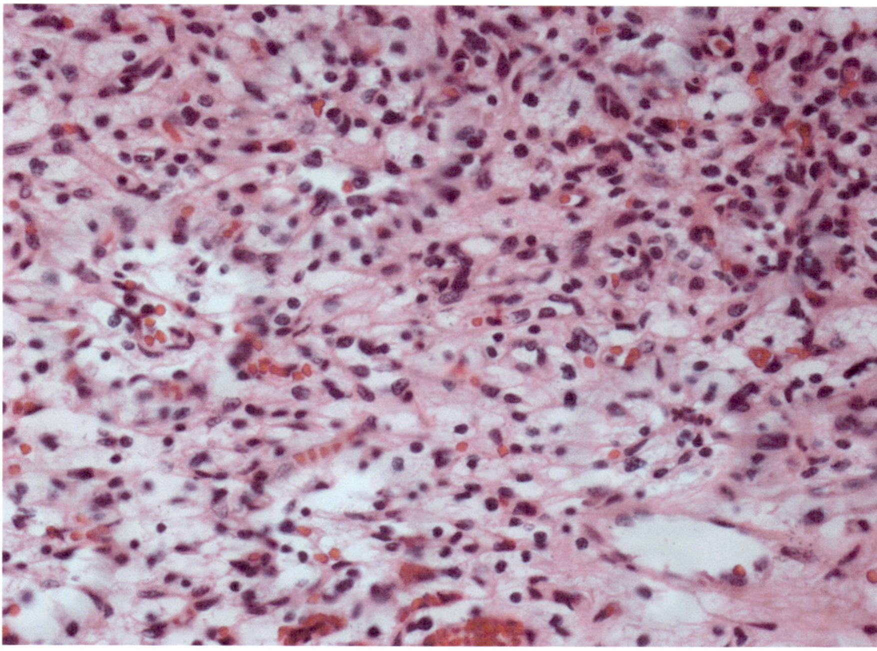

Fig. 31.4 Higher magnification shows that the stromal cells have clear to foamy cytoplasm and vascular channels are present within the tumor (hematoxylin and eosin, ×100)

regions lacking intercellular contact. The intracytoplasmic vacuoles are thought to represent phagocytized lipid originating from a leaky capillary network. The polyhedral cells demonstrate intracytoplasmic intermediate filaments and large nuclei with prominent nucleoli. These findings, coupled with the immunohistochemical staining profiles of retinal hemangioblastomas, support a glial origin of the intrinsic tumor cells, as is the case with central nervous system hemangioblastomas. This is in contrast with the previously held theory that retinal hemangioblastomas are tumors of vascular origin.

Differential Diagnosis

The differential diagnosis includes acquired retinal hemangioma, Coats disease, retinal cavernous hemangioma, racemose hemangioma, retinal macroaneurysm, retinal astrocytoma, retinal gliosis, and toxocariasis.

Prophylaxis

None.

Therapy

Treatment options depend on the size and location of the lesion. They include observation, laser photocoagulation, cryotherapy, photodynamic therapy, and radiotherapy. Laser therapy with light application of argon green or yellow is recommended. Several applications may be necessary.

Prognosis

The visual prognosis depends on the location, size, and number of retinal capillary hemangiomas. Lesions with extensive exudation or that cause tractional retinal detachments often result in permanent visual impairment.

Epidemiology

The incidence of isolated retinal capillary hemangioma is unknown. The birth incidence of VHL is approximately one in 36,000.

Cross-References

Retinal vascular tumors, Coats disease, retinal astrocytoma, phakomatosis

Further Reading

Chang JH, Spraul CW, Lynn ML, Drack A, Grossniklaus HE (1998) The two-stage mutation model in retinal hemangioblastoma. Ophthalmic Genet 19(3):123–130

Grossniklaus HE, Thomas JW, Vigneswaran N, Jarrett WH 3rd (1992) Retinal hemangioblastoma. A histologic, immunohistochemical, and ultrastructural evaluation. Ophthalmology 99(1):140–145

Hinz BJ, Schachat AP (2006) Capillary hemangioma of the retina and von Hippel-Lindau disease. In: Ryan S (ed) Retina. Elsevier Mosby, Philadelphia, pp 615–624

Wong WT, Chew EY (2008) Ocular von Hippel–Lindau disease: clinical update and emerging treatments. Curr Opin Ophthalmol 19:213–217

Intraocular Leukemia

32

Qing Zhang, G. Baker Hubbard III,
and Hans E. Grossniklaus

Synonyms

Retinal leukemia

Definition

Intraocular leukemia describes leukocytic malignancies that manifest within various ocular tissues.

Q. Zhang, M.D. (✉)
Department of Ophthalmology,
Emory University School of Medicine,
Atlanta, GA, USA
e-mail: qzhang7@emory.edu

G.B. Hubbard III, M.D.
Department of Ophthalmology,
Emory University School of Medicine,
Atlanta, GA, USA

The Emory Eye Center,
Atlanta, GA, USA
e-mail: ghubba2@emory.edu

H.E. Grossniklaus, M.D.
Emory University School of Medicine,
Emory Eye Center,
Department of Ophthalmology,
Atlanta, GA, USA
e-mail: ophtheg@emory.edu

H.E. Grossniklaus (ed.), *Pocket Guide to Ocular Oncology and Pathology*,
DOI 10.1007/978-3-642-29782-3_32, © Springer-Verlag Berlin Heidelberg 2013

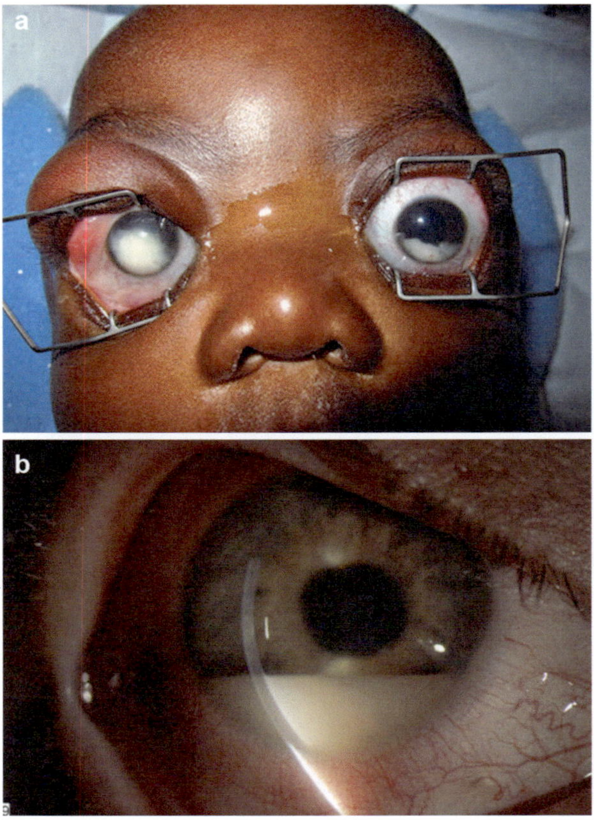

Fig. 32.1 (**a**) A 1-year-old child with AML and leukemic infiltration of the anterior chamber of both eyes. Also note the lacrimal gland enlargement due to leukemic infiltration. (**b**) Teenager with recurrent ALL and pseudohypopyon

Etiology

Leukemia is a neoplasm of the hematopoietic system. Various ocular tissues may become infiltrated by malignant cells in leukemia. In addition, the retina may manifest secondary complications of the disease.

Clinical Presentation

Various case series report leukemic involvement with virtually all ocular structures. Ocular manifestations are more common in acute rather than chronic leukemias. Patients have been described with leukemic infiltrates of the anterior chamber (pseudohypopyon), iris, ciliary body, vitreous, retina, choroid, and optic nerve. Direct infiltration often results in a yellowish white mass lesion (Fig. 32.1). In addition to direct infiltration, secondary complications of leukemia have also been well described. These complications are usually related to anemia, thrombocytopenia, or

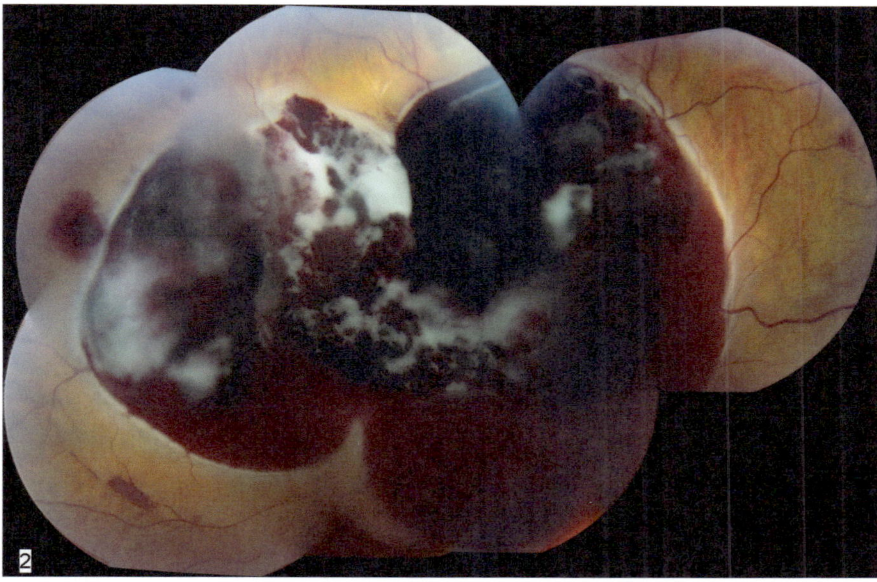

Fig. 32.2 A 19-year-old with sudden vision loss due to preretinal hemorrhage from ALL. Along with red hemorrhage, note the white appearance that may represent leukemic cells

hyperviscosity and typically manifest as retinal hemorrhages, vitreous hemorrhages, vascular sheathing, or retinal venous occlusive disease (Fig. 32.2). Finally, immunosuppression related to neutropenia or related to treatment with antineoplastic agents increases susceptibility to opportunistic infections that may involve the eye. Infectious choroidal infiltrates, retinal infiltrates, and endophthalmitis have all been described.

Diagnostics

For patients presenting with pseudohypopyon, anterior chamber paracentesis should be performed, and the specimen should undergo cytologic and molecular studies. Vitreous or chorioretinal biopsy can be considered to establish the nature of more posterior intraocular processes.

Pathology

The leukemic infiltrate is composed of loosely coherent sheets of small round blue cells with scanty cytoplasm. Pathologically, the infiltrated ocular tissues contain leukemia cells in various quantities. Choroidal involvement with leukemia is diffusedly thickened with tumor cells and reaches its greatest thickness at the posterior

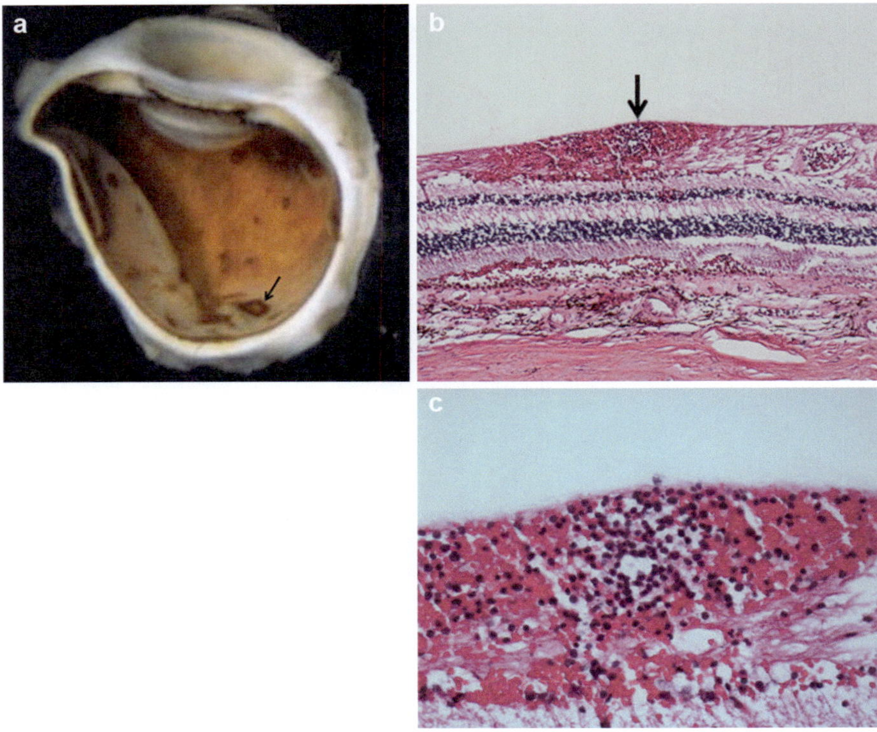

Fig. 32.3 Leukemic infiltration of the retina. (**a**) Gross photograph of leukemic infiltrate with retinal hemorrhages (*arrow*). (**b**) Low-power photomicrograph leukemic infiltrate with associated hemorrhage in on the retinal surface corresponding to gross appearance of infiltrate in **a** (hematoxylin and eosin, ×2).(**c**) A combination of leukemic cells and erythrocytes has accumulated underneath the internal limiting membrane (hematoxylin and eosin, ×100)

pole, showing a salmon pink or cream appearance. Leukemic infiltrate can display marked intravascular involvement so that the neoplastic cells are commonly observed in the lumen of choroidal and retinal blood vessels. The retinal hemorrhage is commonly seen on gross examination and presents a combination of leukemic blast cells and erythrocytes that are accumulated underneath the internal limiting membrane (Fig. 32.3). Leukemic infiltrate in the RPE shows clumps of pigment-containing tumor cells resembling macrophages. Conjunctival infiltrates occur rarely and show abundant leukemic cells, leading to a diffuse tumor-like swelling with a salmon color. Nodular lesions of the bulbar conjunctiva also rarely occur. Histochemical stains are used to classify intraocular leukemia because different blasts are well recognized for demonstrating considerable immunophenotypic heterogeneity. Ultrastructural features by electron microscopy are consistent with the specific type of systemic leukemia. The shape of nuclei and nucleoli, the distribution of nuclear chromatin, the ratio of the cytoplasm and nucleus, and the development of cytoplasmic materials are different depending on the type of systemic leukemia.

Differential Diagnosis

The possibility of retinoblastoma should be considered in young patients when the diagnosis is not otherwise established. In patients with retinal infiltrates and leukemia, distinguishing between neoplasia and infection can be difficult. These patients require systemic and CNS evaluation looking for other evidence of disease. Retinal infiltration in the setting of blast crisis is suggestive of neoplastic cause. In the setting of immunosuppression after bone marrow transplantation, infection may be more likely.

Prophylaxis

There are no known strategies to prevent intraocular manifestations of leukemia.

Therapy

The eye is a sanctuary site with respect to antineoplastic drugs, and therefore the internal structures of the eye can be difficult to treat for leukemic infiltration. Intravitreal methotrexate has been described, but its exact role is not established. For the secondary complications such as vascular occlusion and vitreous hemorrhage, standard techniques may be utilized when the patient is stable.

Prognosis

Prognosis varies considerably with the type of leukemia and the systemic status of the patient.

Epidemiology

Ocular abnormalities have been reported in 8–89% of leukemia cases. Autopsy series find higher rates and clinical series find lower rates. In one study that prospectively performed ophthalmic examinations on 120 patients at the time of diagnosis with leukemia, leukemic infiltrates were present in 3%, and secondary complications of leukemia were found in 39%.

Cross-References

Intraocular lymphoma, choroidal lymphoma

Further Reading

Gordon KB, Hope SR, Duncan JL et al (2001) Ocular manifestations of leukemia: leukemic infiltration versus infectious process. Ophthalmology 108:2293

Lee MH, Park MY, Lee JW (2010) Leukemic glaucoma in a patient with chronic myeloid leukemia treated with intracameral methotrexate. Jpn J Ophthalmol 54:362–364

Schachat AP, Markowitz JA, Guyer DR et al (1989) Ophthalmic manifestations of leukemia. Arch Ophthalmol 107:697–700

Spencer, WH (1996) Ophthalmic pathology, 4th edn. Saunders, Philadelphia, pp 2736–2743

Primary Intraocular Lymphoma 33

Brian J. Lee and Arun D. Singh

Synonyms

Primary lymphoma of the retina and central nervous system

Definition

Primary lymphoma of the retina and central nervous system is an extranodal non-Hodgkin's B-cell lymphoma involving the retina, choroid, or vitreous with or without brain involvement. Primary central nervous system lymphoma (PCNSL) is accompanied by ocular manifestations in 15–25% of patients. Ocular manifestations can occur independent of central nervous system (CNS) disease and is termed primary lymphoma of the central nervous system-ophthalmic (PCNSL-O).

Etiology

The majority of PCNSL are diffuse large B-cell lymphomas. The monoclonal proliferation of cells probably arises from lymphocytes that normally traffic through the CNS. Immunosuppression, iatrogenic or acquired, is a risk factor for PCNSL.

B.J. Lee, M.D.
Department of Ophthalmology, Cole Eye Institute, Cleveland Clinic, Cleveland, OH, USA

A.D. Singh, M.D. (✉)
Department of Ophthalmic Oncology,
Cole Eye Institute, Cleveland Clinic Foundation,
9500 Euclid Ave, Desk i-329, Cleveland, OH 44195, USA
e-mail: singha@ccf.org

H.E. Grossniklaus (ed.), *Pocket Guide to Ocular Oncology and Pathology*,
DOI 10.1007/978-3-642-29782-3_33, © Springer-Verlag Berlin Heidelberg 2013

Clinical Presentation

Typical symptoms may include painless, bilateral, asymmetric visual blurring, and floaters. Common findings are vitreous cells (Fig. 33.1) with or without anterior segment inflammation, perivascular chorioretinitis, and creamy yellow infiltrates below the retinal pigment epithelium (Fig. 33.2). Exudative retinal detachment, choroidal mass, papilledema, and retinal artery occlusion are rare but have been

Fig. 33.1 Vitreous cells in a patient with PCNSL-O

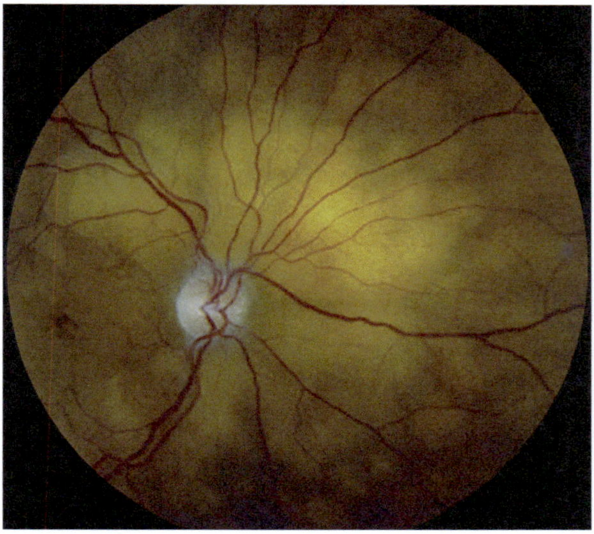

Fig. 33.2 Creamy yellow subretinal infiltrates in a patient with PCNSL-O

reported. Often, patients with PCNSL-O are followed for some time for nonspecific uveitis refractory to treatment before the correct diagnosis is made. Symptoms and findings of CNS involvement are variable depending on the area of the brain affected. Symptoms may vary from mild personality changes to focal neurologic deficits. PCNSL is typically more advanced upon diagnosis, grows quickly, and may be multifocal.

Diagnostics

Diagnosis of PCNSL-O requires a high index of suspicion. Onset of unilateral or bilateral posterior uveitis in patients over the age of 50 should raise the possibility of lymphoma. Diagnostic confirmation of ocular involvement requires vitreous biopsy and occasionally subretinal biopsy. Cytologic evaluation of the specimen is essential in establishing the diagnosis. Flow cytometry and PCR analysis for gene rearrangements are ancillary studies that can support the diagnosis.

Pathology

The cytologic features of the tumor cells are large pleomorphic lymphocytes with scan cytoplasm. The nuclei are round or oval with conspicuous nuclear membranes andmultiple,prominent,eccentricallylocatednucleoli(Fig33.3).Immunohistochemical staining and flow cytometry show a monoclonal proliferation of cells.

Differential Diagnosis

Other causes of panuveitis include syphilis, tuberculosis, sarcoidosis, Vogt-Koyanagi-Harada syndrome, infectious endophthalmitis, sympathetic ophthalmia, and Behcet's disease. Other infectious etiologies of posterior uveitis include fungal, viral, and toxoplasmosis. Choroidal metastases or amelanotic melanoma can present similar to PCNSL and should be considered. Additional entities involving the posterior segment include birdshot chorioretinopathy, multifocal choroiditis, multiple evanescent white-dot syndrome, punctuate inner choroidopathy, acute posterior multifocal placoid pigment epitheliopathy, and diffuse unilateral subacute neuroretinitis.

Clinical Evaluation

1. Brain MRI shows lesions that enhance with gadolinium.
2. Lumbar puncture for cytology.
3. Diagnostic vitrectomy if CSF not diagnostic.

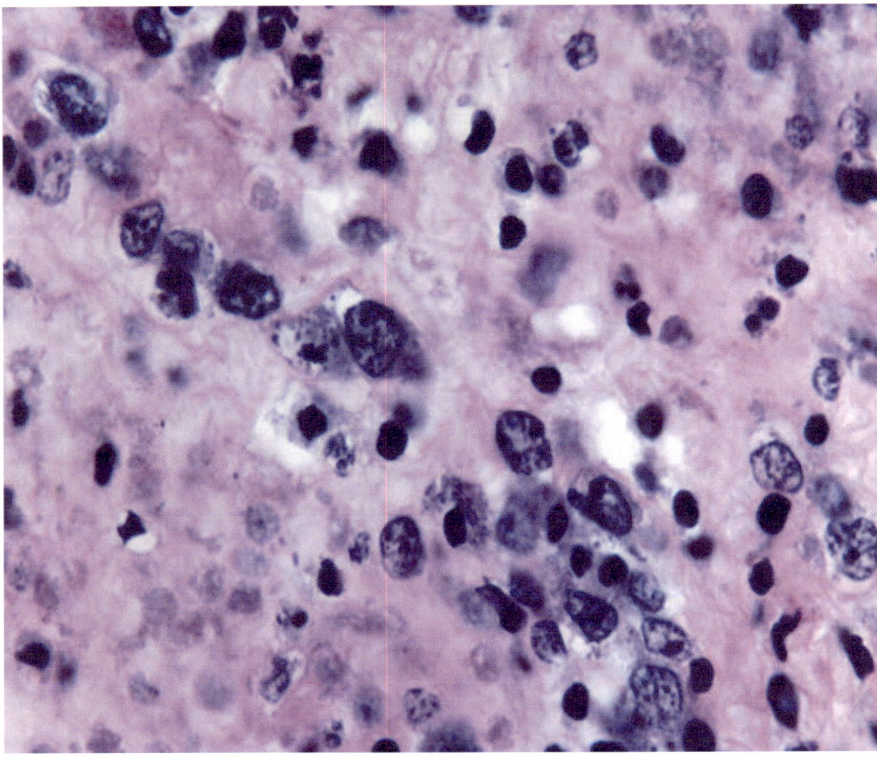

Fig. 33.3 Vitreous biopsy specimen showing large pleomorphic lymphocytes in this patient with primary intraocular lymphoma

4. Retinal or subretinal biopsy may be recommended if vitreous sample is negative for lymphoma.
5. Stereotactic brain biopsy may be needed if all other evaluations are negative and brain lesions are present.

Patients with PCNSL-O require oncologic evaluation for CNS involvement, and patients with PCNSL require ophthalmic examinations during initial diagnosis and during posttreatment follow-up. Up to 12% of patients may have extraneural involvement, so computed tomography of the chest, abdomen, and pelvis along with bone marrow biopsy is recommended.

Prophylaxis

There is no prophylaxis for PCNSL-O.

Therapy

The mainstay of treatment for PCNSL-O is radiation therapy. Because of the frequency of asymmetric, bilateral disease, treatment of both eyes should be considered. Possible treatment of the CNS with high-dose methotrexate can be considered as prophylactic therapy. Methotrexate delivered as an intravitreal injection has been used in cases of recurrence after radiation. Some ocular oncologists are now using intravitreal rituximab in addition to methotrexate. The optimal treatment for CNS disease is the subject of ongoing studies. Because of its significant side-effect profile, whole brain radiation is no longer the mainstay of treatment. Chemotherapy with methotrexate has shown to be as effective. Current treatment modalities include intrathecal reservoirs or blood-brain barrier disruption.

Prognosis

The prognosis for patients with PCNSL and PCNSL-O is poor. Most patients will die within 2 years from central nervous system disease. Cellular markers associated with poor prognosis include p53, c-Myc, and Bcl-6.

Epidemiology

Patients with PCNSL-O usually present in the sixth or seventh decade. Males and females are affected equally. The incidence of primary lymphoma of the central nervous system (PCNSL) is 5/1,000 person-years in AIDS patients and 0.3/100,000 person-years in immunocompetent patients.

Cross-References

Retinal leukemia

Further Reading

Batchelor T, Loeffler JS (2006) Primary CNS lymphoma. J Clin Oncol 24(8):1821–1828

Levy-Clarke GA, Chan CC, Nussenblatt RB (2005) Diagnosis and management of primary intraocular lymphoma. Hematol Oncol Clin North Am 19:739–749

Singh AD, Lewis H, Schachat AP (2005) Primary lymphoma of the central nervous system. Ophthalmol Clin North Am 18:199–207

Retinal Vascular Tumors

34

Hajir Dadgostar, Arun D. Singh, and Hans E. Grossniklaus

Retinal Cavernous Hemangioma

Synonyms

None

Definition

Cavernous hemangioma of the retina is a benign tumor consisting of multiple dilated, thin-walled vascular spaces, which can occur sporadically or in association with an autosomal dominant syndrome featuring cerebral vascular malformations.

H. Dadgostar, M.D., Ph.D. (✉)
Valley Retina Associates Medical Group,
16500 Ventura Blvd, Suite 250, Encino, CA 91436, USA
e-mail: vision@doctor.com

A.D. Singh, M.D.
Department of Ophthalmic Oncology,
Cole Eye Institute, Cleveland Clinic Foundation,
9500 Euclid Ave, Desk i-329, Cleveland, OH 44195, USA
e-mail: singha@ccf.org

H.E. Grossniklaus, M.D.
Emory University School of Medicine, Emory Eye Center,
Department of Ophthalmology,
Atlanta, GA, USA
e-mail: ophtheg@emory.edu

H.E. Grossniklaus (ed.), *Pocket Guide to Ocular Oncology and Pathology*,
DOI 10.1007/978-3-642-29782-3_34,

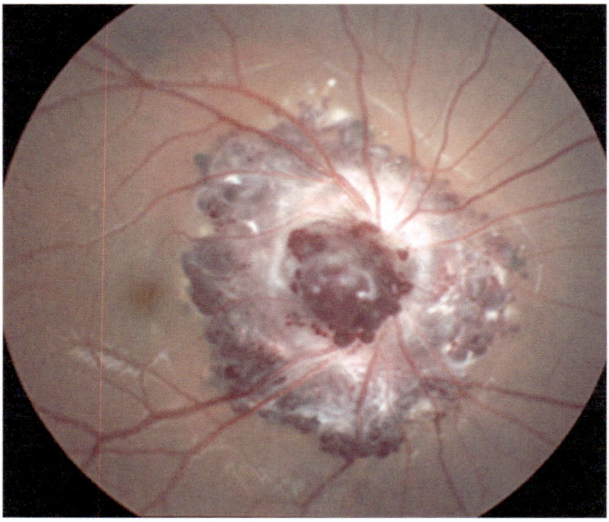

Fig. 34.1 Retinal cavernous hemangioma. A grape-like cluster of vascular channels within the retina (Reproduced with permission from Patikulsila et al. (2007))

Etiology

Cavernous hemangiomas are considered congenital hamartomas. The familial form has been linked to loci on chromosomes 3q, 7p, and 7q.

Clinical Presentation

This tumor can vary in size and location and is classically described as a grapelike cluster of vascular channels within the retina (Fig. 34.1). Epiretinal membranes are common. These lesions do not have prominent feeder vessels and are not exudative. Vitreous hemorrhage can rarely occur.

Diagnosis

The funduscopic appearance is characteristic. Fluorescein angiography demonstrates a slowly filling low-flow system of saccular channels with hyperfluorescent plasma overlying dark sediments representing cellular blood elements. Leakage is typically absent. CT and/or MRI imaging should be performed to rule out intracranial hamartomas.

Pathology

On histopathology, the lesion is composed of numerous thin-walled vascular channels (Fig. 34.2). The lesion occupies the inner retina, and telangiectatic vessels are

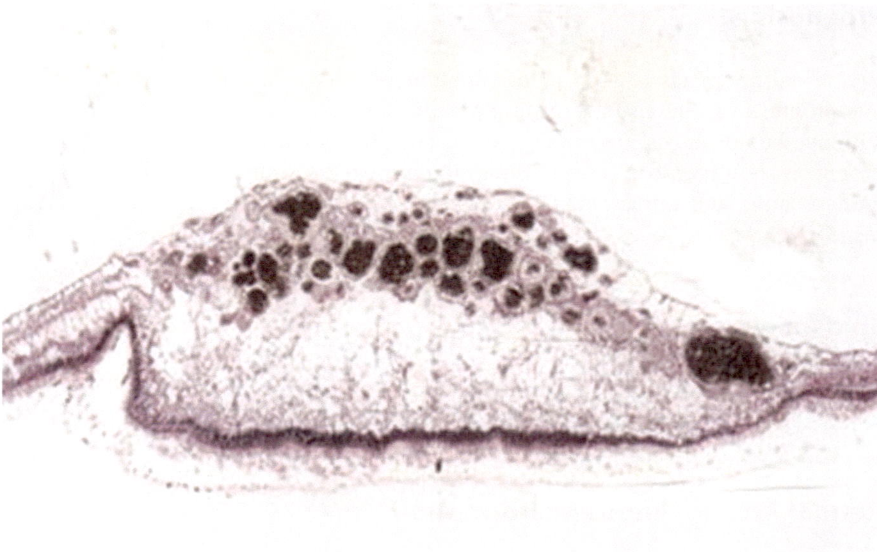

Fig. 34.2 A retinal cavernous hemangioma is composed of a collection of dilated thin-walled vascular channels that are congested with blood (hematoxylin and eosin, ×25)

separated by thin fibrous septae. Neither proteinaceous exudates nor foamy histiocytes are typically present. Ultrastructurally, nonfenestrated, flat endothelial cells that possess terminal bars on the luminal side line the vessel walls. This feature explains the absence of leakage on fluorescein angiography.

Differential Diagnosis

Important diagnostic alternatives include capillary hemangioma, macroaneurysms, and vasoproliferative tumor as well as vascular malformations including Coats' disease. The absence of feeder vessels and exudation is a distinguishing feature of cavernous hemangiomas.

Prophylaxis

There is no known prophylactic treatment for cavernous hemangioma of the retina.

Therapy

Most cases are self-limited and asymptomatic, requiring no treatment.

Prognosis

The visual prognosis is good unless the tumor is in the macula. These lesions are not progressive, are usually asymptomatic, and often undergo autothrombosis. Vitreous hemorrhages may rarely occur, but often clear spontaneously. Systemic prognosis, however, can be variable in the presence of intracranial hemangiomas, with seizures and intracranial hemorrhages reported in 44% and 48% of cases, respectively.

Epidemiology

This is a rare lesion with an average age at diagnosis of 23 years. In a review of reported cases, 60% occurred in women.

Retinal Arteriovenous Malformation

Synonyms

Racemose hemangioma
Wyburn-Mason syndrome

Definition

The retinal arteriovenous malformations (AVMs) represent a spectrum of congenital retinal vascular malformations with a diminished or often absent capillary plexus between abnormal arterial and venous channels in the retina, orbit, and brain.

Etiology

Retinal AVMs are a developmental abnormality of vascular mesoderm.

Clinical Presentation

Fundus examination reveals an abnormal arteriovenous anastomosis with variable degrees of dilation and tortuosity (Fig. 34.3). With larger lesions, exudates and hemorrhage may also occur and can compromise vision. Retinal ischemia and neovascular glaucoma may occur as a result of occlusions or steal phenomena. These malformations may present as isolated lesions or as part of the Wyburn-Mason syndrome.

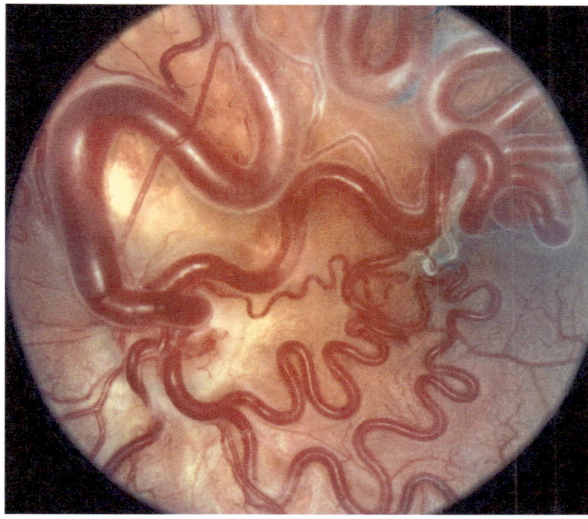

Fig. 34.3 Retinal arteriovenous malformation. Arteriovenous anastomosis with dilation and tortuosity of retinal vessels (Reproduced with permission from Singh et al. (2007))

Diagnosis

Diagnosis is made based on ophthalmoscopic features. Fluorescein angiography may demonstrate ischemia in cases with an occlusion. CT and/or MRI imaging should be used to rule out the presence of orbital and intracranial lesions.

Pathology

Histopathologically, this lesion consists of large dilated retinal vessels that are otherwise normal.

Differential Diagnosis

Capillary and cavernous hemangiomas can usually be distinguished based on clinical and angiographic features.

Prophylaxis

There is no known prophylactic treatment for retinal arteriovenous malformations.

Therapy

Treatment is usually not necessary for ocular lesions. Neovascular glaucoma is managed by medical or surgical measures to reduce intraocular pressure. For CNS lesions, embolization and radiotherapy have been attempted with variable success; however, many CNS lesions are inoperable because of their location.

Prognosis

Vision may be compromised by ischemia and exudation in some cases; however, the majority of retinal lesions do not cause vision loss. Intracranial AVMs have been reported in 23% to 80% of cases and can lead to serious morbidity as a result of intracranial hemorrhage.

Epidemiology

Arteriovenous malformations of the retina are rare. Most cases present before 30 years of age.

Vasoproliferative Retinal Tumor

Synonyms

Presumed acquired retinal hemangioma
- Angiomatous mass
- Peripheral retinal telangiectasis
- Reactive Retinal Glial Tumor

Definition

Vasoproliferative tumors are peripheral, solitary, unilateral, and vascular retinal masses that can occur as primary tumors or in association with an underlying uveitic or degenerative disease.

Etiology

The majority of cases are idiopathic in origin. However, about one-fourth are associated with other ocular diseases such as intermediate uveitis, ocular toxoplasmosis, and retinitis pigmentosa.

Clinical Presentation

A solitary raised, dome-shaped, yellowish pink mass in the retinal periphery (Fig. 34.4). There is a predilection for the inferotemporal quadrant. Normal-sized

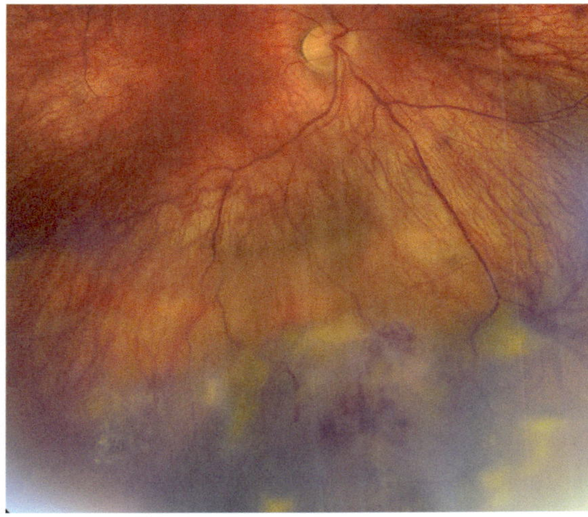

Fig. 34.4 Retinal vasoproliferative tumor. A solitary raised, dome-shaped, yellowish pink mass in the retinal periphery with surrounding exudation

retinal vessels, as opposed to the dilated feeder vessels associated with retinal capillary hemangioma, supply most lesions. About 80% feature some degree of exudation. Serous retinal detachment, vitreous hemorrhage, preretinal membranes, and macular edema are associated findings.

Diagnosis

Fundus examination is usually diagnostic. Fluorescein angiography reveals a peripheral hyperfluorescent lesion with prominent late leakage.

Pathology

This lesion likely represents a reactive process containing retinal blood vessels, glial cells, and retinal pigment epithelial cells. It is in the spectrum of massive retinal gliosis (Fig. 34.5). There is recent evidence that this is likely a retinal glial tumor with associated prominent vascular channels.

Differential Diagnosis

Capillary hemangioblastoma can have a similar appearance, but vasoproliferative tumors are typically unilateral and solitary, present in adulthood, and lack dilated feeder vessels.

Prophylaxis

There is no known prophylactic treatment for retinal vasoproliferative tumor.

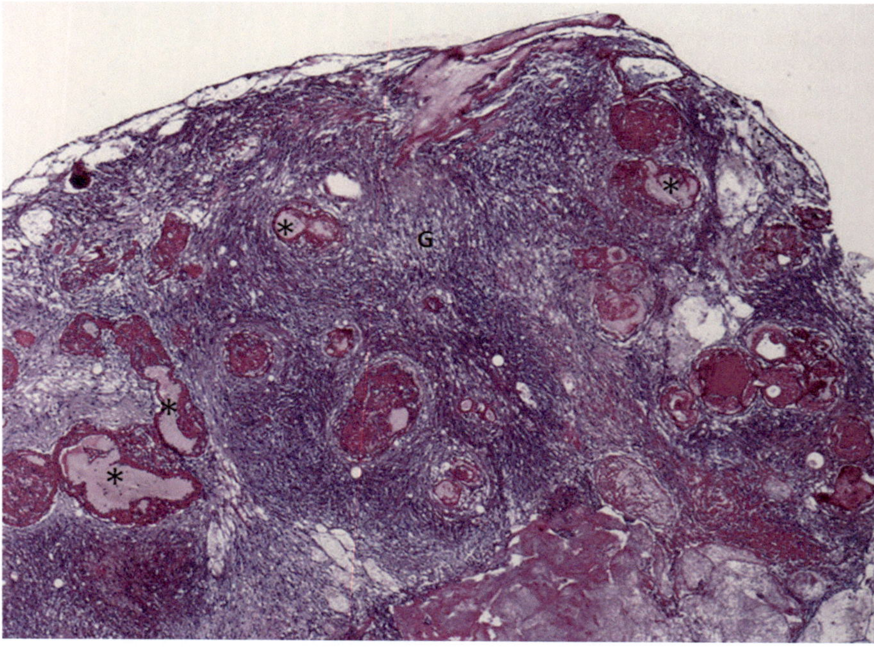

Fig. 34.5 A retinal vasoproliferative tumor is composed of hyalinized vascular channels (*) and intervening gliosis (*G*) (periodic acid Schiff, ×25)

Therapy

Asymptomatic lesions can be observed. In cases with significant exudation or macular edema, the lesion can be treated by cryotherapy, laser therapy, photodynamic therapy, or plaque brachytherapy.

Prognosis

The visual prognosis is variable and depends on the degree of exudation, hemorrhage, and edema. Macular preretinal fibrosis and edema have been reported in 31% and 18% of cases, respectively. In secondary cases, the visual prognosis is also dependent on the underlying diagnosis (e.g., retinitis pigmentosa).

Epidemiology

These tumors are rare, are usually present in the third or fourth decade of life, and have no gender predilection.

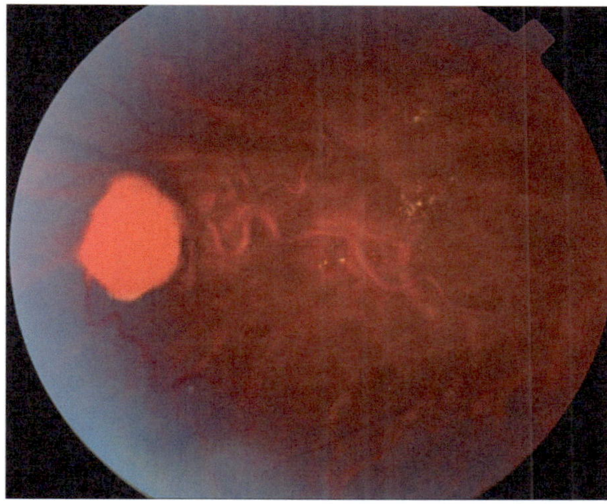

Fig. 34.6 Retinal hemangioblastoma appears as a red to pink tumor with a feeding artery and draining vein

Cross-References

Phakomatoses

Retinal Hemangioblastoma

This entity is covered in a separate entry and in phakomatoses. An example is provided in Fig. 34.6.

Further Reading

Chan CC, Collins ABD, Chew EY (2007) Molecular pathology of eye with von Hippel-Lindau (VHL) disease: a review. Retina 27:1–7

Dayani PN, Sadun AA (2007) A case report of Wyburn-Mason syndrome and review of the literature. Neuroradiology 49(5):445–456

Messmer E, Font RL, Laqua H et al (1984) Cavernous hemangioma of the retina: immunohistochemical and ultrastructural observations. Arch Ophthalmol 102:413–418

Patikulsila D, Visaetsilpanonta S, Sinclair SH et al (2007) Cavernous hemangioma of the optic disk. Retina 27:391–392

Shields CL, Shields JA, Barrett J et al (1995) Vasoproliferative tumors of the ocular fundus. Classification and clinical manifestations in 103 patients. Arch Ophthalmol 113:615–623

Singh AD, Nouri M, Shields CL et al (2001a) Retinal capillary hemangioma: a comparison of sporadic cases and cases associated with von Hippel-Lindau disease. Ophthalmology 108:1907–1911

Singh AD, Shields CL, Shields JA (2001b) von Hippel-Lindau disease. Surv Ophthalmol 46:117–142

Singh AD, Rundle PA, Rennie I (2005) Retinal vascular tumors. Ophthalmol Clin North Am 18:167–176

Singh AD, Rundle PA, Rennie I (2007) Retinal vascular tumors. In: Singh AD, Damato BE, Pe'er J, Murphree AL, Perry JD (eds) Clinical ophthalmic oncology. Saunders-Elsevier, Philadelphia, pp 341–347

Adenoma and Adenocarcinoma of the Retinal Pigment Epithelium (RPE) 35

Martin Heur, Arun D. Singh, Chris Bergstrom, and Hans E. Grossniklaus

Synonyms

None

Definition

Neoplastic proliferation of RPE cells.

Etiology

Acquired neoplastic transformation of RPE cells.

M. Heur, M.D., Ph.D.
Department of Ophthalmology, University of Southern California Keck School of Medicine, 1450 San Pablo St., DEI 5702, Los Angeles, CA 90033, USA
e-mail: heur@usc.edu

A.D. Singh, M.D. (✉)
Department of Ophthalmic Oncology,
Cole Eye Institute, Cleveland Clinic Foundation,
9500 Euclid Ave, Desk i-329, Cleveland, OH 44195, USA
e-mail: singha@ccf.org

C. Bergstrom, M.D.
Department of Ophthalmology, Emory University School of Medicine,
Atlanta, GA, USA
e-mail: cbergs2@emory.edu

H.E. Grossniklaus, M.D.
Emory University School of Medicine,
Emory Eye Center,
Department of Ophthalmology,
Atlanta, GA, USA
e-mail: ophtheg@emory.edu

H.E. Grossniklaus (ed.), *Pocket Guide to Ocular Oncology and Pathology*,
DOI 10.1007/978-3-642-29782-3_35, © Springer-Verlag Berlin Heidelberg 2013

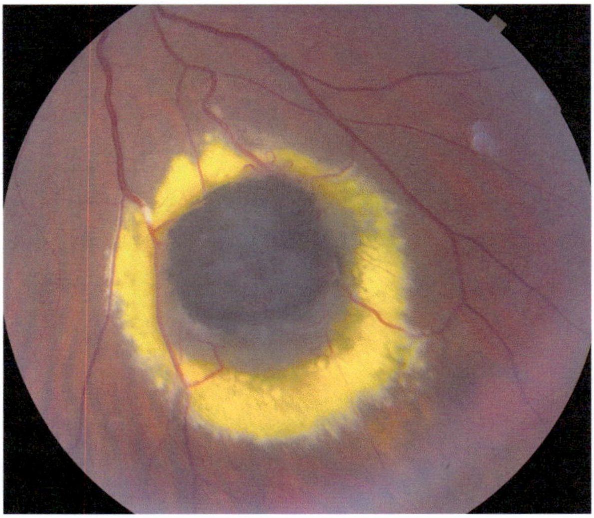

Fig. 35.1 RPE adenoma (adenocarcinoma) is a black lesion often associated with prominent feeder vessels, hard exudates, and serous retinal detachment (Reproduced with permission from Mosby-Elsevier)

Clinical Presentation

Adenomas and adenocarcinomas of the RPE are rare tumors appearing as very dark brown or black lesions often associated with prominent feeder vessels, hard exudates, and serous retinal detachment (Fig. 35.1). They may appear similar to retinal capillary hemangioblastoma except that they are black instead of red. The tumor appears as an abruptly elevated dome-shaped mass arising from the RPE, and they do not display a mushroom configuration. RPE tumors may produce vitreous cells or vitreous hemorrhage.

Diagnostics

The diagnosis can often be made based on clinical examination, but ancillary testing may be helpful. Fluorescein angiography shows relative hypofluorescence in the early phase, and this finding is distinct from melanoma that tends to have early hyperfluorescence. No intrinsic circulation is seen with the RPE tumor as is seen in melanoma. Ultrasonography reveals an acoustically solid lesion with high internal reflectivity and abrupt elevation from the RPE.

Pathology

Histopathology reveals the tumors to arise abruptly from the adjacent normal RPE (Fig. 35.2). The cells may show a solid or vacuolated pattern. Vacuolated tumors show round, clear vacuoles that contain a hyaluronidase-resistant acid, mucopolysaccharide. The solid tumors contain ribbons or tubules of cells separated by connective

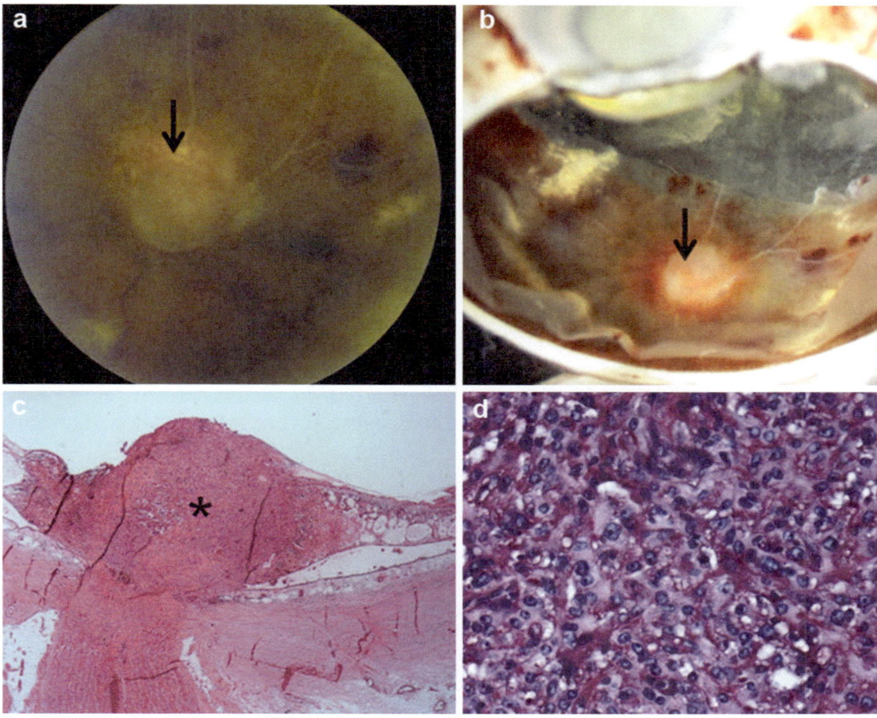

Fig. 35.2 (**a**) A nodular tumor (*arrow*) is present, extending over the optic nerve head. The retina contains hemorrhages, exudates, and a branch vein occlusion. (**b**) The enucleated eye contains the tumor (*arrow*) and surrounding retinal hemorrhages and exudates. (**c**) The tumor (*) overlies the optic nerve head. (**d**) The tumor is composed of chords of cells with vesiculated nuclei, prominent nucleoli, and PAS-positive basement membrane production ((**c**) hematoxylin and eosin, 10×; (**d**) periodic acid Schiff, 100×)

tissue septa with abundant basement membrane visible on PAS staining. Differentiation between adenoma and adenocarcinoma can be difficult and is based on the degree of nuclear atypia and local invasiveness.

Differential Diagnosis

Lesions to consider in the differential include pigmented lesions of the RPE, such as CHRPE, and simple or combined hamartoma. The latter, however, are not associated with feeder vessels, hard exudates, or serous retinal detachment. Melanoma may be considered, but again the presence of exudates and dilated feeder vessels distinguishes RPE adenoma/adenocarcinoma. Ultrasound features can also be very helpful in distinguishing melanoma from RPE adenoma and adenocarcinoma. Adenomas and adenocarcinomas of the RPE can only be differentiated from each other by histopathologic examination.

Prophylaxis

There is no known prophylaxis for RPE adenoma or adenocarcinoma.

Therapy

Management options include surgical resection, brachytherapy, and enucleation. Photocoagulation can be considered for smaller lesions.

Prognosis

These lesions may be locally invasive and may cause severe loss of vision. They are not known to metastasize.

Epidemiology

The prevalence of RPE adenomas and adenocarcinomas is unknown, but it is believed to be extremely rare.

Cross-References

CHRPE
RPE hamartoma
Choroidal nevus
Choroidal melanoma
Retinal exudates
Serous retinal detachment

Further Reading

Shields JA, Shields CL, Gunduz K, Eagle RC Jr (1999) Neoplasms of the retinal pigment epithelium: the 1998 Albert Ruedemann, Sr, memorial lecture, part 2. Arch Ophthalmol 117:601–608
Singh AD (2006) CHRPE and other pigmented RPE lesions. In: Huang D, Kaiser P, Lowder CY, Traboulsi EI (eds) Retinal imaging. Mosby-Elsevier, Philadelphia, pp 519–552

Benign Tumors of the Retinal Pigment Epithelium (RPE)

36

Martin Heur, Arun D. Singh, and Hans E. Grossniklaus

Congenital Hypertrophy of the RPE (CHRPE)

Synonyms

Retinal nevus, Benign melanoma of the RPE, Bear tracks, Polar bear tracks, Atypical CHRPE, Pigmented ocular fundus lesion (POFL)

Definition

This lesion is a well-circumscribed area of congenital hypertrophy and hyperpigmentation of retinal pigment epithelial cells.

M. Heur, M.D., Ph.D.
Department of Ophthalmology, University of Southern California Keck School of Medicine, 1450 San Pablo St., DEI 5702, Los Angeles, CA 90033, USA
e-mail: heur@usc.edu

A.D. Singh, M.D. (✉)
Department of Ophthalmic Oncology,
Cole Eye Institute, Cleveland Clinic Foundation,
9500 Euclid Ave, Desk i-329, Cleveland, OH 44195, USA
e-mail: singha@ccf.org

H.E. Grossniklaus, M.D.
Emory University School of Medicine, Emory Eye Center,
Department of Ophthalmology,
Atlanta, GA, USA
e-mail: ophtheg@emory.edu

H.E. Grossniklaus (ed.), *Pocket Guide to Ocular Oncology and Pathology*,
DOI 10.1007/978-3-642-29782-3_36, © Springer-Verlag Berlin Heidelberg 2013

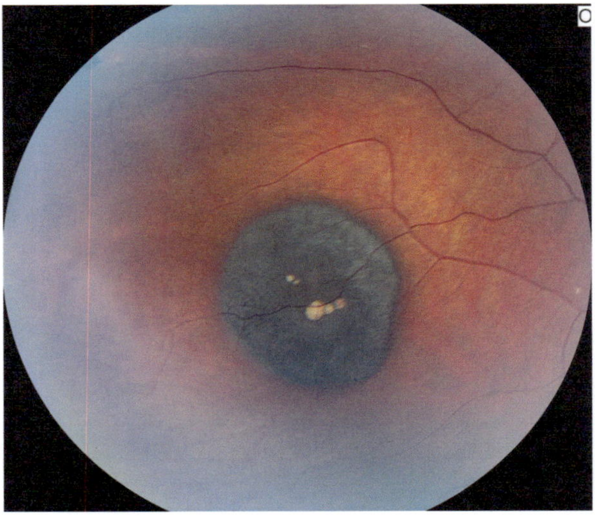

Fig. 36.1 CHRPE is a flat, pigmented lesion with sharp borders at the levels of RPE. Note areas of hypopigmentation or depigmentation known as lacunae

Etiology

Multiple bilateral lesions have been associated with a mutation in adenomatous polyposis coli (APC) gene on chromosome 5q21.

Clinical Presentation

CHRPE is a flat, pigmented lesion with sharp borders at the level of RPE. The lesions are usually unilateral with round, dark pigmentation, but can contain areas of depigmentation known as lacunae (Fig. 36.1). They can also be completely depigmented in rare instances. Solitary CHRPEs are isolated findings with no known systemic associations. CHRPE can be seen in groups, commonly occurring unilaterally in a single sector. These lesions are called bear tracks because of their resemblance to paw prints. Like CHRPE, bear tracks are not associated with systemic conditions. Pigmented ocular fundus lesions (POFL) are groups of atypical CHRPE that occur bilaterally and appear oval, often with a depigmented tail oriented toward the optic disc. They can be associated with familial adenomatous polyposis (FAP). Patients with FAP have gastrointestinal polyposis with an increased risk of colon cancer and an increased risk of neuroepithelial tumors of the CNS (Turcot syndrome).

Diagnostics

Diagnosis is clinically based on recognition of characteristic features identified by indirect ophthalmoscopy. When multiple bilateral lesions are present, the patient should be evaluated for familial adenomatous polyposis and should be tested for mutations in the APC gene.

Pathology

On histopathology, hypertrophic RPE cells with hyperpigmentation and macromelanosomes are seen in the center or dark part of the lesion, and hypopigmented RPE cells filled with lipofuscin are at the margin or forming the lacunae of the lesion (Fig. 36.2). The CHRPE-like lesions seen with FAP exhibit RPE hyperplasia and hamartomatous changes such as tubule formations in addition to RPE hypertrophy.

Differential Diagnosis

Pigmented lesions of the RPE such as hamartoma, adenoma, or adenocarcinoma. Pigmented lesions of the choroid such as nevus or melanoma.

Prophylaxis

There is no known prophylaxis for CHRPE.

Therapy

Because of their benign nature, CHRPE lesions can be observed.

Prognosis

The prognosis is excellent in most cases because of the benign nature of CHRPE. Patients with multiple bilateral CHRPE need further evaluation because of its association with FAP.

Epidemiology

The prevalence of CHRPE in the general population is estimated to be around 1%, while the prevalence of CHRPE in Gardner syndrome is estimated to be around 37%.

Cross-References

RPE adenoma and adenocarcinoma

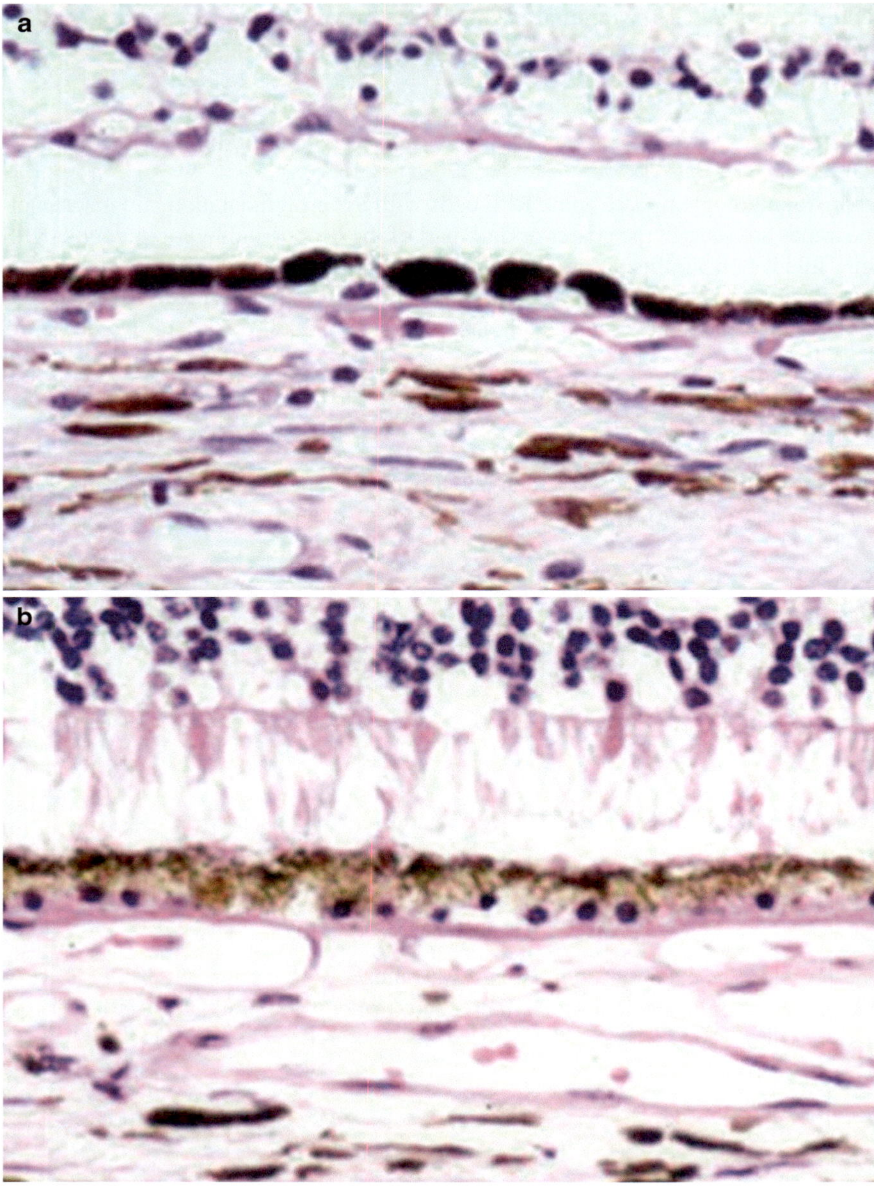

Fig. 36.2 The pathology of CHRPE includes hyperpigmented RPE cells with abundant intracytoplasmic melanin pigment granules (**a**) in the dark center of the lesion and lightly pigmented RPE with intracytoplasmic lipofuscin (**b**) forming the light rim surrounding the lesion (hematoxylin and eosin, ×100)

Hamartoma of the Retinal Pigment Epithelium (RPE)

Synonyms

None

Definition

Benign proliferation of tissues normally found in and around the RPE. Simple hamartomas are isolated to the RPE while combined hamartomas involve the RPE and retina. Combined hamartomas can contain RPE, glial, and vascular elements.

Etiology

The etiology of RPE hamartoma is unknown, but it is believed to be a congenital lesion.

Clinical Presentation

Simple hamartomas of the RPE appear as small black nodules under the neurosensory retina and are histologically different from CHRPE in that hamartomas consist of proliferation rather than hypertrophy of RPE cells. Combined hamartomas appear as gray-black lesions and may have membranous components causing retinal striae or traction (Fig. 36.3). Several systemic diseases have been associated with combined hamartomas, but the most common association is with neurofibromatosis 2 (NF2).

Diagnostics

The diagnoses of simple hamartoma and combined hamartoma are based on the clinical features seen with indirect ophthalmoscopy.

Pathology

Histopathologic features of combined hamartoma have been described in a few cases. Thickened and disorganized retinal tissue intermixed with vascular and glial elements along with tubules of proliferating RPE are present adjacent to normal retina (Fig. 36.4). It is unknown if this is a congenital or acquired abnormality.

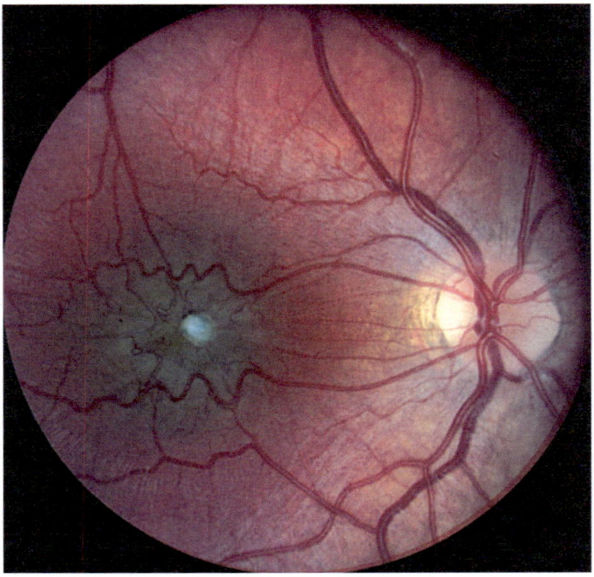

Fig. 36.3 Combined hamartoma is a gray-black lesion causing retinal striae or traction (reproduced with permission from Saunders-Elsevier)

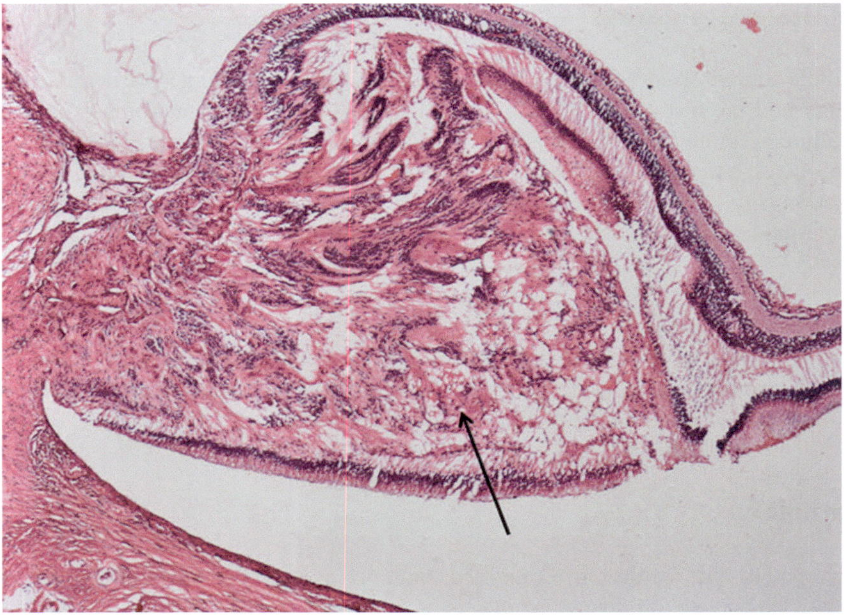

Fig. 36.4 The combined hamartoma (*arrow*) is adjacent to normal retina and is composed of disorganized retina, vascular channels, and RPE forming tubules (hematoxylin and eosin, ×25)

Differential Diagnosis

Pigmented lesions of the RPE including CHRPE, adenoma, and adenocarcinoma. Pigmented lesions of the choroid such as nevus or melanoma.

Prophylaxis

There is no known prophylaxis for RPE hamartomas.

Therapy

Because of the benign nature of these lesions, no treatment for simple or combined hamartomas is usually necessary. The benefit of vitrectomy for epiretinal membranes in combined hamartomas is controversial. The lesion is known to involve all layers of the retina, and removal of the epiretinal tissue is of unproven benefit. Patients with associated systemic involvement, such as deafness in NF2, need appropriate intervention.

Prognosis

The prognosis is usually excellent for simple hamartomas of the RPE. For combined hamartomas, visual prognosis is guarded, particularly when the macula is involved. In one large series, mean visual acuity after 4 years of follow-up was 20/800 for such lesions.

Epidemiology

The prevalence of RPE hamartomas is unknown, but it is believed to be rare.

Cross-References

Phakomatoses, choroidal nevus, choroidal melanoma

Further Reading

Font RL, Moura RA, Shetlar DJ et al (1989) Combined hamartoma of sensory retina and retinal pigment epithelium. Retina 9:302–311
Gass JD (1973) An unusual hamartoma of the pigment epithelium and retina simulating choroidal melanoma and retinoblastoma. Trans Am Ophthalmol Soc 71:171–185
Gass JD (1989) Focal congenital anomalies of the retinal pigment epithelium. Eye (Lond) 3:1–18
Parsons MA, Rennie IG, Rundle PA et al (2005) Congenital hypertrophy of retinal pigment epithelium: a clinico-pathologic case report. Br J Ophthalmol 89:920–921
Shields CL et al (2003a) Solitary congenital hypertrophy of the retinal pigment epithelium: clinical features and frequency of enlargement in 330 patients. Ophthalmology 110:1968–1976
Shields CL, Shields JA, Marr BP et al (2003b) Congenital simple hamartoma of the retinal pigment epithelium: a study of 5 cases. Ophthalmology 110:1005–1011
Shields CL, Thangappan A, Hartzell K et al (2008) Combined hamartoma of the retina and retinal pigment epithelium in 77 consecutive patients: visual outcome based on macular versus extramacular tumor location. Ophthalmology 115:2246–2252

Tiret A, Parc C (1999) Fundus lesions of adenomatous polyposis. Curr Opin Ophthalmol 10:168–172

Traboulsi EI et al (1987) Prevalence and importance of pigmented ocular fundus lesions in Gardner's syndrome. N Engl J Med 316:661–667

Traboulsi ET et al (2007) Tumors of the retinal pigment epithelium. In: Singh AD, Damato BE, Pe'er J, Murphree AL, Perry JD (eds) Clinical ophthalmic oncology. Saunders-Elsevier, Philadelphia, pp 358–365

Ciliary Body-Fuchs Adenoma

37

Sumitra Khandewal and Hans E. Grossniklaus

Synonyms

"Pseudoepitheliomatous hyperplasia" of nonpigmented epithelium of ciliary body

Definition

A benign pseudo-adenomatous proliferation of ciliary body nonpigmented epithelium that may be pedunculated, countersunk, or buried.

Etiology

There is no known etiology, although this likely represents a reactive process.

S. Khandewal, M.D. (✉)
Department of Ophthalmology, Emory Eye Center,
Atlanta, GA, USA

Department of Ophthalmology,
Emory University School of Medicine,
Atlanta, GA, USA
e-mail: ssubra9@emory.edu

H.E. Grossniklaus, M.D.
Emory University School of Medicine, Emory Eye Center,
Department of Ophthalmology,
Atlanta, GA, USA
e-mail: ophtheg@emory.edu

H. Grossniklaus (ed.), *Pocket Guide to Ocular Oncology and Pathology*,
DOI 10.1007/978-3-642-29782-3_37, © Springer-Verlag Berlin Heidelberg 2013

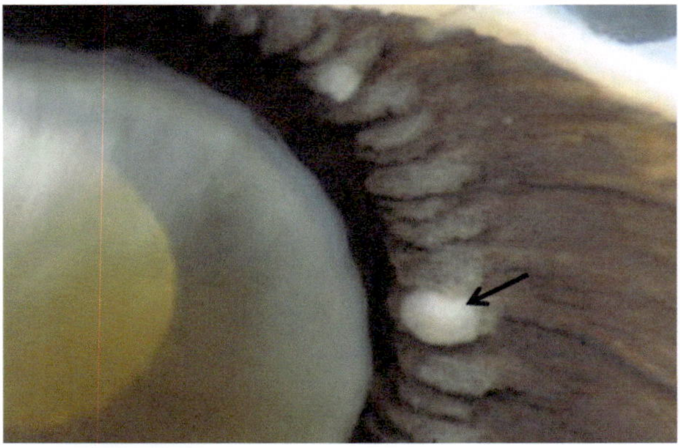

Fig. 37.1 Gross appearance of Fuchs adenoma (*arrow*) appearing as small, white nodule in pars plicata

Clinical Presentation

Often not seen clinically and only noted as incidental finding in eye bank or autopsy eye. Occasionally, a Fuchs adenoma may be observed adjacent to a focal cataract or during a routine dilated examination. The adenoma appears as a small, 1 mm or less in diameter, nodule in the pars plicata of the ciliary body.

Pathology

A Fuchs adenoma may be an incidental finding in eye bank eyes and appear as a small, white nodule in the pars plicata of the ciliary body (Fig. 37.1). Microscopic examination shows a pedunculated, countersunk, or buried island of nonpigmented ciliary epithelium arranged in chords with associated extracellular basement membrane-like material (Fig. 37.2).

Diagnosis

The diagnosis may be suspected clinically and confirmed by biopsy if indicated.

Differential Diagnosis

The differential diagnosis includes adenoma, adenocarcinoma, nevus, and melanoma of the ciliary body.

Prophylaxis

There is no known prophylaxis.

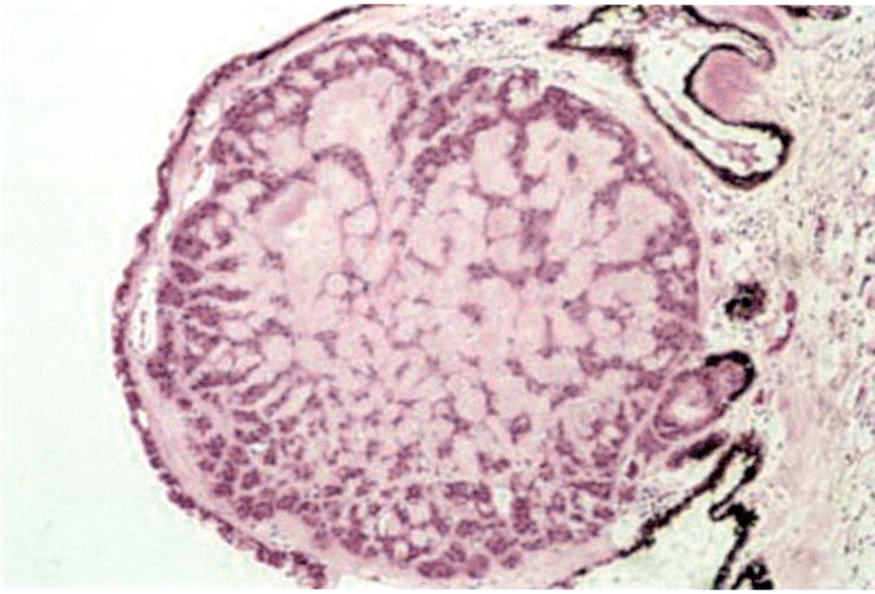

Fig. 37.2 Microscopic appearance of Fuchs adenoma showing hyperplasia of nonpigmented ciliary epithelium forming pedunculated nodule (hematoxylin and eosin, ×25)

Therapy

A suspected Fuchs adenoma may be clinically followed with direct visualization with B and A scan ultrasound examination. If an adenoma/adenocarcinoma or melanoma is suspected, a biopsy or resection may be performed.

Prognosis

The prognosis is excellent for vision, and there is no risk of malignant change.

Epidemiology

Approximately 18–20% of eye bank eyes have a Fuchs adenoma. The adenomas are equally found in men and women, usually in persons greater than 50 years old.

Cross-Reference

Ciliary body nonmelanocytic tumors

Further Reading

Bateman JB, Foos RY (1979) Coronal adenomas. Arch Ophthalmol 97(12):2379–2384
Iliff WJ, Green WR (1972) The incidence and histology of Fuchs's adenoma. Arch Ophthalmol 88(3):249–254
Shields JA, Shields CL, Eagle RC Jr, Friedman ES, Wheatley HM (2009) Age-related hyperplasia of the nonpigmented ciliary body epithelium (Fuchs adenoma) simulating a ciliary body malignant neoplasm. Arch Ophthalmol 127(9):1224–1225
Zaidman GW, Johnson BL, Salamon SM, Mondino BJ (1983) Fuchs' adenoma affecting the peripheral iris. Arch Ophthalmol 101(5):771–773

Ciliary Body Adenocarcinoma 38

Hans E. Grossniklaus

Synonyms

Epithelioma, adenocarcinoma of nonpigmented epithelium, adenocarcinoma of pigmented epithelium

Definition

This tumor is an acquired malignant neoplasm that arises from the epithelium of the ciliary body.

Etiology

There is often a history of trauma, and these tumors may be found in blind, painful eyes.

Clinical Presentation

Adenocarcinoma of the ciliary body epithelium may appear as an amelanotic or minimally pigmented nodular tumor of the ciliary body that transmits light on transillumination (see entry *Nonmelanocytic Tumors of Ciliary Body*). They may also

H.E. Grossniklaus, M.D.
Emory University School of Medicine,
Emory Eye Center,
Department of Ophthalmology,
Atlanta, GA, USA
e-mail: ophtheg@emory.edu

H.E. Grossniklaus (ed.), *Pocket Guide to Ocular Oncology and Pathology*,
DOI 10.1007/978-3-642-29782-3_38, © Springer-Verlag Berlin Heidelberg 2013

present as a solid intraocular mass that is found by ultrasound examination of a blind, painful eye or an incidental finding in an enucleated blind, painful eye (Fig. 38.1). In this instance, the tumor may appear as a glandular configuration of epithelial cells within a collagenous matrix (Fig. 38.2). These tumors may fill the globe, extending into the anterior chamber and eroding the cornea to form an epibulbar mass.

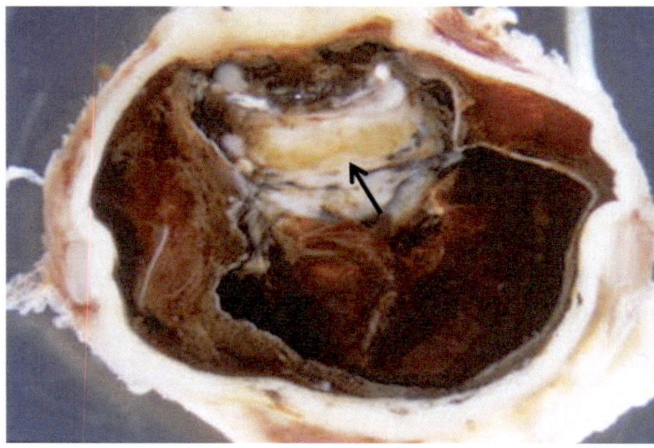

Fig. 38.1 This enucleated blind, painful eye contains a whitish-yellow mass in the ciliary body (*arrow*) adjacent to an intraocular lens

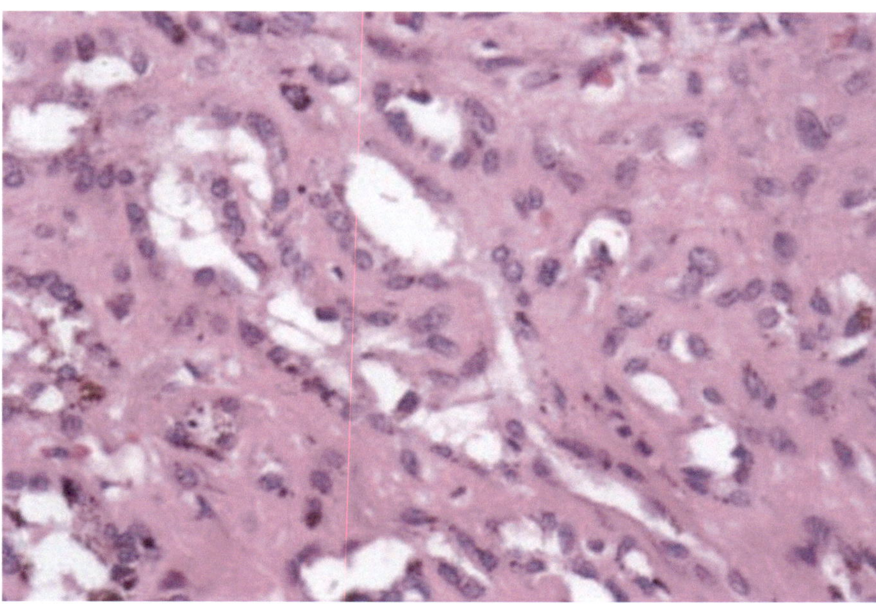

Fig. 38.2 The mass is composed of glandular configurations of epithelial cells within a collagenous matrix (hematoxylin and eosin, ×100)

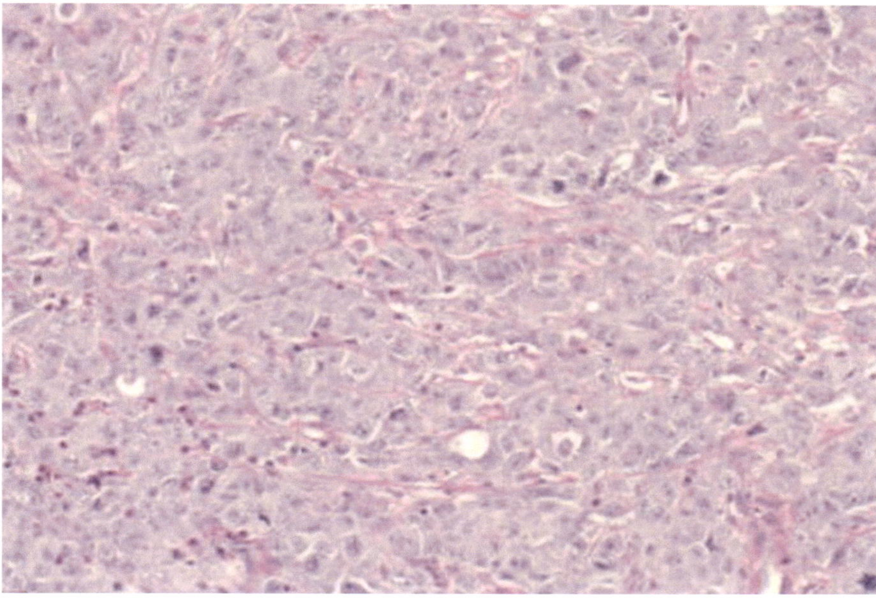

Fig. 38.3 The epibulbar component of the tumor is composed of a solid sheet of cells with malignant cytology features (periodic acid Schiff, ×150)

Diagnosis

The diagnosis is made by histologic examination of an excisional biopsy specimen obtained by a partial sclerouveactomy eye wall or enucleation specimen.

Pathology

Biopsy of the epibulbar component of a ciliary body adenocarcinoma that extends onto the ocular surface may show histologic findings that simulate melanoma or carcinoma (Fig. 38.3). Examination of the intraocular component of the tumor shows glandular configurations of neoplastic cells (Fig. 38.4). There is a spectrum of histologic growth patterns of the tumor, including papillary, pleomorphic, and anaplastic. The pleomorphic variety simulates the histology of a pleomorphic adenoma.

Differential Diagnosis

The differential diagnosis, especially of the extensive variety of this tumor found in blind, painful eyes, is mainly metastatic adenocarcinoma. Immunohistochemical staining should be positive for EMA and possibly S100 or NSE in ciliary body adenocarcinoma, and cytokeratins in metastatic adenocarcinoma.

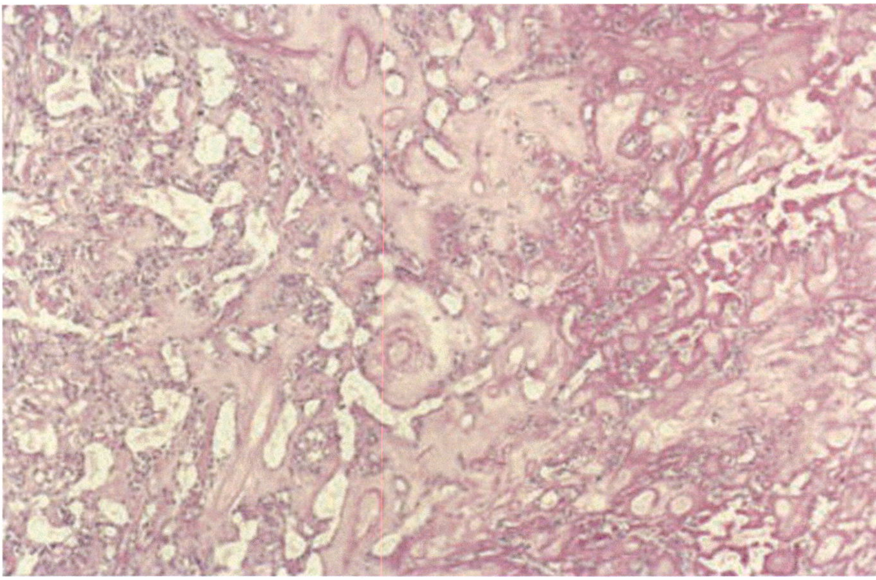

Fig. 38.4 The intraocular component of the tumor forms tubules within a collagenous matrix simulating a pleomorphic adenoma (periodic acid Schiff, ×100)

Prophylaxis

There is no prophylaxis for these tumors.

Therapy

Therapy is surgical excision via a partial eye wall resection in localized tumors and enucleation of blind, painful eyes.

Prognosis

The prognosis is excellent for persons with this tumor, as it is unlikely to metastasize.

Epidemiology

There may be some relationship to trauma in the variety of tumors that fill the eye or are found in blind, painful eyes. Hyperplasia of the ciliary epithelium in blind eyes after trauma may be the source of the adenocarcinoma. As ocular trauma is more common in men than women, it is possible that this tumor is more common in men. This is difficult to confirm as these tumors are rare.

Cross-References

Ciliary body nonmelanocytic tumors, surgical techniques

Further Reading

Grossniklaus HE, Zimmerman LE, Kachmer ML (1990) Pleomorphic adenocarcinoma of the ciliary body. Immunohistochemical and electron microscopic features. Ophthalmology 97:673–678

Rodrigues M, Hidayat A, Karesh J (1998) Pleomorphic adenocarcinoma of the ciliary epithelium simulating an epibulbar tumor. Am J Ophthalmol 105:595–600

Shields JA, Eagle RC Jr, Shields CL, De Potter P (1996) Acquired neoplasms of the nonpigmented ciliary epithelium (adenoma and adenocarcinoma). Ophthalmology 103:2007–2016

Ciliary Body Medulloepithelioma (Diktyoma)

39

Qing Zhang, Hans E. Grossniklaus, and G. Baker Hubbard III

Synonyms

Nonteratoid medulloepithelioma (diktyoma), teratoid medulloepithelioma (teratoneuroma)

Definition

Medulloepithelioma is an embryonal neuroepithelial tumor of nonpigmented ciliary epithelium that can be benign or malignant, and both the benign and malignant variants can occur as either a nonteratoid or teratoid type: the nonteratoid type consists of a proliferation of fairly well-differentiated cells of the nonpigmented ciliary epithelium; the teratoid type contains cells from two different embryonic germ layers.

Q. Zhang, M.D. (✉)
Department of Ophthalmology, Emory University School of Medicine,
Atlanta, GA, USA
e-mail: qzhang7@emory.edu

H.E. Grossniklaus, M.D.
Emory University School of Medicine, Emory Eye Center,
Department of Ophthalmology,
Atlanta, GA, USA
e-mail: ophtheg@emory.edu

G.B. Hubbard III, M.D.
Department of Ophthalmology, Emory University School of Medicine,
Atlanta, GA, USA

The Emory Eye Center, Atlanta, GA, USA
e-mail: ghubba2@emory.edu

H.E. Grossniklaus (ed.), *Pocket Guide to Ocular Oncology and Pathology*,
DOI 10.1007/978-3-642-29782-3_39, © Springer-Verlag Berlin Heidelberg 2013

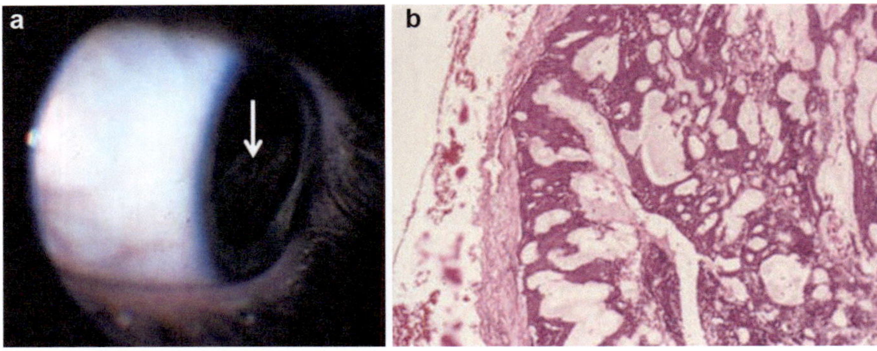

Fig. 39.1 (**a**) A minimally pigmented ciliary body tumor (arrow) is observed through the dilated pupil. (**b**) The tumor is composed of a netlike configuration of chords of medulloepithelium ((**b**) hematoxlyn and eosin, ×25)

Etiology

Medulloepithelioma is a congenital lesion, but the exact etiology is unknown.

Clinical Presentation

The tumor is usually diagnosed in children in their first decade of life. It appears as a nonpigmented vascular mass arising from the ciliary body (Fig. 39.1) and sometimes displacing the iris and lens. The lens may be subluxed or notched and may show localized areas of opacification or advanced cataract. Cysts within the tumor are often visible, and sometimes there are free-floating cysts in the vitreous. A layer of tumor cells may proliferate on the anterior hyaloid face and cause a sheetlike opacification of the retrolental space. In teratoid medulloepithelioma, the tumor may contain clinically visible chalky gray-white opacities that represent foci of cartilage when examined histologically. The tumor has a strong tendency to induce secondary glaucoma resulting from iris neovascularization.

Diagnostics

Medulloepithelioma is generally diagnosed on the basis of characteristic features identified on clinical examination. Ultrasonography may be useful in distinguishing some cases from retinoblastoma or persistent fetal vasculature syndrome (PFV). In addition, anterior chamber paracentesis may yield diagnostic material. Electron microscopic analysis of this flocculent material may reveal a complex apical junctional intercellular attachment apparatus.

Pathology

Histologically, the tumor cells of medulloepithelioma are organized into ribbonlike structures that have a distinct cellular polarity. The ribbonlike structures are composed of multilayered sheets or cords of undifferentiated round to oval cells possessing little cytoplasm (Figs. 39.2a. b). Cell nuclei are stratified in 3–5 layers, and the entire structure is lined on one side by a thin basement membrane. One surface secretes a mucinous substance, rich in hyaluronic acid that resembles primitive vitreous. Stratified sheets of cells are capable of forming mucinous cysts. Homer Wright and Flexner-Wintersteiner rosettes can also be seen. The typical rosettes in medulloepitheliomas are larger than those of retinoblastomas and are composed of multiple layers of elongated neuroepithelial cells, which closely resemble the embryonic ciliary epithelium. Heterologous elements, such as hyaline cartilage, brain-like tissue, and skeletal muscle, may be found in teratoid medulloepitheliomas. Ultrastructural analysis of medulloepithelioma shows neuroepithelial cells forming rosettes with a plethora of microvilli at the luminal surface. A polarized thin basement membrane can be present on the basilar surface of the tubules. The tumor cells have irregular, pleomorphic nuclei that cluster centrally within the lobule. Striated muscle cells with sarcomeric organization may be present in the teratoid medulloepitheliomas. Tumors that have substantial amounts of undifferentiated cells with high mitotic rates are considered malignant, although they rarely exhibit distant metastasis and patients treated with enucleation have high survival rates.

Differential Diagnosis

Entities to consider in the differential include retinoblastoma and persistent fetal vasculature syndrome (PFV). Clinical features evident on examination can usually distinguish these entities. In cases where there is a retrolental membrane with or without cataract, ultrasound may be useful to identify a ciliary body mass and to exclude a fibrovascular stalk between disc and lens as would be seen with PFV.

Prophylaxis

There is no known prophylaxis for medulloepithelioma.

Therapy

Enucleation is generally the treatment of choice. Local resection with or without combined brachytherapy may be considered in select cases where the tumor is small and well circumscribed.

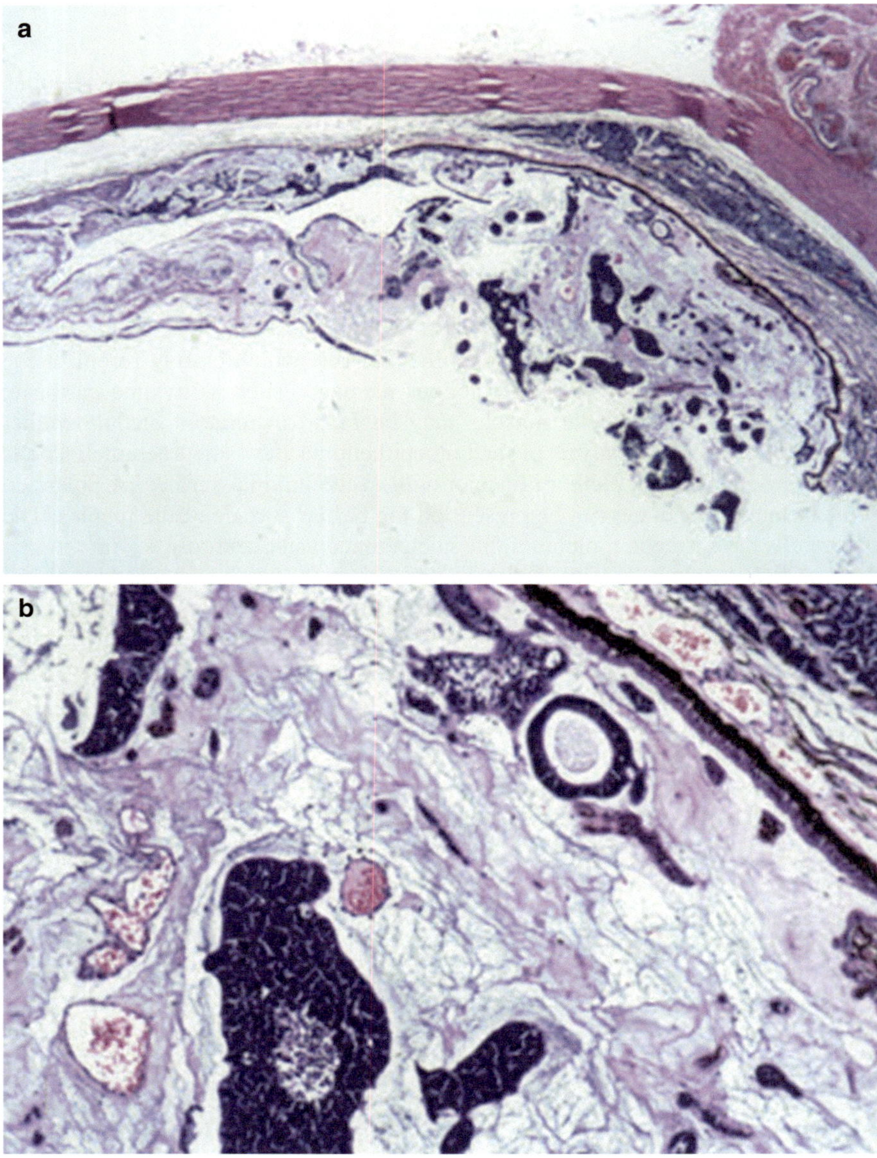

Fig. 39.2 (**a**) Ribbonlike structures of medulloepithelioma are present in the area of the ciliary body. (**b**) The cords and sheets of tumor cells that seem to recapitulate the morphology of the ciliary epithelium ((**a**) hematoxylin and eosin, ×25; (**b**) hematoxylin and eosin, ×100)

Prognosis

Tumors treated with local resection frequently relapse and usually require secondary enucleation. Medulloepithelioma may rarely metastasize. Most cases of fatal metastatic disease occur after orbital extension.

Epidemiology

This tumor is extremely rare.

Cross-References

Retinoblastoma, retinocytoma, ciliary body non-melanocytic tumors.

Further Reading

Broughton WL, Zimmerman LE (1978) A clinicopathologic study of 56 cases of intraocular medulloepitheliomas. Am J Ophthalmol 85:407–418

Cassoux N, Charlotte F, Sastre X et al (2010) Conservative surgical treatment of medulloepithelioma of the ciliary body. Arch Ophthalmol 128:380–381

Jakobiec FA (1978) Ocular and adnexal tumors. Aesculapius, Birmingham, pp 367–369, 181–196

Shields JA, Eagle RC, Shields CL, De Potter P (1996) Congenital neoplasms of the nonpigmented ciliary epithelium (medulloepithelioma). Ophthalmology 103:1998–2006

Spencer WH (1996) Ophthalmic pathology, 4th edn. Saunders, Philadelphia, pp 1316–1323

Tasman W, Jaeger EA (2000). Foundations of clinical ophthalmology. Lippincott Williams and Wilkins, Philadelphia; 2000(3) 11, pp 14–17, 21: pp 16–17

Part IV

Retinal Tumors: Retinoblastoma

Retinoblastoma: Brachytherapy

40

Carryn Anderson and Hans E. Grossniklaus

Synonyms

Eye plaque, eye plaque brachytherapy, eye plaque radiotherapy, episcleral plaque radiotherapy.

Definition

Brachytherapy is a technique that utilizes a radioactive source implanted within or next to a tumor.

Indication

This technique can be used for definitive therapy but is most often used for salvage treatment of retinoblastoma.

C. Anderson, M.D. (✉)
Department of Radiation Oncology,
University of Iowa,
Iowa City, IA, USA
e-mail: carryn-anderson@uiowa.edu

H.E. Grossniklaus, M.D.
Emory University School of Medicine, Emory Eye Center,
Department of Ophthalmology,
Atlanta, GA, USA
e-mail: ophtheg@emory.edu

H.E. Grossniklaus (ed.), *Pocket Guide to Ocular Oncology and Pathology*,
DOI 10.1007/978-3-642-29782-3_40,

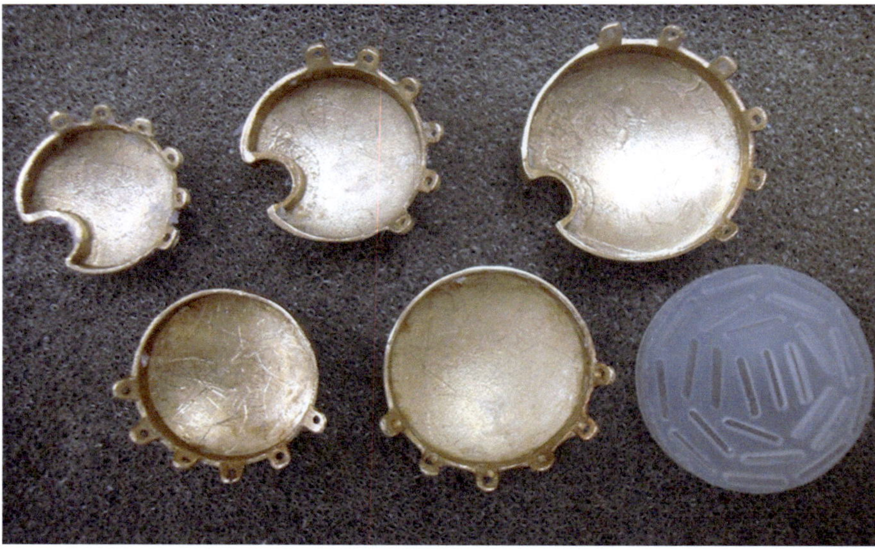

Fig. 40.1 Iodine-125 gold shield plaques of varying sizes, notched and unnotched, shown with a Silastic carrier

Contraindications

Contraindications include tumors with the largest basal diameter of >16 mm, tumors with thickness that exceeds 6–10 mm (depends upon isotope used), multiple tumors that cannot be encompassed by a single plaque, and tumors that have seeded the vitreous. Relative contraindications include tumors that involve the optic disc or fovea.

Techniques and Principles

A retinal drawing is created to specify location, diameter, and height of the tumor. The size, shape, isotope, dose, and time required for delivery are then determined for the plaque. The size is large enough to provide a 2-mm margin around the base of the tumor. The shape can be round or notched if near the optic nerve. The isotope is usually I-125 in the USA, but in Europe, some use Ru-106. The half-life of I-125 is 60 days while that of Ru-106 is 374 days. I-125 seeds fit into a Silastic carrier within a gold shield (Fig. 40.1). Flexible dose delivery is facilitated by the ability to use individual seeds with specified levels of activity and also by variable use of slots within the carrier (Fig. 40.2). Ru-106 plaques come manufactured with the isotope coated on the inner surface of a silver shield (Fig. 40.3). Ru-106 has a steep dosimetric falloff due to shallow penetration of the beta particles it emits. This allows for

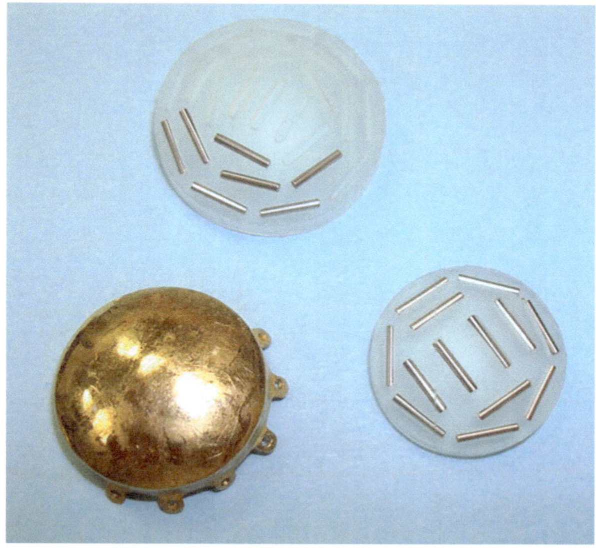

Fig. 40.2 Iodine plaques allow flexible dosimetry because activity and loading pattern of seeds within the silastic carrier can be modified

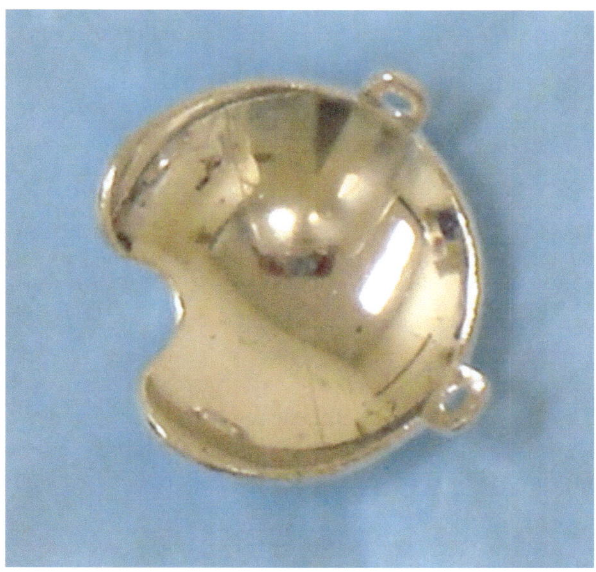

Fig. 40.3 Notched silver shield with ruthenium-106 coated on the inner surface

reduced dose to nearby structures but also means that the limit on tumor thickness treatable with Ru-106 is 6–6.5 mm (Fig. 40.4). The time required for delivery of the prescribed dose is usually several days. Placement of the plaque is performed by the ocular oncologist and confirmed with ultrasonography.

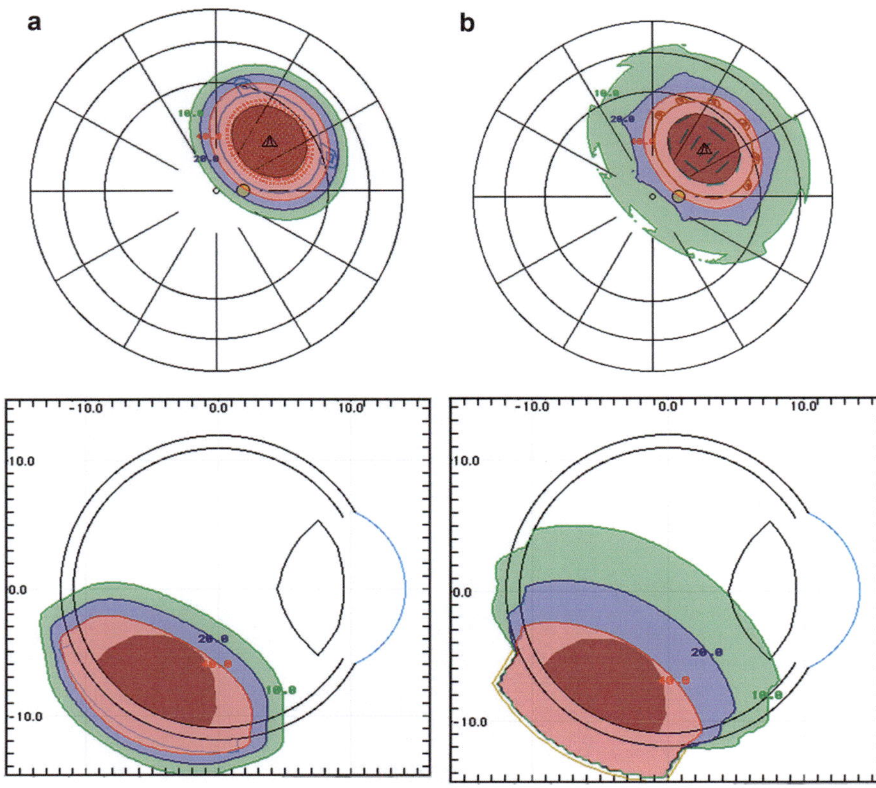

Fig. 40.4 Comparison of ruthenium-106 dosimetry (**a**) to iodine-125 dosimetry (**b**) for a 6-mm-thick tumor, showing steeper falloff of dose with ruthenium-106. *Red* = 40 Gy, *Blue* = 20 Gy, *Green* = 10 Gy (Plaque Simulator software v.5.3.6, BEBIG GmbH, Berlin, Germany)

Pathology

The pathology of failed brachytherapy for retinoblastoma (Fig. 40.5) generally shows well-differentiated tumor, including areas containing fleurettes. The cells in this area are not cycling, therefore they may be resistant to radiation.

Outcome

There is a 5-year tumor control of 80–95%.

Complications

Complications include retinopathy, maculopathy, optic neuropathy, cataract, neovascularization, glaucoma, vitreous hemorrhage, retinal detachment, scleral necrosis, and secondary malignancy.

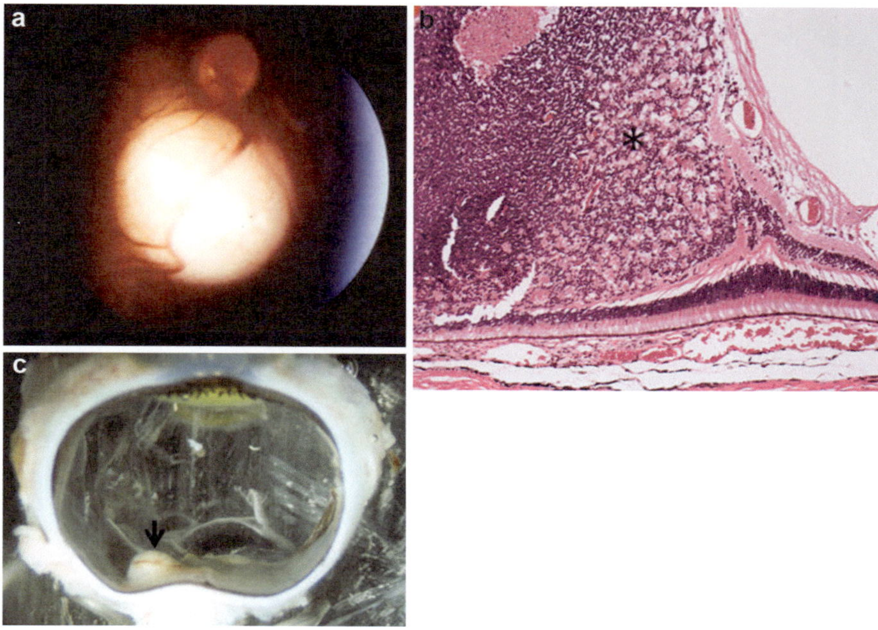

Fig. 40.5 (**a**) A local retinoblastoma is present near the optic nerve. (**b**) The tumor failed to respond to brachytherapy, and the eye was removed. The residual tumor (*arrow*) is present posteriorly. (**c**) The residual tumor contains a well-differentiated area (*) containing numerous fleurettes ((**c**) hematoxylin and eosin, ×25)

Cross-References

Retinoblastoma-teletherapy

Further Reading

Linn MA (2007) Local therapy, brachytherapy, and enucleation. In: Singh A et al (eds) Clinical ophthalmic oncology with CD-ROM. Saunders, Philadelphia, pp 454–461

Schueler AO, Flühs D, Anastassiou G et al (2006) Beta-ray brachytherapy with 106Ru plaques for retinoblastoma. Int J Radiat Oncol Biol Phys 65:1212–1221

Shields CL, Shields JA, Cater J et al (2001) Plaque radiotherapy for retinoblastoma: long-term tumor control and treatment complications in 208 tumors. Ophthalmology 108:2116–2121

Shields CL, Mashayekhi A, Sun H et al (2006) Iodine 125 plaque radiotherapy as salvage treatment for retinoblastoma recurrence after chemoreduction in 84 tumors. Ophthalmology 113:2087–2092

Spraul CW, Lim JI, Lambert SR, Grossniklaus HE (1996) Retinoblastoma recurrence after iodine 125 plaque application. Retina 16(2):135–138

Retinoblastoma: Chemoreduction 41

Michael Levien, Arun D. Singh, and G. Baker Hubbard III

Synonym

Neoadjuvant chemotherapy

Definitions

Chemoreduction is the use of intravenous chemotherapy to achieve tumor volume reduction in order to increase the efficacy of local therapies. Local therapies (focal therapies) include: photocoagulation, thermotherapy, cryotherapy, or brachytherapy. The following contains an outline for chemoreduction therapy based on the International Classification System of Retinoblastoma shown in Table 41.1 and Fig. 41.1.

M. Levien, M.D.
Department of Pediatric Oncology, Cleveland Clinic Children's Hospital,
Cleveland, OH, USA
e-mail: levienm@ccf.org

A.D. Singh, M.D. (✉)
Department of Ophthalmic Oncology,
Cole Eye Institute, Cleveland Clinic Foundation,
9500 Euclid Ave, Desk i-329, Cleveland, OH 44195, USA
e-mail: singha@ccf.org

G.B. Hubbard III, M.D. (✉)
Department of Ophthalmology, Emory University School of Medicine,
Atlanta, GA, USA

The Emory Eye Center, Atlanta, GA, USA
e-mail: ghubba2@emory.edu

H.E. Grossniklaus (ed.), *Pocket Guide to Ocular Oncology and Pathology*,
DOI 10.1007/978-3-642-29782-3_41,

Table 41.1 International classification system for intraocular retinoblastoma

Group A: small intraretinal tumors away from the foveola and disc
All tumors are 3 mm or smaller in greatest dimension, confined to the retina:
1. All tumors are located farther than 3 mm from the foveola and 1.5 mm from optic disc.
Group B: all remaining discrete tumors confined to the retina:
1. All other tumors confined to the retina not in Group A
2. Tumor-associated subretinal fluid less than 3 mm from the tumor with no subretinal seeding
Group C: discrete local disease with minimal subretinal or vitreous seeding:
1. Tumor(s) are discrete.
2. Subretinal fluid, present or past, without seeding involving up to ¼ of the retina.
3. Local fine vitreous seeding may be present close to discrete tumor.
4. Local subretinal seeding less than 3 mm (2DD) from the tumor.
Group D: diffuse disease with significant vitreous or subretinal seeding:
1. Tumor(s) may be massive or diffuse.
2. Subretinal fluid, present or past without seeding, involving up to total retinal detachment.
3. Diffuse or massive vitreous disease may include "greasy" seeds or avascular tumor masses.
4. Diffuse subretinal seeding may include subretinal plaques or tumor nodules.
Group E: presence of any or more of these poor prognostic features
1. Tumor touching the lens
2. Tumor anterior to anterior vitreous face involving ciliary body or anterior segment
3. Diffuse infiltrating retinoblastoma
4. Neovascular glaucoma
5. Opaque media from hemorrhage
6. Tumor necrosis with septic orbital cellulitis
7. Phthisis bulbi

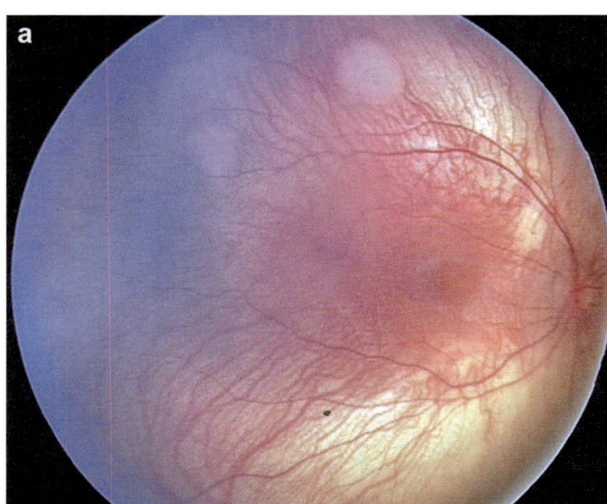

Fig. 41.1 See Table 41.1. Groups (**a**–**e**) are shown

Fig. 41.1 (continued)

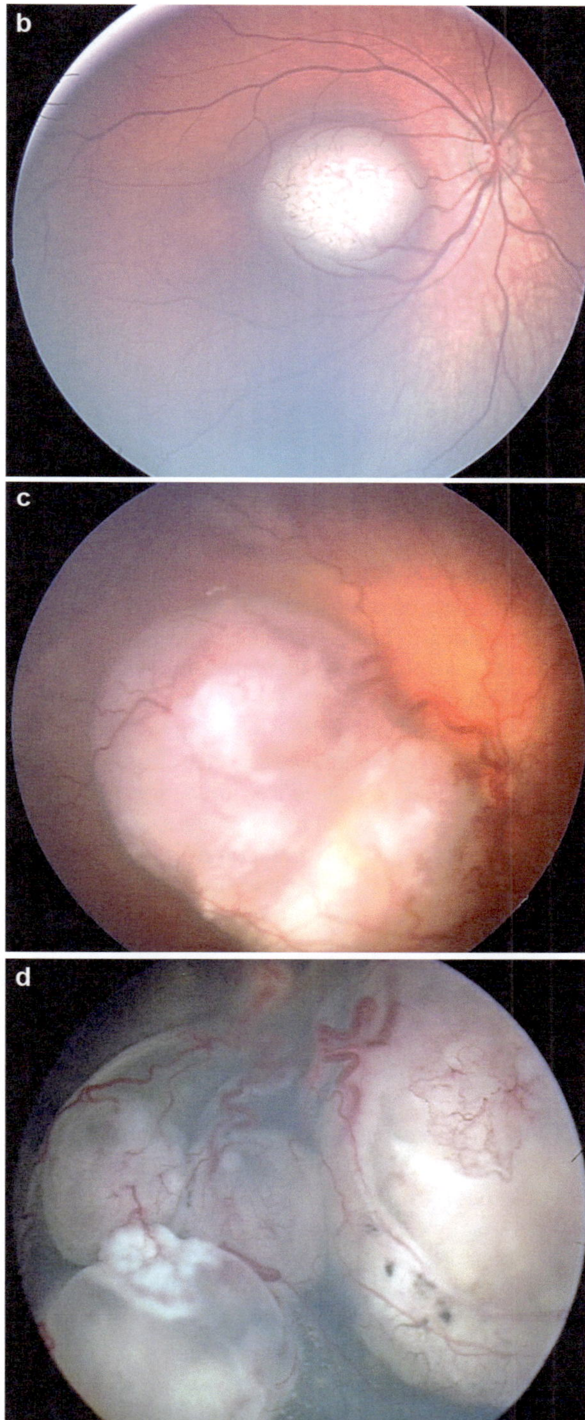

Fig. 41.1 (continued)

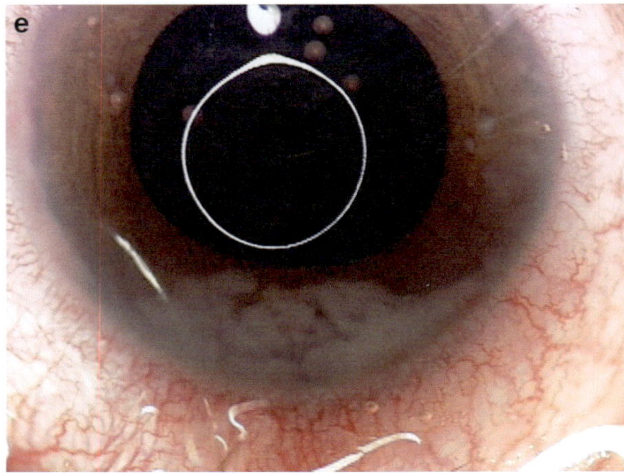

Indications

The following are indications for chemoreduction in retinoblastoma (Fig. 41.2):

(A) Newly diagnosed bilateral retinoblastoma in which at least one eye has Group B or worse disease (International Classification System of Intraocular Retinoblastoma).
(B) Select cases of newly diagnosed unilateral retinoblastoma (Groups B and C).
(C) In bilateral cases, if one eye is Group E, enucleation of the Group E eye should be considered before chemotherapy to identify high-risk histopathologic features that may not be evident after chemotherapy.
(D) Chemoreduction is used in conjunction with focal therapies:
   1. Usually laser thermotherapy using 810-nm infrared laser.
   2. Also laser photocoagulation using green or yellow wavelength lasers.
   3. Cryotherapy is sometimes used.
   4. Laser and cryotherapy improve penetration of systemic chemotherapy into retinoblastoma.
   5. Local periocular injections of carboplatin are sometimes used.

Contraindications

The following are contraindications to chemoreduction therapy:

(A) Unacceptable hypersensitivity to the chemotherapy drugs vincristine, carboplatin, or etoposide (VP-16):
   1. Anaphylaxis is possible.
   2. Reactions can worsen on subsequent exposures to drug.
   3. Desensitizing protocols are available for carboplatin.
(B) Unacceptable peripheral neuropathies associated with vincristine:
   1. Can decrease the dose or frequency or delay dosing
(C) Liver or renal toxicity:
   1. Doses must be modified or doses omitted until patient recovers.

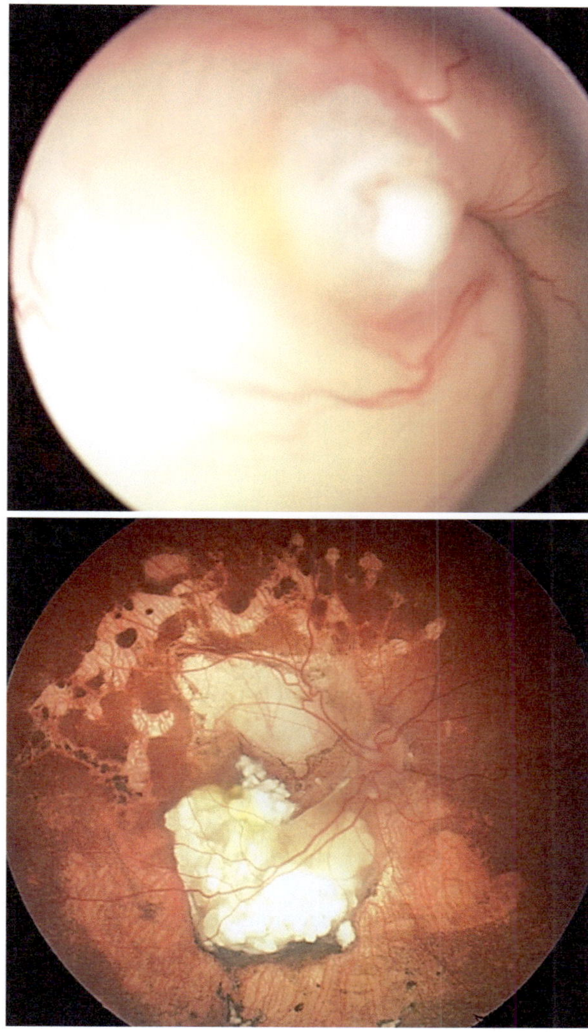

Fig. 41.2 A child with bilateral retinoblastoma treated with chemotherapy (VEC protocol) and adjuvant thermotherapy. (**top**) Pretreatment appearance of right eye (**bottom**). Note dramatic regression of the tumors after three cycles of chemotherapy

Use and Dosage

The dosage and timing of the most common chemoreduction protocol is as follows:

(A) Six courses of VEC (vincristine, etoposide, and carboplatin):

1. Each course is repeated every 28 days upon adequate recovery of blood counts and resolution of toxicities.
2. Local ophthalmic therapy is not given until response to chemotherapy is assessed after the first course.
3. EUAs are done and local therapy is delivered (usually laser thermotherapy) in conjunction with cycle 2–6 at the discretion of the ophthalmologist.

(B) Usual dosage of systemic chemotherapy for intraocular Rb:

Vincristine	Patients	<36 months: 0.05 mg/kg
		>36 months: 1.5 mg/M^2 (maximum dose 2 mg)
		IV on day # 1 only
Etoposide (VP16)	Patients	<36 months: 6 mg/kg
		>36 months: 180 mg/M^2
		IV daily × 2 days (day 1 and 2)
Carboplatin	Patients	<36 months: 18.6 mg/kg
		>36 months: 560 mg/M^2
		IV on day # 1

(C) If periocular carboplatin is given, systemic dosage of carboplatin may be adjusted as follows:

Carboplatin	Patients	<36 months: 14 mg/kg
		>36 months: 420 mg/M^2
		IV daily × 2 days (day 1 and 2)

(D) Patients less than 6 months of age will have a 25% dose reduction on the first course with escalation of doses on subsequent courses if patient tolerates the chemotherapy.

(E) SubTenon carboplatin:
1. Utilized in selected cases of Groups C and D retinoblastoma.
2. Administered on the day before or the day of course number 2–4.
3. Dose is 20 mg (10 mg/ml – give 2 ml).

(F) High-risk histopathologic features in enucleated eye:
1. Posterior uveal invasion (includes choroidal invasion: 3 mm of tumor in contact with the sclera)
2. Any degree of concomitant choroid and optic nerve involvement
3. Tumor involving the optic nerve posterior to the lamina cribosa as an independent finding
4. Scleral invasion
5. Anterior chamber seeding
6. Ciliary body infiltration
7. Iris infiltration

Adverse Reactions

The following are adverse reactions to chemoreduction agents:

Vincristine: alopecia, constipation, loss of deep tendon reflexes (common), jaw pain, headaches, muscle weakness, abdominal pain, anemia (occasional), peripheral paresthesias (numbness, tingling and pain in finger tips and toes), wrist-drop, foot drop, abnormal gait (occasional), paralytic ileus, ptosis, diplopia, night blindness, hoarseness, vocal cord paralysis, SIADH, and seizure (rare)

Etoposide (VP-16): nausea, vomiting, myelosuppression (common); anorexia, abdominal pain, asthenia, malaise, rash, urticaria (occasional); transient hypotension during infusion if given rapidly; anaphylaxis (rare); peripheral neuropathy, mucositis, hepatotoxicity, chest pain, thrombophlebitis (give through central venous catheter to avoid this problem); congestive heart failure, Stevens-Johnson syndrome (rare); secondary malignancy (preleukemia or leukemia syndromes) (highly unlikely if total cumulative dose is <2 g/M^2)

Carboplatin: nausea, vomiting, constipation, diarrhea; myelosuppression (thrombocytopenia, anemia, leucopenia, and neutropenia) (common); hypersensitivity reactions; renal (decreased GFR, increased creatinine) and hepatic toxicities (liver enzyme elevations, increased bilirubin) (occasional); ototoxicity (rhinitis, hearing loss); metallic taste, rash, mucositis; peripheral neuropathy (rare)

SubTenon carboplatin: periorbital swelling and erythema (common), restriction of ocular rotation, peripheral fat atrophy resulting in mild retraction of the globe (occasional), optic nerve atrophy (rare)

Interactions

The following are drug-drug interactions that may occur with chemoreduction agents:

Vincristine: cytochrome P450 isoenzyme CYP3A3/4 and CYP3A5–7 substrate and isoenzyme CYP2D6 inhibitor

Asparaginase may decrease vincristine clearance; acute pulmonary reactions may occur with concomitant use of mitomycin C; concurrent administration with itraconazole may result in an increased severity of neuromuscular side effects. CYP3A4 inhibitors (i.e., azole antifungals, ciprofloxacin, clarithromycin, diclofenac, doxycycline, erythromycin, imatinib, isoniazid, nefazodone, nicardipine, propofol, protease inhibitors, quinidine, and verapamil) may decrease vincristine metabolism.

Carboplatin: aminoglycosides (increased ototoxicity and nephrotoxicity), nephrotoxic drugs (increased renal toxicity), decreases phenytoin serum levels

Etoposide (*VP16*): cytochrome P450 isoenzyme CYP3A3/4 substrate Cyclosporine may increase plasma levels of etoposide.

Cross-References

Retinoblastoma brachytherapy, retinoblastoma cryotherapy, retinoblastoma thermotherapy, retinoblastoma laser photocoagulation

Further Reading

Jubran RF, Villablanca JG, Meadows AT (2007) Chemotherapy for retinoblastoma: an overview. In: Singh AD, Damato BE, Pe'er J, Murphree AL, Perry JD (eds) Clinical ophthalmic oncology. Saunders-Elsevier, Philadelphia, pp 449–453

Kiss S, Leiderman Y, Mukal S (2008) Diagnosis, classification and treatment of retinoblastoma. Retina 48(2):135–147

Meadows AT, Chintagumpala M, Dunkel IJ, Friedman DL, Stoner JA, Villablanca JG (2007) Children's Oncology group (COG) trials for retinoblastoma. In: Singh AD, Damato BE, Pe'er J, Murphree AL, Perry JD (eds) Clinical ophthalmic oncology. Saunders-Elsevier, Philadelphia, pp 491–495

Shields C, Meadows A et al (2004) Continuing challenges in the management of retinoblastoma with chemotherapy. Retina 24(6):849–862

Retinoblastoma: Enucleation

42

Masood Naseripour and Arun D. Singh

Synonym

None.

Definition

Removal of the eye from the orbit involving the transection of the optic nerve and severing of the extraocular muscles and all soft tissues around it.

Indications

Any eye classified as Group E or unilateral disease classified as Group D by the International Classification.

M. Naseripour (✉)
Eye Research Center,
Iran University of Medical Sciences, Tehran, Iran
e-mail: masoodnp@yahoo.com

A.D. Singh, M.D.
Department of Ophthalmic Oncology,
Cole Eye Institute, Cleveland Clinic Foundation,
9500 Euclid Ave, Desk i-329, Cleveland, OH 44195, USA
e-mail: singha@ccf.org

H.E. Grossniklaus (ed.), *Pocket Guide to Ocular Oncology and Pathology*,
DOI 10.1007/978-3-642-29782-3_42, © Springer-Verlag Berlin Heidelberg 2013

Techniques and Principles

The primary goal of enucleation in the setting of retinoblastoma is to remove the diseased globe with cosmetically acceptable result and to prevent the extraocular dissemination of tumor. Informed consent and examination under anesthesia are necessary before making the incision.

Under general anesthesia, a 360° limbal peritomy is performed, and conjunctiva and Tenon's capsule are dissected gently. The rectus muscles are then isolated and tagged with absorbable sutures. All rectus and oblique muscles are cut at their insertion except for horizontal rectus muscles that are cut 3–4 mm proximal to the insertion into the sclera. This leaves a stump of muscle that can be used for traction while cutting the optic nerve with a curved scissor. This maneuver facilitates obtaining of a long section of optic nerve, which is very important in enucleating the eyes for retinoblastoma. It is crucial to avoid perforation of the globe. Hemostasis is achieved by direct compression of the orbit. To replace the orbital volume, an integrated implant (wrapped in processed or banked sclera, synthetic mesh, or autologous tissue) is placed in the socket. The rectus muscles are attached to the implant to impart good motility to the prosthesis. Tenon's capsule is meticulously closed in a purse-string fashion, and the conjunctiva is closed separately with running or interrupted absorbable sutures. A mixture of antibiotic and steroid ointment is instilled, and after insertion of a conformer, a firm pressure patch is applied for 1–2 days. Once the eye has been removed from the field and taken to a separate table, it can be opened to obtain fresh tissue for genetic analysis. After opening the eye, care must be taken not to contaminate the operative field with tumor. Any instruments used to open the globe should be discarded for the remainder of the case, and gowns and gloves should be changed.

Complications

Removal of the wrong eye is the most catastrophic and feared complication. It can be avoided by marking of the eye to be enucleated, review of the chart, and fundus examination just before enucleation. It is important to take appropriate measures to prevent the accidental perforation of globe, which could result in orbital extension of tumor. The likelihood of extraocular muscle loss is minimized by careful placement of traction sutures. Irrigating the retrobulbar space before cutting the optic nerve with mixture of 1% lidocaine with epinephrine and 0.5% bupivacaine and adequate tamponade of orbital apex can reduce the chance of orbital hemorrhage. Implant exposure and extrusion can be avoided by meticulous closure of Tenon's layer and conjunctiva. Postenucleation orbital infection is rare.

Outcome

It is very important to review the histopathology report of enucleated eyes with intraocular retinoblastoma. Any extraocular extensions of tumor, involvement of optic nerve beyond the lamina cribrosa, or massive choroidal invasion are indications for adjuvant chemotherapy. Prosthesis fitting is usually performed about 2 months after enucleation to allow for resolution of edema before fitting. Long-term follow-up after enucleation is necessary to monitor for orbital recurrence of tumor or metastatic disease.

Contraindications

Evidence of extraocular extension of tumor on clinical examination or neuroimaging is a contraindication to enucleation.

Cross-References

Retinoblastoma thermotherapy, retinoblastoma chemotherapy, retinoblastoma brachytherapy, retinoblastoma teletherapy, surgical techniques

Further Reading

Harbour JW (2001) Retinoblastoma: treatment. In: Char DH (ed) Tumors of the eye and ocular adnexa. BC Decker Inc., Hamilton, Ontario pp 266–284

Murphree AL (2007a) Local therapy, brachytherapy, and enucleation. In: Singh AD, Damato BE, Pe'er J, Murphree AL, Perry JD (eds) Clinical ophthalmic oncology. Philadelphia, Saunders-Elsevier, WB Saunders, Philadelphia, PA pp 454–461

Murphree AL (2007b) In: Singh AD, Singh AD (eds) Clinical Ophthalmic Oncology. Saunders-Elsevier Co, Philadelphia, pp 458–461

Murphree AL, Sammuel MA, Harbour JW, Mansfield NC (2006) Retinoblastoma. In: Ryan SJ (ed) Retina, 4th edn. Mosby, Philadelphia, pp 557–607

Perman KI, Baylis HI (1988) Evisceration, enucleation, and exenteration. Otolaryngol Clin North Am 21:171–182

Shields JA, Shields CL (1999) Atlas of intraocular tumors. WB Saunders Co, Philadelphia, pp 208–231

Singh AD, Shields CL, Shields JA (2000) Prognostic factors in retinoblastoma. J Pediatr Ophthalmol Strabismus 37:134–141

Retinoblastoma: Epidemiology

43

Luke Peterson and Hans E. Grossniklaus

Overview

Retinoblastoma (RB) is the most common primary intraocular cancer in children. Study of retinoblastoma identified the first known tumor suppressor gene, RB1, which was localized to chromosome 13q14. Using retinoblastoma as a model, Knudson first proposed the classic "two-hit" model of tumorigenesis in 1971, which was later confirmed when RB tumor cells were demonstrated to have loss of both RB1 alleles. Research increasingly suggests that retinoblastoma arises from near terminally differentiated retinal cells in the inner nuclear layer of the developing retina.

Epidemiology/Prevalence

Retinoblastoma comprises 4% of all pediatric malignancies. The cumulative lifetime incidence is 1 in 16,000–18,000 live births worldwide. There are 250–350 cases per year in the USA (7,000–8,000 cases worldwide). Approximately 60% of cases are unilateral and 40% are bilateral or hereditary. Bilateral and familial cases have a germline RB mutation and are inherited in an autosomal dominant fashion. Ninety percent of hereditary RB mutations develop bilateral disease, but they may

L. Peterson, M.D. (✉)
Department of Ophthalmology, Emory University School of Medicine,
Atlanta, GA, USA
e-mail: ltpeter@emory.edu

H.E. Grossniklaus, M.D.
Emory University School of Medicine,
Emory Eye Center,
Department of Ophthalmology,
Atlanta, GA, USA
e-mail: ophtheg@emory.edu

H.E. Grossniklaus (ed.), *Pocket Guide to Ocular Oncology and Pathology*,
DOI 10.1007/978-3-642-29782-3_43, © Springer-Verlag Berlin Heidelberg 2013

also develop unilateral RB or no tumors. The mean number of separate tumors in each affected eye is 3–4. Germline mutations place patients at significant risk for second and third nonocular primary tumors. The incidence of second tumors is 4.4% at 10 years follow-up, 18.3% at 20 years, and 26.1% at 30 years. These tumors are most commonly osteogenic sarcoma, spindle cell sarcoma, chondrosarcoma, rhabdomyosarcoma, neuroblastoma, glioma, leukemia, sebaceous cell carcinoma, squamous cell carcinoma, and malignant melanoma. Recurrence of disease can be seen in 24% of hereditary RB patients by 5 years of follow-up. The mean interval to new tumor development is 5 months.

Fifty percent of hereditary RB patients have been found to already have paramacular or macular tumors when delivered prematurely at 36 weeks gestation. Trilateral retinoblastoma (bilateral RB + pinealoblastoma or other parasellar tumor) occurs in about 3% of children and 10% of bilateral or familial cases. The median time from diagnosis of RB to diagnosis of the neuroblastic tumor is 21 months. Pinealoblastoma is nearly universally fatal. A 2001 retrospective analysis by Shields and colleagues showed that chemoreduction may reduce the risk of intracranial neuroblastic tumors. Of the 142 patients treated with chemoreduction, none developed pinealoblastoma. It was estimated that 5–15 of these patients should have manifested pinealoblastoma. Patients at highest risk for metastatic spread included those with high-risk histopathologic features, including invasion of tumor beyond the lamina cribrosa and invasion to the choroid, sclera, orbit, or anterior chamber. Metastasis typically develops within 1 year of diagnosis of the intraocular tumor.

Survival and Ocular Salvage Rates

There is a 95–99% survival rate and 90% ocular salvage rate in developed countries.

	Latin America	Iran	China	India	Africa
Survival rate (%)	80–89	83	81	48	20–46

From Houston et al. (2011)

	U-MIC	L-MIC	LIC
Estimated survival	79% (54–93%)	77% (60–92%)	40% (23–70%)
% presenting with metastatic disease	9.5% (3–24%)	12% (3–31%)	32% (12–50%)
% of patients refusing treatment	5% (1–25%)	11% (2–37%)	35% (30–50%)

From Canturk et al. (2010)
LICs lower-income countries (GNI<US $755), *MICs* middle-income countries, Upper-MICs (GNI US $2996–9265), Lower MICs (GNI US $756–2995)

Enucleation is required in 75% of unilateral retinoblastoma cases. Bilateral enucleation is necessary in only 1% of heritable cases. The World Retinoblastoma Survey documents 1,949 affected eyes from 1,487 children from 1997 to 2001. This survey includes 25 treatment centers in 5 continents. Enucleation was the primary treatment for 84% of unilaterally affected eyes. Chemotherapy with focal therapy was the primary treatment for 57% of eyes of bilaterally affected children. The mortality rate is 50–85% if tumor cells reach the surgical resection line of the optic nerve, 13–69% if tumor is posterior to the lamina cribrosa but anterior to the surgical margin, and insignificant if cells are anterior to the lamina cribrosa. There are no differences in the risk of metastatic disease between germline and sporadic RB. A delay in diagnosis is the major risk factor for metastatic spread, and there are 3,000–4,000 deaths worldwide yearly.

Diagnosis

Cases are diagnosed by age 5 years in 90% of cases. The average age at presentation for germline RB is 3–18 months. Patients with known family history typically undergo screening examinations at birth and then every 2–3 months after for the first 3 years. The oldest age at which a child with a family history of RB was reported to develop a tumor in a previously tumor-free eye is 48 months, and the average age at presentation for sporadic RB is 18–24 months. Per the Worldwide Retinoblastoma Survey, the median age at diagnosis is 22 months in Asia, 12 months in North America, and 9 months in Europe.

Shields et al. evaluated 249 eyes with RB treated with chemoreduction in an interventional case series. They found that avoidance of enucleation or EBRT was directly related to severity at diagnosis. Group E patients were excluded from the study as they were treated with primary enucleation.

ICRB major group	% of patients	Chemoreduction success (avoidance of EBRT or enucleation) (%)
A	9	100
B	39	93
C	8	90
D	44	47

From Shields et al. (2006)

Presenting Symptoms

Leukocoria is by far the most common presenting sign. Nearly 60% of cases in the USA are diagnosed after the observation of leukocoria, most often by a family member. Leukocoria correlates with the presence of advanced disease, and there is a poorer prognosis for globe salvage than without leukocoria. There is an approximately 88% survival rate at 5 years with leukocoria as the presenting sign. Strabismus occurs in approximately 20% of cases and is associated with higher survival and globe salvage rates than without strabismus. The remaining 20% of cases present with atypical symptoms, including a red, painful eye with glaucoma; cloudy cornea; poor vision; vitreous hemorrhage; and signs of orbital inflammation mimicking cellulitis. Studies of retinoblastoma referrals indicate that 52–68% of cases referred for suspected RB proved to be retinoblastoma. Approximately 10% of those referred had persistent fetal vasculature and 9% had Coats disease. Any child with unexplained, atraumatic hyphema or vitreous hemorrhage should be evaluated for retinoblastoma. Vitrectomy or retinal detachment repair should be avoided until the diagnosis of RB is reliably ruled out. If vitrectomy is performed in an eye with unsuspected RB, enucleation combined with adjuvant chemotherapy and/or radiotherapy should be performed without delay to prevent systemic tumor dissemination.

Growth Patterns

Endophytic growth occurs in 60% of cases. In this case, there is tumor growth toward the vitreous cavity as a result of cell division within the inner retinal layers, and there is a tendency for vitreous seeding. Exophytic growth occurs in 39% of cases. In exophytic growth, the tumor develops in the outer retinal layers with expansion beneath the retina into the subretinal space. These patients often present with retinal detachment surrounding the tumor, and the eye is more likely to develop glaucoma than with endophytic growth. Choroidal invasion is also more common in exophytic growth compared to endophytic growth. The remaining 1–2% of cases exhibit a diffuse, infiltrating, plaque-like growth pattern. Diffuse retinoblastoma typically presents with signs of inflammation, is often misdiagnosed as uveitis, and has an average age at diagnosis of 6 years. There is >95% survival after enucleation of the affected eye.

Risk Factors

There is no sex or racial predilection and no environmental or socioeconomic risk factors identified for heritable RB. Sporadic retinoblastoma is more common in poorer tropical or subtropical regions than developed regions of the world. A possible viral etiology (human papillomavirus) has been implicated for this finding. Other possibilities include a diet deficient in fruits and vegetables. Advanced paternal age has also been associated with new sporadic RB gene mutations and sporadic RB.

Surveillance and Strategies to Optimize Worldwide RB Management

The American Academy of Pediatrics recommends that all infants have an examination of the red reflex during the first 2 months of life performed by a pediatrician or other trained clinician. Honduras in 2003 initiated an awareness campaign linked to yearly vaccination campaigns. This included posters, fliers, and education of healthcare workers regarding retinoblastoma. They noted a significant decrease in the number of extraocular cases (from 73% to 35%) since initiation of the campaign. Brazil initiated strategies to optimize RB care, including fliers and posters distributed in São Paolo, training of primary school teachers, and specific RB training for medical students and primary physicians. Extraocular retinoblastoma decreased from 56% in 1985 to <10% in 2003.

Further Reading

Abramson DH, Schefler AC (2004) Update on retinoblastoma. Retina 24:828–848
Canturk S, Qaddoumi I, Khetan V et al (2010) Survival of retinoblastoma in less-developed countries impact of socioeconomic and health-related indicators. Br J Ophthalmol 94:1432–1436
Chantada GL, Qaddoumi I, Canturk S et al (2011) Strategies to manage retinoblastoma in developing countries. Pediatr Blood Cancer 56:341–348
Gallie B, Zhao J, Vandezande K et al (2007) Global issues and opportunities for optimized retinoblastoma care. Pediatr Blood Cancer 49:1083–1090
Houston S, Murray T, Wolfe S, Fernandes CE (2011) Current update on retinoblastoma. Int Ophthalmol Clin 51(1):77–91
Kiss S, Leiderman Y, Mukai S (2008) Diagnosis, classification and treatment of retinoblastoma. Int Ophthalmol Clin 48(2):135–147
Mastrangelo D, De Francesco S, Leonardo A et al (2007) Retinoblastoma epidemiology: does the evidence matter? Eur J Cancer 43(10):1596–1603
Orjuela M, Castaneda VP, Ridaura C et al (2000) Presence of human papilloma virus in tumor tissue from children with retinoblastoma: an alternative mechanism for tumor development. Clin Cancer Res 6:4010–4016
Rodriguez-Galindo C, Wilson M, Chantada G et al (2008) Retinoblastoma: one world, one vision. Pediatrics 122:e763–e770
Schefler AC, Abramson DH (2008) Retinoblastoma: what is new in 2007–2008. Curr Opin Ophthalmol 19(6):526–534
Shields CL, Meadows AT, Shields JA et al (2001) Chemoreduction for retinoblastoma may prevent intracranial neuroblastic malignancy (trilateral retinoblastoma). Arch Opthalmol 119:1269–1272
Shields CL, Mashayekhi A, Au AK et al (2006) The international classification of retinoblastoma predicts chemoreduction success. Ophthalmology 113:2276–2280

Metastatic Retinoblastoma

44

Guillermo L. Chantada

Synonym

Extraocular retinoblastoma.

Definition

Metastatic retinoblastoma occurs after dissemination to distant organs such as the CNS, bone, or bone marrow among others.

Etiology

In developing countries, metastatic Rb usually results from delayed diagnosis. Patients may have a long-standing history of ocular complaints, and overt disease is often obvious at diagnosis. In more affluent nations, metastatic Rb is usually seen as a consequence of relapse after failed attempt at globe salvage or after enucleation of eyes with high-risk histopathologic features.

Clinical Presentation

Metastatic Rb may result from dissemination through the optic nerve into the CNS or dissemination through the sclera into the orbit (Fig. 44.1a). Once in the orbit, spread may occur through lymphatic involvement or hematogenous dissemination. Systemic metastasis may also occur after choroidal invasion. Any organ may be a

G.L. Chantada, M.D.
Hemato-oncology Service,
Hospital JP Garrahan, Buenos Aires, Argentina
e-mail: gchantada@yahoo.com

H.E. Grossniklaus (ed.), *Pocket Guide to Ocular Oncology and Pathology*,
DOI 10.1007/978-3-642-29782-3_44,

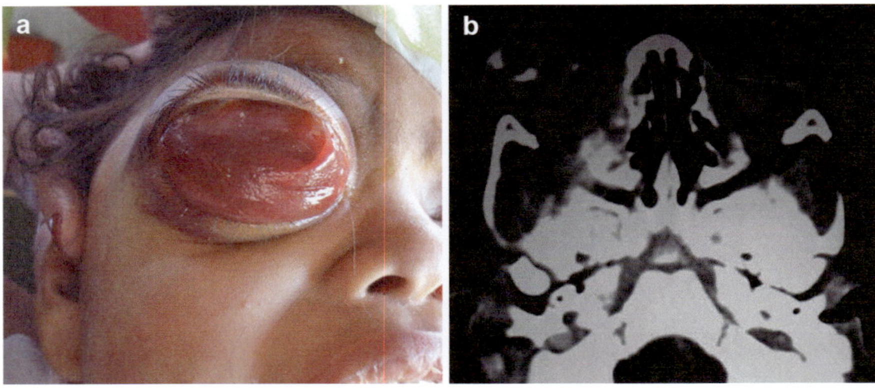

Fig. 44.1 Massive orbital extension in a child with bilateral retinoblastoma (**a**). CT scan of the same patient showing massive orbital extension with bony invasion and tumor calcification (**b**)

site for metastasis, but Rb most commonly goes to CNS, bone marrow, and bone. Liver and distant lymph nodes are less common sites. Presenting signs and symptoms depend on the site of involvement. Orbital involvement is common in developing nations, while CNS disease is more commonly found in developed countries. CNS disease may be found on routine MRI for intraocular disease or may be identified as the result of symptoms such as headache, seizures, irritability, nausea, vomiting, or focal neurologic signs. Bone disease may manifest as a palpable mass or as bone pain.

Diagnostics

All patients with Rb should undergo neuroimaging for staging (MRI brain and orbits preferred) (Fig. 44.1b). A complete metastatic evaluation should be performed for patients with overt extraocular dissemination or high-risk histopathologic features on enucleated eyes. The metastatic work-up consists of bone marrow and CSF evaluation along with bone scintigraphy in selected cases.

Pathology

The pathology of metastatic Rb is essentially the same as intraocular Rb.

Differential Diagnosis

Secondary neuroectodermal tumors in patients with germ line RB1 mutations may be difficult to distinguish from metastatic Rb.

Prophylaxis

Timely diagnosis is the best prophylaxis for metastatic Rb.

Therapy

When the CNS is involved, metastatic Rb is virtually incurable with any modality. When the CNS is not involved, some are curable with high-dose chemotherapy and autologous stem cell rescue (ASCR). Chemosensitivity renders heroic surgical resection (like orbital exenteration) unnecessary in most cases. The current recommended approach utilizes induction chemotherapy, including a platinum compound, etoposide, an alkylating agent, and eventually anthracyclines. The benefit of including intrathecal chemotherapy in this regimen is unproven. The choice of the induction regimen may vary depending on the previous exposure to chemotherapy in cases of relapsing metastatic disease. In chemotherapy naïve patients where a beneficial response is observed, the addition of high-dose chemotherapy with ASCR is associated with improved survival for patients without CNS involvement. After ASCR, the use of radiotherapy for the treatment of bulky metastatic sites is controversial. The Children's Oncology Group has recently launched a consensus protocol including multimodality therapy for extraocular retinoblastoma (COG ARET 0321) designed to allow for other cooperative groups or major centers around the world to join.

Prognosis

The prognosis for metastatic Rb is generally dismal. Those without CNS involvement may be cured with high-dose chemotherapy and ASCR.

Epidemiology

Metastatic retinoblastoma occurs in less than 5% of the patients in developed countries but represents a significant challenge in less developed nations.

Cross-References

Retinoblastoma brachytherapy, retinoblastoma chemoreduction, retinoblastoma enucleation, retinoblastoma teletherapy, retinoblastoma transpupillary thermotherapy

Further Reading

Chantada G, Fandino A, Manzitti J et al (1999) Late diagnosis of retinoblastoma in a developing country. Arch Dis Child 80:171–174

Chantada G, Doz F, Antoneli CB et al (2006) A proposal for an international retinoblastoma staging system. Pediatr Blood Cancer 47:801–805

Dunkel IJ, Aledo A, Kernan NA et al (2000) Successful treatment of metastatic retinoblastoma. Cancer 89:2117–2121

MacKay CJ, Abramson DH, Ellsworth RM (1984) Metastatic patterns of retinoblastoma. Arch Ophthalmol 102:391–396

Namouni F, Doz F, Tanguy ML et al (1997) High-dose chemotherapy with carboplatin, etoposide and cyclophosphamide followed by a haematopoietic stem cell rescue in patients with high-risk retinoblastoma: a SFOP and SFGM study. Eur J Cancer 33:2368–2375

Retinoblastoma: Orbital Involvement 45

Santosh G. Honavar and Arun D. Singh

Synonym

Extraocular retinoblastoma.

Definition

Clinically, radiologically, or histopathologically detected orbital extension of an intraocular retinoblastoma.

Etiology and Clinical Presentation

Orbital retinoblastoma can manifest in several different ways. Primary orbital retinoblastoma is orbital extension of an intraocular retinoblastoma noted at the initial presentation, with or without proptosis or a fungating mass. Secondary orbital retinoblastoma is an orbital recurrence following uncomplicated enucleation for intraocular retinoblastoma. Accidental orbital retinoblastoma results from inadvertent perforation, fine needle aspiration biopsy, or intraocular surgery in an eye with unsuspected intraocular retinoblastoma. Overt orbital retinoblastoma may be discovered at the time of enucleation in cases of previously unrecognized extrascleral

S.G. Honavar, M.D. (✉)
Department of Ocular Oncology, LV Prasad Eye Institute,
Hyderabad, Andhra Pradesh, India
e-mail: honavar@lvpei.org

A.D. Singh, M.D.
Department of Ophthalmic Oncology,
Cole Eye Institute, Cleveland Clinic Foundation,
9500 Euclid Ave, Desk i-329, Cleveland, OH 44195, USA
e-mail: singha@ccf.org

H.E. Grossniklaus (ed.), *Pocket Guide to Ocular Oncology and Pathology*,
DOI 10.1007/978-3-642-29782-3_45,

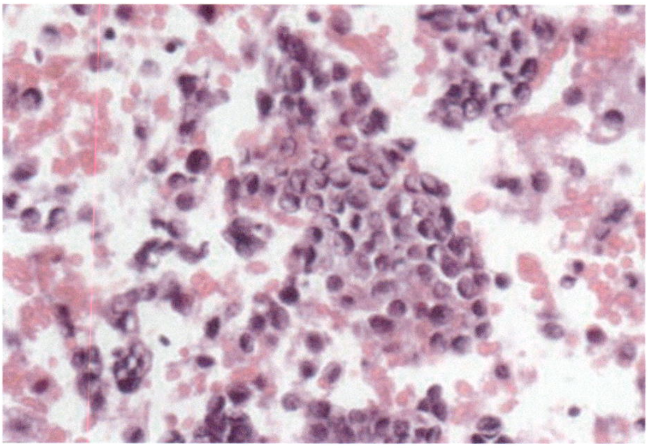

Fig. 45.1 A fine needle aspiration biopsy of orbital retinoblastoma shows a small, round blue cell tumor (hematoxylin and eosin, ×100)

or optic nerve extension. Finally, microscopic orbital retinoblastoma is not evident clinically but is observed histopathologically.

Diagnostics

Magnetic resonance imaging (MRI) or computed tomography (CT) scan of the orbit and brain in axial and coronal orientations with 2-mm slice thickness helps confirm the presence of orbital retinoblastoma and determine its extent. Detailed physical examination including palpation of the regional lymph nodes, chest X-ray, abdominal ultrasound, bone marrow biopsy, and cerebrospinal fluid cytology may all be performed to evaluate a patient with orbital retinoblastoma.

Pathology

The histopathology of orbital retinoblastoma is the same as intraocular retinoblastoma. It is composed of small, round blue cells with high nuclear to cytoplasmic ratios and hyperchromatic nuclei. There may be Flexner-Wintersteiner and/or Homer-Wright rosettes present. Fine needle aspiration biopsy will show a small, round blue cell tumor (Fig. 45.1).

Differential Diagnosis

If the diagnosis of intraocular retinoblastoma is certain clinically or radiologically, the main differential diagnosis is proptosis secondary to orbital inflammation induced by spontaneous tumor necrosis. In the absence of evidence of intraocular retinoblastoma, all major causes of rapidly evolving proptosis in children including orbital cellulitis, orbital lymphangioma with hemorrhage, rhabdomyosarcoma, Burkitt's lymphoma, primitive neuroectodermal tumor, and orbital metastasis (from Wilm's tumor) may be considered. Imaging modalities (CT or MRI) will help in establishing the diagnosis.

Prophylaxis

Awareness about early diagnosis and appropriate treatment can minimize the incidence of primary orbital retinoblastoma. While enucleating eyes with advanced primary retinoblastoma, manipulations should be minimal, accidental ocular perforation avoided, and a long (at least 15 mm) optic nerve stump should be obtained. Adjuvant therapy to a child with histopathologic high-risk features following enucleation may minimize the risk of orbital retinoblastoma. Adjuvant therapy is comprised of: triple-drug chemotherapy (vincristine, etoposide, and carboplatin) and external beam radiation for those with inadvertent intraocular surgery, accidental perforation, full-thickness scleral infiltration, extrascleral extension, or optic nerve involvement to the surgical margin.

Therapy

Orbital retinoblastoma has been managed in the past with orbital exenteration, chemotherapy, or external beam radiotherapy with each modality used as monotherapy or in sequential combination. Results of these treatments have been variable. It is well known that local treatments have a limited effect on the course of this advanced disease. We have developed the following treatment protocol: initial triple-drug (vincristine, etoposide, carboplatin) high-dose chemotherapy (3–6 cycles), followed by surgery (enucleation, extended enucleation, or orbital exenteration as appropriate), orbital radiotherapy, and then continued chemotherapy for a total of 12 cycles chemotherapy (Fig. 45.2).

Prognosis

With the protocol outlined above, there is over 90% survival in patients with orbital retinoblastoma.

Epidemiology

The incidence of retinoblastoma is reported to be 1 in 10,000–15,000 live births. The incidence of orbital retinoblastoma varies from 6% to 40%, being higher in the developing countries.

Cross-References

Retinoblastoma enucleation, metastatic.

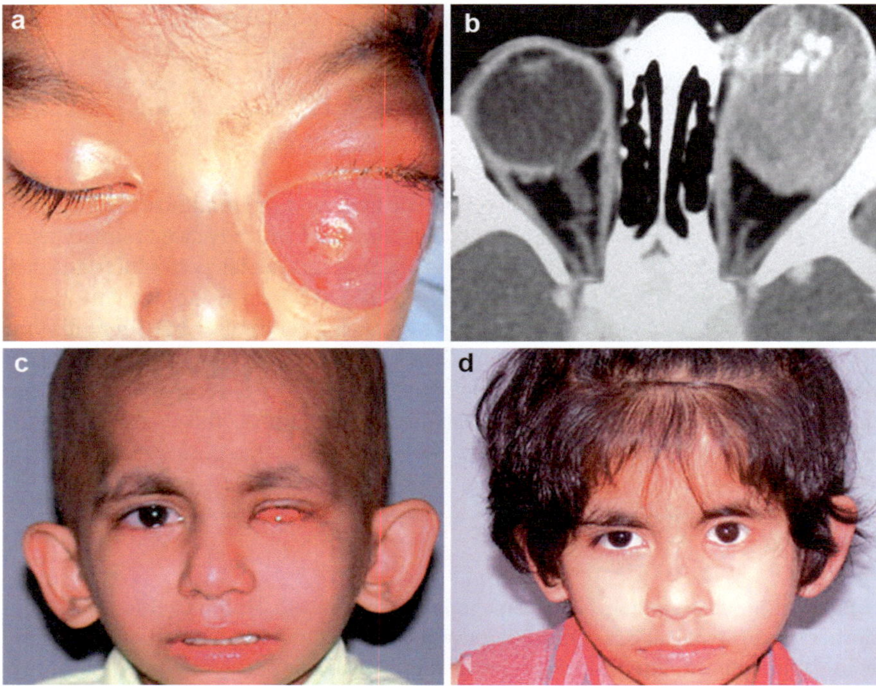

Fig. 45.2 Outcome in a case of primary orbital retinoblastoma. A 2-year-old child with primary orbital retinoblastoma in the left eye (**a**). CT scan showing massive orbital tumor (**b**). Following three cycles of neoadjuvant chemotherapy, enucleation, orbital external beam radiotherapy, and an additional nine cycles of chemotherapy, the orbital tumor is completely resolved (**c**). Three years later, the child is free of local and systemic recurrence and has an acceptable cosmetic appearance (**d**) (Reproduced with permission from Honavar ((2007))

Further Reading

Doz F, Khelfaoui F, Mosseri V et al (1994) The role of chemotherapy in orbital involvement of retinoblastoma: the experience of a single institution with 33 patients. Cancer 74:722–732

Goble RR, McKenzie J, Kingston JE et al (1990) Orbital recurrence of retinoblastoma successfully treated by combined therapy. Br J Ophthalmol 74:97–98

Honavar SG (2007) Orbital retinoblastoma. In: Singh AD, Damato BE, Pe'er J, Murphree AL, Perry JD (eds) Clinical ophthalmic oncology. Saunders-Elsevier, Philadelphia, pp 477–483

Honavar SG, Singh AD (2005) Management of advanced retinoblastoma. Ophthalmol Clin North Am 18:65–73

Kiratli H, Bilgic S, Ozerdem U (1998) Management of massive orbital involvement of intraocular retinoblastoma. Ophthalmology 105:322–326

Leal-Leal C, Flores-Rojo M, Medina-Sanson A et al (2004) A multicentre report from the Mexican retinoblastoma group. Br J Ophthalmol 88:1074–1077

Retinoblastoma: Teletherapy

46

Carryn Anderson and Arun D. Singh

Synonyms

External beam radiation therapy (EBRT)

Definition

Teletherapy describes a technique of using radiation beams from an external source to treat a tumor.

Indications

This technique can be used for definitive therapy, adjuvant therapy after enucleation, or salvage treatment of retinoblastoma. EBRT is useful when a tumor does not meet criteria for plaque brachytherapy.

C. Anderson, M.D. (✉)
Department of Radiation Oncology,
University of Iowa,
Iowa City, IA, USA
e-mail: carryn-anderson@uiowa.edu

A.D. Singh, M.D.
Department of Ophthalmic Oncology,
Cole Eye Institute, Cleveland Clinic Foundation,
9500 Euclid Ave, Desk i-329, Cleveland, OH 44195, USA
e-mail: singha@ccf.org

H.E. Grossniklaus (ed.), *Pocket Guide to Ocular Oncology and Pathology*,
DOI 10.1007/978-3-642-29782-3_46,

Contraindications

Contraindications include that the patient (or the family) does not desire globe preservation, media opacity, neovascular glaucoma, and anterior chamber seeding.

Techniques and Principles

Teletherapy sources include cobalt (photons), linear accelerator (both photons and electrons), and charged particle accelerators (most commonly protons). The radiation target is the entire retina. The dose is 36–45 Gy at 1.8–2 Gy/day. Delivery techniques include two-dimensional, three-dimensional conformal, intensity-modulated (IMRT), and stereotactic radiotherapy. Patient is anesthetized, and a mask is used to immobilize the head for more precise delivery of the radiation. Reisner et al. reproduced 13 EBRT delivery techniques and evaluated the dosimetry on a 2-year-old patient with unilateral retinoblastoma (Reisner et al. 2007). IMRT allowed the greatest reduction of dose to the orbit and lacrimal gland, while maintaining the therapeutic dose to the ora serrata and vitreous. One of the great concerns about using teletherapy in children with retinoblastoma is the risk of secondary malignancy. Patients with retinoblastoma often carry a genetic mutation that makes them more likely to develop additional tumors. With teletherapy, the radiation must go through normal tissues in order to reach the tumor within the eye. The most common radiation-induced tumor is osteosarcoma. Several measures have been employed to decrease the radiation-related sequelae: delay of radiation therapy until the patient is 12 months old, decreasing the radiation dose, employing plaque brachytherapy when possible, and using conformal techniques such as IMRT and protons.

Outcome

Ocular preservation at 10 years is approximately 80%. The rate of secondary malignancy in patients with bilateral retinoblastoma treated with EBRT is 30% at 10 years.

Complications

Orbital and midfacial growth retardation, cataract, keratitis, dry eye, temporary loss of eye lashes, and second malignant neoplasms. Radiation retinopathy, radiation maculopathy, and radiation optic neuropathy are less common than with plaque brachytherapy.

Cross-References

Retinoblastoma: Brachytherapy

Further Reading

Abramson DH, Beaverson KL, Chang ST et al (2004) Outcome following initial external beam radiotherapy in patients with Reese-Ellsworth group Vb retinoblastoma. Arch Ophthalmol 122:1316–1323

Merchant TE (2007) Teletherapy: indications, risks, and new delivery options. In: Singh AD, Damato BE, Pe'er J, Murphree AL, Perry JD (eds) Clinical ophthalmic oncology. Saunders-Elsevier, Philadelphia, pp 462–467

Merchant TE, Gould CJ, Hilton NE et al (2002) Ocular preservation after 36 Gy external beam radiation therapy for retinoblastoma. J Pediatr Hematol Oncol 24:246–249

Reisner ML, Viégas CM, Grazziotin RZ et al (2007) Retinoblastoma – comparative analysis of external radiotherapy techniques, including an IMRT technique. Int J Radiat Oncol Biol Phys 67:933–941

Retinoblastoma: Transpupillary Thermotherapy

47

Evelyn X. Fu and Arun D. Singh

Synonym

Transpupillary thermotherapy

Definition

Transpupillary thermotherapy (TTT) uses an 810-nm infrared diode laser to apply heat to the tumor at a sub-photocoagulation temperature (45–60°C) to induce apoptosis.

Indication

TTT is one of the most commonly used modalities for the treatment of posterior lesions less than 3 mm in diameter without evidence of vitreal or subretinal seeding. It can be used as the primary treatment or as a part of a consolidation treatment.

Contraindication

TTT should not be used for tumors larger than 3 mm in basal diameter unless it is combined with systemic chemotherapy as part of a chemoreduction protocol. In addition, TTT should not be used for vitreous seeding.

E.X. Fu, M.D.
Cole Eye Institute, Cleveland Clinic Foundation,
Cleveland, OH, USA

A.D. Singh, M.D. (✉)
Department of Ophthalmic Oncology,
Cole Eye Institute, Cleveland Clinic Foundation,
Cleveland, OH, USA
e-mail: singha@ccf.org

H.E. Grossniklaus (ed.), *Pocket Guide to Ocular Oncology and Pathology*,
DOI 10.1007/978-3-642-29782-3_47, © Springer-Verlag Berlin Heidelberg 2013

Techniques and Principles

Hyperthermia is applied with the infrared diode laser (810 nm), a large spot size (2–3 mm), and low power settings (300–600 mW) to achieve gentle whitening of the treatment spot. The duration of treatment for each tumor is adapted to the size of the lesion for blanching of the tumor and associated surrounding retinal edema (Fig. 47.1). Delivery systems for the laser include a pediatric laser gonioscopy lens and an adaptor on the operating microscope, an adaptor on the indirect ophthalmoscope and a 20-D or 28-D lens for transpupillary delivery, and a DioPexy probe (IRIDEX) for transconjunctival delivery. TTT is frequently utilized for chemoreduction.

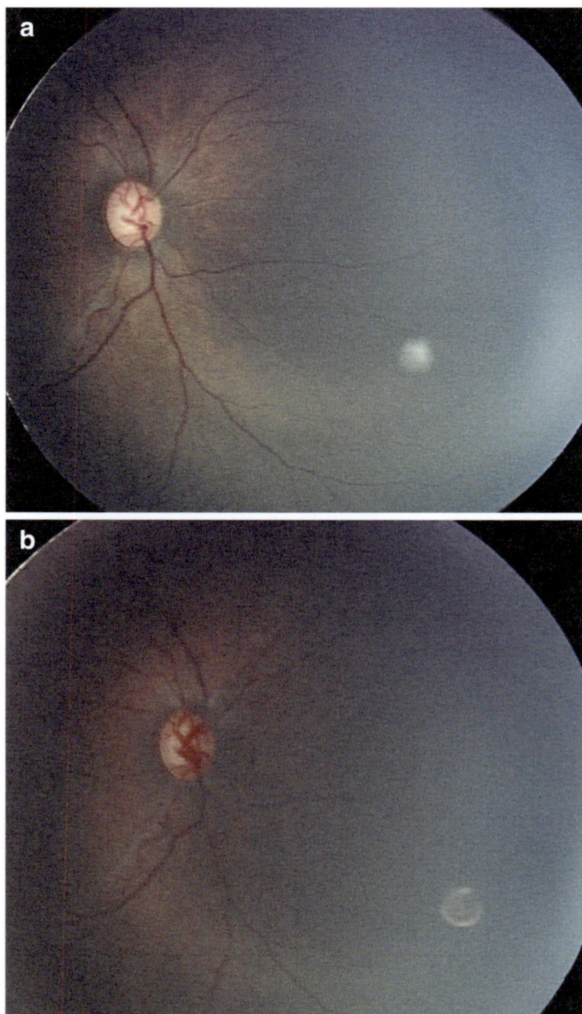

Fig. 47.1 A 0.5-mm retinoblastoma OS noted on screening examination because of positive family history. Note blanching of the tumor at the end of TTT (**a**). Four weeks later, chorioretinal atrophy is noted at the site of treated tumor (**b**)

Outcome

Since Lagendijk's first description of TTT for retinoblastoma, studies have shown this technique is effective in inducing regression in relatively small retinoblastomas without associated vitreous or subretinal seeds. Shields et al. demonstrated in 188 retinoblastomas with a mean tumor base of 3.0 mm and tumor thickness of 2.0 mm that complete tumor regression was achieved in 161 tumors (85.6%). In a more recent study of 91 tumors with a mean tumor base of 1.01 mm, 84 tumors (92%) underwent complete regression and 95% of eyes were preserved. Larger tumors may be treated when TTT is used for chemoreduction.

Complications

Complications of TTT include focal iris atrophy, peripheral focal lens opacity, retinal traction, retinal vascular obstruction, and transient localized serous retinal detachment.

Cross-References

Retinoblastoma brachytherapy, retinoblastoma radiotherapy, retinoblastoma thermotherapy, retinoblastoma chemoreduction

Further Reading

Abramson DH, Schefler AC (2004) Transpupillary thermotherapy as initial treatment for small intraocular retinoblastoma: technique and predictors of success. Ophthalmology 111:984–991

Lagendijk JJ (1982) A microwave heating technique for the hyperthermic treatment of tumours in the eye, especially retinoblastoma. Phys Med Biol 27:1313–1324

Murphree AL (2007) Local therapy, brachytherapy, and enucleation. In: Singh AD, Damato BE, Pe'er J, Murphree AL, Perry JD (eds) Clinical Ophthalmic Oncology. Saunders-Elsevier, Philadelphia, pp 454–461

Shields CL, Santos MC, Diniz W et al (1999) Thermotherapy for retinoblastoma. Arch Ophthalmol 117:885–893

Retinoblastoma: Trilateral

48

Sonia Mehta and G. Baker Hubbard III

Synonyms

Intraocular retinoblastoma with pineoblastoma, pinealoblastoma, pinealoma, pineal neuroblastic tumor (PNT), primitive neuroectodermal tumor (PNET), ectopic intracranial neuroblastic tumor (EINT).

Definition

Trilateral retinoblastoma is the occurrence of intraocular retinoblastoma in association with a primary midline intracranial neuroblastic tumor. Midline intracranial tumors are typically found in the pineal gland, but these tumors may also occur in the sellar or suprasellar spaces and more rarely in the third and fourth ventricles.

Etiology

Theories on the development of trilateral retinoblastoma are based on Knudson's "two-hit" hypothesis which describes the occurrence of two genetic events in hereditary retinoblastoma. The first mutation is inherited, and the second mutation

S. Mehta, M.D.
Department of Ophthalmology,
Emory University School of Medicine, Atlanta, GA, USA
e-mail: sonia.mehta@emory.edu

G.B. Hubbard III, M.D. (✉)
Department of Ophthalmology,
Emory University School of Medicine, Atlanta, GA, USA

The Emory Eye Center, Atlanta, GA, USA
e-mail: ghubba2@emory.edu

H.E. Grossniklaus (ed.), *Pocket Guide to Ocular Oncology and Pathology*,
DOI 10.1007/978-3-642-29782-3_48, © Springer-Verlag Berlin Heidelberg 2013

occurring in the retina is acquired during life. Cells in the pineal gland may also be susceptible to this second mutation due to its ontogenetic similarities to the retina. The pineal gland is often referred to as the "third eye" based on its role as a photosensitive organ in nonmammalian vertebrates. Cells compromising the pineal gland in nonmammalian vertebrates have a strong resemblance to the photoreceptor cells of the retina. Many evolutionary biologists believe that the vertebrate pineal cells share common evolutionary ancestry with the retinal cells. There are two hypotheses for the occurrence of trilateral retinoblastoma in the suprasellar region. In addition to the optic primordia, the diencephalon also gives rise to the pineal gland and suprasellar region. Therefore, germinal matrix cells in the central nervous system may share susceptibility to the Rb gene mutation. Alternatively, presence of ectopic photoreceptor cells in the suprasellar area may be susceptible to the Rb gene mutation.

Clinical Presentation

In the largest meta-analysis reviewing all reported cases of trilateral retinoblastoma, median age at diagnosis of trilateral retinoblastoma was 26 months ranging from 1 month to 12 years. Median time from intraocular retinoblastoma to development of trilateral retinoblastoma was 21 months ranging from 6 months before to 11 years after diagnosis of intraocular retinoblastoma. Most commonly, intracranial lesions develop after diagnosis of intraocular retinoblastoma. Less frequently, intracranial and intraocular retinoblastomas are detected at the same time. Rarely, intracranial tumors have been found before the development of intraocular retinoblastoma. The majority of patients with trilateral retinoblastoma are detected after symptoms of intracranial pressure develop such as headaches, seizures, irritability, nausea, vomiting, and focal neurologic signs. Less frequently, trilateral retinoblastoma cases are detected during screening of intraocular retinoblastoma patients. Intracranial tumors diagnosed by screening tend to be smaller and are associated with a better prognosis than tumors found after symptom development. The term trilateral retinoblastoma can be misleading. While the majority of trilateral retinoblastoma cases occur in association with bilateral retinoblastoma, primary midline intracranial neuroblastic tumor can also occur in patients with unilateral retinoblastoma.

Diagnostics

All patients with retinoblastoma should, at the time of diagnosis, undergo neuroimaging for the evaluation of trilateral retinoblastoma and also for detection of tumor extension into the optic nerve, sclera, orbit, and cerebrospinal metastases. The authors suggest magnetic resonance imaging (MRI) of the brain and orbits with and without gadolinium (Fig. 48.1). MRI of intracranial tumors in trilateral retinoblastoma typically reveals a solid lesion isointense with gray matter on T1-weighted images with homogeneous and intense contrast enhancement. Patients diagnosed

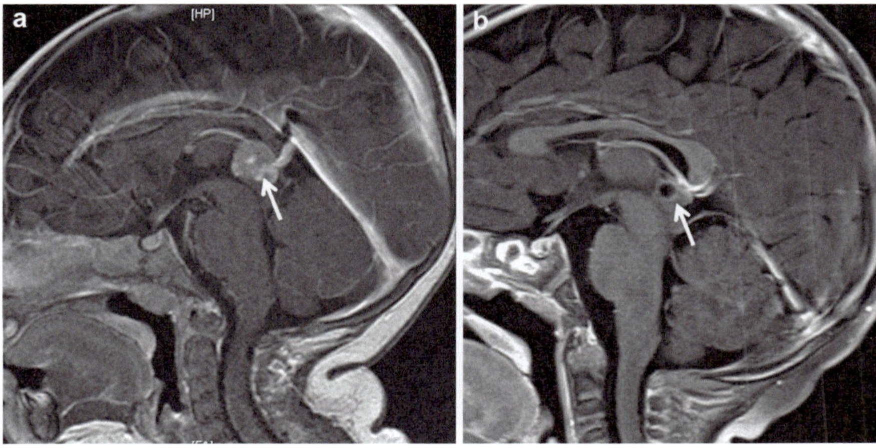

Fig. 48.1 A child with family history of retinoblastoma diagnosed with trilateral retinoblastoma at 6 months of age. (**a**) Pretreatment appearance of the tumor on T1 postcontrast sagittal MRI shows an enhancing solid lesion in the pineal gland (*arrow*) measuring 14 × 13 × 12 mm. (**b**) Note regression of the pineal tumor (*arrow*) with a cystic cavity after intensive chemotherapy with COG ARET 0321 protocol

with trilateral retinoblastoma should also undergo metastatic evaluation with MRI of the spinal cord, abdominal imaging, bone scan, lumbar puncture with cerebrospinal fluid analysis, and bone marrow aspiration. In some cases, biopsy of the lesion may be needed for confirmation of the diagnosis.

Pathology

Histopathologic analysis of primary intracranial midline neuroblastic tumors is similar to that seen in intraocular retinoblastoma. Microscopic analysis reveals a proliferation of small round blue cells with a high nucleus to cytoplasmic ratio, hyperchromatic nuclei, and mitotic figures. Tumors may contain Flexner-Wintersteiner rosettes, Homer-Wright rosettes, calcifications, and areas of necrosis. Diffuse immunoreactivity to the neuronal marker synaptophysin in the cytoplasm of tumor cells is characteristic.

Differential Diagnosis

Trilateral retinoblastoma should be distinguished from intraocular retinoblastoma associated with simple pineal cysts and metastatic retinoblastoma. Pineal cysts can be distinguished from pinealoblastoma based on neuroimaging features. MRI of a pineal cyst reveals a round or oval-shaped pineal gland, hypointense to white matter on T1, isointense to cerebrospinal fluid on T2, and surrounded by a thin wall not measuring more than 2 mm with rim contrast enhancement on T1. In addition, these cysts show no lobularity of the margin or nodular contrast enhancement. Metastatic intracranial retinoblastoma can be distinguished from primary intracranial lesions seen in trilateral retinoblastoma based on neuroimaging and pathology. Neuroimaging of cerebral metastasis from retinoblastoma typically shows multiple intracranial lesions; midline location for metastatic lesions is not characteristic. Metastatic intracranial retinoblastoma is also often associated with skull vault, long bone, and pulmonary metastases. In addition, metastatic retinoblastoma is histopathologically characterized by undifferentiated small round cells without Flexner-Wintersteiner rosettes, whereas primary intracranial lesions are morphologically similar to ocular retinoblastoma.

Prophylaxis

In patients with intraocular retinoblastoma, there is evidence that chemoreduction reduces the risk of developing trilateral retinoblastoma. One study reviewed 214 consecutive patients with intraocular retinoblastoma. Of the 142 that received chemoreduction, no trilateral retinoblastoma developed. In the nonchemoreduction group (72 patients), one developed trilateral disease. The authors conclude that chemoreduction was protective against trilateral disease in their patients. Several studies have recommended routine neuroimaging of patients with familial retinoblastoma or bilateral sporadic retinoblastoma until the age of 4 in order to detect asymptomatic primary intracranial tumors as prognosis for asymptomatic lesions is better than for symptomatic patients. Magnetic resonance imaging is advisable to reduce radiation exposure, reduce risk of secondary cancers, and for enhanced ability to detect tumors of the pineal, sellar, and suprasellar region. Various screening programs have been suggested. The authors suggest MRI brain and orbits with and without gadolinium every 3 months during the first year after diagnosis of familial or bilateral retinoblastoma followed by every 6 months for the next 3 years. In most patients with trilateral retinoblastoma, intracranial lesions are detected at the same time or after development of intraocular tumors. However, cases of trilateral retinoblastoma in which the intracranial tumors were detected prior to the intraocular tumor have also been reported. Based on this, it has been suggested that children below 4 years of age with primary intracranial midline tumors should undergo careful ophthalmologic examination for evaluation of retinoblastoma.

Therapy

Despite treatment of trilateral retinoblastoma with conventional chemotherapy, radiation therapy, and/or surgery, survival is often poor. One series reported good results in patients with trilateral retinoblastoma treated with intensive chemotherapy. The Children's Oncology Group has recently opened a prospective multicenter trial (COG ARET 0321) in which patients with trilateral retinoblastoma will receive intensive chemotherapy consisting of four cycles of induction chemotherapy with vincristine, cisplatin, cyclophosphamide, and etoposide followed by one cycle of high-dose carboplatin, thiotepa, and etoposide with autologous hematopoietic stem cell rescue. Radiation therapy will be omitted for patients achieving a complete response with intensive chemotherapy.

Prognosis

While the survival rate for intraocular retinoblastoma is generally good in the United States, the prognosis for trilateral disease is significantly worse due to cerebrospinal metastasis. Mean survival time reported in the literature for trilateral retinoblastoma is 9–13 months from diagnosis. Patients with small intracranial tumors measuring less than 15 mm in size, asymptomatic intracranial tumors, or tumors detected by screening have better prognosis.

Epidemiology

Trilateral retinoblastoma can occur in patients with familial or sporadic retinoblastoma. Data from large centers estimate the chances of trilateral retinoblastoma developing to be less than 0.5% in unilateral retinoblastoma, 5–13% in sporadic bilateral retinoblastoma, and 5–15% in familial bilateral retinoblastoma.

Cross-Reference

Retinoblastoma metastasis.

Further Reading

Bader JL, Miller RW, Meadows AT, Zimmerman LE, Champion LA, Voute PA (1980) Trilateral retinoblastoma. Lancet 2:582–583

Dunkel IJ, Jubran RF, Gururangan S, Chantada GL, Finlay JL, Goldman S, Khakoo Y, O'Brien JM, Orjuela M, Rodriguez-Galindo C, Souweidane MM, Abramson DH (2010) Trilateral retinoblastoma potentially curable with intensive chemotherapy. Pediatr Blood Cancer 54:384–387

Jakobiec FA, Tso MO, Zimmerman LE, Danis P (1977) Retinoblastoma and intracranial malignancy. Cancer 39:2048–2058

Jurkiewicz E, Pakula-Kosciesza I, Rutynowska O, Nowak K (2010) Trilateral retinoblastoma: an institutional experience and review of the literature. Childs Nerv Syst 26:129–132

Karatza E, Shields CL, Flanders AE et al (2006) Pineal cyst simulating pinealoblastoma in 11 children with retinoblastoma. Arch Ophthalmol 124:595–597

Kivela T (1999) Trilateral retinoblastoma: a meta-analysis of hereditary retinoblastoma associated with primary ectopic intracranial retinoblastoma. J Clin Oncol 17:1829–1837

Knudson AG Jr (1971) Mutation and cancer: statistical study of retinoblastoma. Proc Natl Acad Sci USA 68:820–823

Popovic MB, Balmer A, Maeder P, Braganca T, Munier FL (2006) Benign pineal cysts in children with bilateral retinoblastoma: a new variant of trilateral retinoblastoma? Pediatr Blood Cancer 46:755–761

Provenzle JM, Weber AL, Klintworth GK, McLendon RE (1995) Radiologic-pathologic correlation: bilateral retinoblastoma with coexistent pinealoblastoma (trilateral retinoblastoma). AJNR Am J Neuroradiol 16:157–165

Shields JA, Pesin SP, Shields CL (1989) Trilateral retinoblastoma. J Clin Neuroophthalmol 9:222–223

Shields CL, Meadows AT, Shields JA, Carvalho C, Smith AF (2001) Chemoreduction for retinoblastoma may prevent intracranial neuroblastic malignancy (trilateral retinoblastoma). Arch Ophthalmol 119:1269–1272

Tateishi U, Hasegawa T, Miyakawa K, Sumi M, Moriyama N (2003) CT and MRI features of recurrent tumors and second primary neoplasms in pediatric patients with retinoblastoma. Am J Roentgenol 181:879–884

Retinocytoma

49

Sunir Joshi and Curtis E. Margo

Synonyms

Retinoma, spontaneously arrested retinoblastoma.

Definition

Retinocytoma describes the benign variant of retinoblastoma. Initially referred to as retinoma, retinocytoma is a histologically bland, nonprogressive primary retinal tumor. It is conceptually distinguished from the rare condition in which a typical retinoblastoma undergoes spontaneous total necrosis (spontaneously regressed retinoblastoma). The designation of "spontaneously arrested retinoblastoma" may aptly describe retinocytoma in light of the function of the retinoblastoma protein in cell proliferation and differentiation.

Etiology

This tumor is a manifestation of the retinoblastoma gene.

Clinical Presentation

Retinocytoma is usually diagnosed in older children, is usually unilateral, and is usually located outside of the macula. Leukocoria is a presenting symptom only rarely.

S. Joshi
Beraja Medical Institute, Coral Gambles, FL, USA
e-mail: sunirjoshi@gmail.com

C.E. Margo, M.D., MPH
Department of Ophthalmology, University of South Florida, Tampa, FL, USA
e-mail: cmargo@health.usf.edu

H.E. Grossniklaus (ed.), *Pocket Guide to Ocular Oncology and Pathology*,
DOI 10.1007/978-3-642-29782-3_49, © Springer-Verlag Berlin Heidelberg 2013

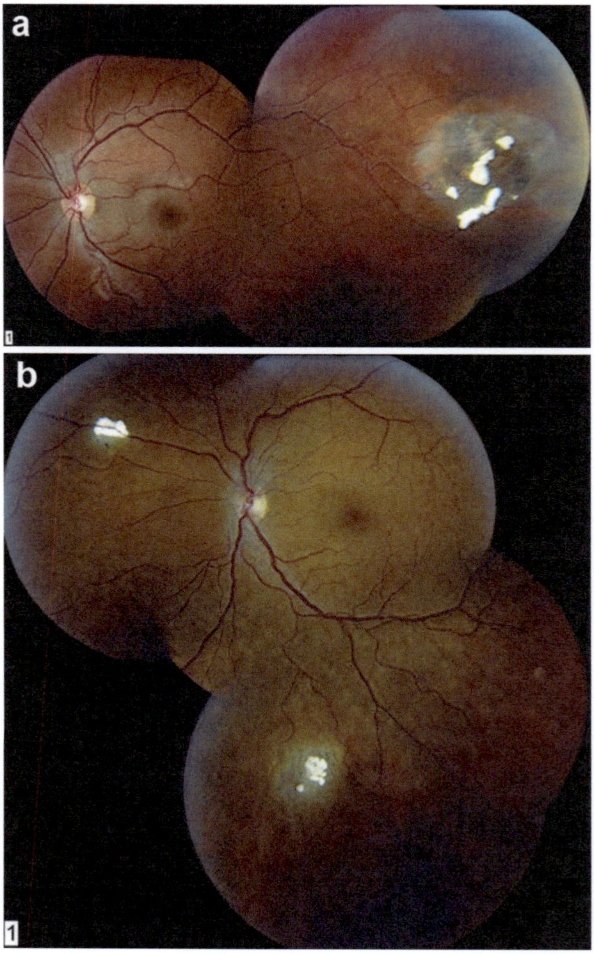

Fig. 49.1 Retinocytoma. Mother (**a**) and grandmother (**b**) of a patient with bilateral retinoblastoma. Note the areas of calcification and zone of chorioretinal atrophy around each lesion that simulates type 1 and type 4 regression

Ophthalmoscopic features characteristic of retinocytoma generally mimic the patterns of regression seen after irradiation and include the presence of a translucent retinal mass, calcification, and retinal pigment epithelial alteration (Fig. 49.1a and b). A zone of chorioretinal atrophy may be observed in approximately half of tumors.

Diagnostics

Retinocytoma is diagnosed based on its ophthalmoscopic features and by lack of growth documented with longitudinal follow-up.

Pathology

Retinocytoma is a primary retinal tumor composed of cells showing signs of photoreceptor differentiation admixed with varying amounts of glial cells. At low magnification, retinocytoma appears pink when stained with hematoxylin and eosin, rather than the blue tone of retinoblastoma. Individual cells have more cytoplasm than their malignant counterpart in retinoblastoma. Nuclear chromatin is less dense, and mitotic figures are absent or rare. Photoreceptor differentiation manifests in the form of "fleurettes," a term based on the resemblance of the structure to a bouquet of flowers and rosettes (Flexner-Wintersteiner type) (Fig. 49.2a and b). Most retinocytomas consist of a mixture of fleurettes, rosettes, and individual cells showing photoreceptor differentiation (Fig. 49.3). Areas of necrosis and calcification can often be found. The diagnosis of retinocytoma is based on the absence of typical cellular findings of retinoblastoma. Ultrastructural studies of retinocytoma confirm the arrested photoreceptor development and the presence of glial cells. The structures referred to as "fleurettes" correspond to clusters of inner segments of photoreceptors attached by zonula adherens. Evidence of widespread photoreceptor differentiation can be seen in individual cells as well.

Differential Diagnosis

Spontaneously regressed retinoblastoma is usually a phenomenon associated with large tumors and inflammation. Features of phthisis bulbi are usually present. Medulloepithelioma, a tumor arising from the nonpigmented ciliary epithelium, is characterized by ribbons of primitive medullary epithelium. The so-called massive gliosis or reactive gliosis can mimic a primary retinal tumor but shows no evidence of photoreceptor differentiation.

Prophylaxis

There is no known prophylaxis for retinocytoma. However, molecular testing plays an important role in the management of retinocytoma just as it does for retinoblastoma. The justification for and implications of molecular testing are the same for retinocytoma as they are for retinoblastoma. A sporadic, unifocal retinocytoma carries the same clinical implications as a sporadic, unifocal retinoblastoma. Similarly, if a retinocytoma is associated with a retinoblastoma in the opposite eye, it has the same implications as bilateral retinoblastoma (i.e., affected patients have one germline RB1 mutant allele and an autosomal dominant pattern of transmission). One practical strategy recommended for genetic testing in patients with sporadic, unilateral retinoblastoma is adaptable for retinocytoma. This involves harvesting tumor DNA (fresh tissue from tumor) for identification of the two mutant RB1 alleles, followed by analysis of blood DNA for each of those mutations. A negative result

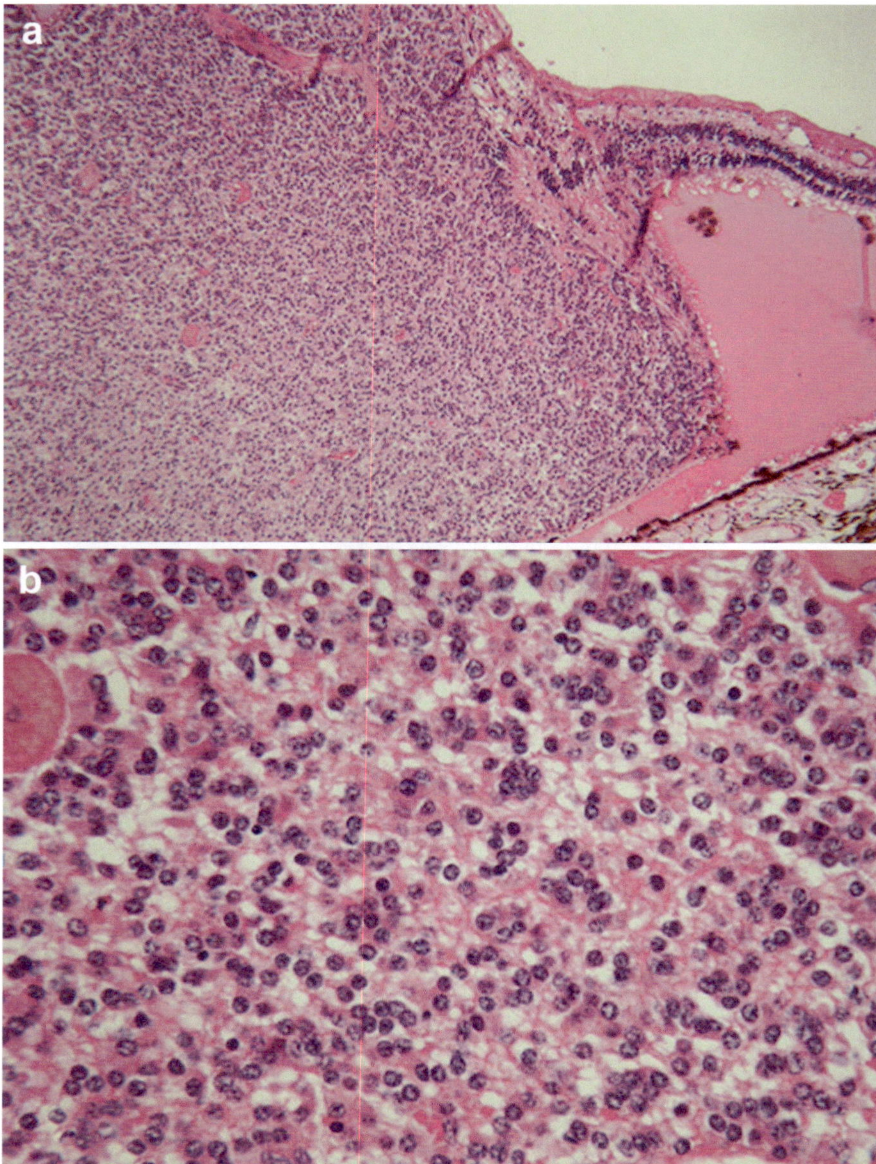

Fig. 49.2 Retinocytoma. (**a**) Low magnification shows a pale pink tumor arising from the deep retina. (**b**) Individual cells have abundant cytoplasm, some of which appears clear, and round nucleus with open chromatin. No mitotic figures are present

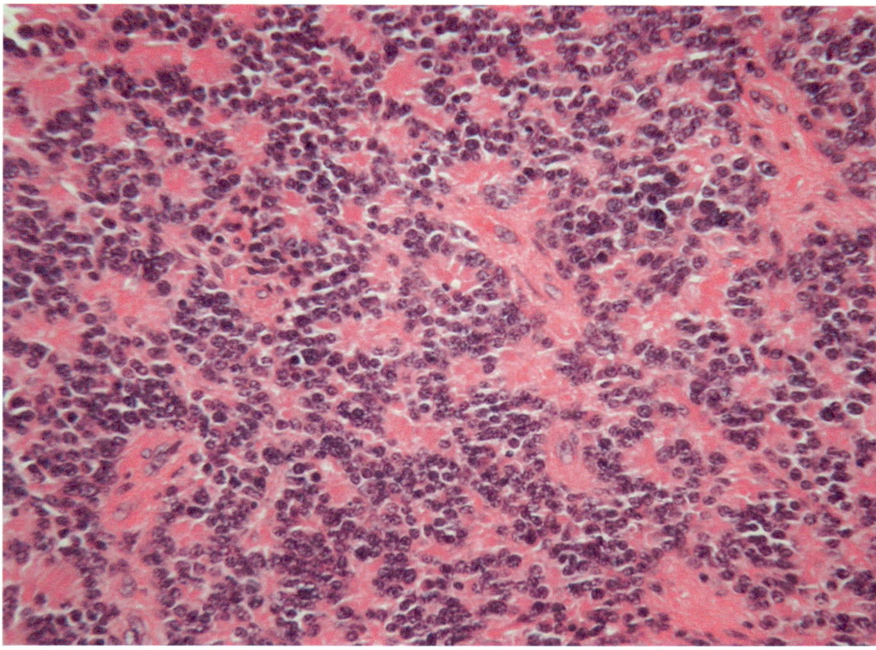

Fig. 49.3 Retinocytoma. This retinocytoma has cells with abundant pink cytoplasm, some of which form rosettes and small fleurettes. Nuclear chromatin is bland and no mitotic activity is present

generally excludes heritable retinoblastoma in the proband, except for the possibility of genetic mosaicism.

Therapy

Management of retinocytoma consists of surveillance to monitor for the possibility of malignant transformation.

Prognosis

The risk of malignant transformation is thought to be approximately 4%. In addition, the risk for developing pineoblastoma likewise seems to be very low. The prognosis for these lesions is therefore good.

Epidemiology

Retinocytoma is very rare and is usually diagnosed in children older than 6 years. In one large series of 920 patients with retinoblastoma, 1.8% were found to have retinocytoma.

Cross-References

Ciliary body medulloepithelioma; retinoblastoma; retinoblastoma: chemoreduction, transpupillary thermotherapy, teletherapy; enucleation.

Further Reading

Brown V, Chan HSLC, Gallie BL (2003) A cascade of genomic changes leads to retinoblastoma. In: Albert DM, Polans A (eds) Ocular oncology. Marcel Dekker, New York, pp 103–128, Ch 7

Eagle RC Jr, Shields JA, Donoso L, Milner RS (1989) Malignant transformation of spontaneously regressed retinoblastoma, retinoma/retinocytoma variant. Ophthalmology 96:1389–1395

Keith CG, Webb GC (1985) Retinoblastoma and retinoma occurring in a child with a translocation and deletion of the long arm of chromosome 13. Arch Ophthalmol 103:941–944

Margo C, Hidayat A, Kopelman J, Zimmerman LE (1983) Retinocytoma. A benign variant of retinocytoma. Arch Ophthalmol 101:1419–1431

Singh AD, Santos CM, Shields CL, Shields JA, Eagle RC Jr (2000) Observations on 17 patients with retinocytoma. Arch Ophthalmol 118:199–205

Part V

Uveal Tumors: Non-melanocytic Tumors

Ciliary Body Non-melanocytic Tumors 50

Qing Zhang and Hans E. Grossniklaus

Synonyms

Neuroepithelial tumors – adenoma, adenocarcinoma, medulloepithelioma (diktyoma, teratoneuroma), teratoid medulloepithelioma; stromal tumors – leiomyoma, mesectodermal leiomyoma, schwannoma (neurilemoma)

Definition

This is a group of non-melanocytic tumors that arise in the ciliary body, including the ciliary epithelium and stroma. Note: ciliary body adenoma (Fuchs adenoma), adenocarcinoma, and medulloepithelioma are also described in separate entries under "retina, RPE, and ciliary epithelial tumors". They are also included in this entry as they are all included in the differential diagnosis of ciliary body melanoma. Table 50.1 shows the classification of this group of tumors.

Table 50.2 summarizes the histologic, immunohistochemical, electron microscopic, and molecular diagnostic features of this group of tumors.

Q. Zhang, M.D. (✉)
Department of Ophthalmology,
Emory University School of Medicine,
Atlanta, GA, USA
e-mail: qzhang7@emory.edu

H.E. Grossniklaus, M.D.
Emory University School of Medicine,
Emory Eye Center,
Department of Ophthalmology,
Atlanta, GA, USA
e-mail: ophtheg@emory.edu

H.E. Grossniklaus (ed.), *Pocket Guide to Ocular Oncology and Pathology*,
DOI 10.1007/978-3-642-29782-3_50,

Table 50.1 Classification of ciliary body non-melanocytic tumors

Neuroepithelial tumors
Congenital
Glioneuroma
Medulloepithelioma (diktyoma, teratoneuroma)
Acquired
Nonpigmented (adenoma, adenocarcinoma)
Pigmented (adenoma, adenocarcinoma)
Neural tumors
Schwannoma (neurilemoma)
Neurofibroma
Myogenic tumors
Leiomyoma
Leiomyosarcoma
Rhabdomyosarcoma
Vascular tumors
Hemangioma
Hemangiopericytoma

Etiology

There is no known cause for most of the tumors in this category. Adenoma and adenocarcinoma may be found in blind eyes after trauma. Leiomyoma occurs generally in young women, and its growth may be hormonally influenced.

Clinical Presentation

These tumors present as asymptomatic, lightly pigmented, or amelanotic tumors of the ciliary body. They may be incidentally found during dilated examination through the pupil (Fig. 50.1). Medulloepithelioma may present as cysts in the anterior chamber or behind the iris.

Diagnosis

The diagnosis is suspected by clinical appearance. Transillumination shows that these tumors will fail to block light and may in fact increase the transmission of light. Ultrasound will usually show medium internal reflectivity and, in some cases of medulloepithelioma or adenoma/adenocarcinoma, cystic spaces. A metastatic evaluation should be performed in patients with ciliary body tumors.

Table 50.2 Histology, immunohistochemistry, electron microscopy, molecular diagnosis, and differential diagnosis of ciliary body non-melanocytic tumors

	Histology	Immunohistochemistry	Electron microscopy	Molecular diagnosis	Differential diagnosis
Glioneuroma	Displays well-differentiated neural tissues that are mixed of neurons and glial cells. Rosette can be seen	(+) for NSE, synaptophysin, S-100, GFAP, vimentin, CK	Many of the neurons possess coarse clumps of Nissl substance and axonal processes		Coloboma Medulloepithelioma
Medulloepithelioma	Contains multilayered sheets and cords of poorly differentiated neuroepithelial cells that organized into ribbonlike structure	(+) for nestin, vimentin, CK, GFAP, S-100, NF protein, NSE, EMA	Shows neuroepithelial cells forming rosettes with a plethora of microvilli at the luminal surface	A karyotype of 46,XX,der(16)t(1;16)(q21;q22)[1]/45,idem,-15[5]/45,idem,del(6)(q2?),-15[5]/46,XX[3] was reported	Retinoblastoma
Adenoma of nonpigmented epithelium	Classified to be solid, papillary, tubuloacinar, or pleomorphic type. Fuchs adenoma is an idiopathic hyperplasia that can occur following injury or chronic inflammation or normal	(+) for vimentin, CK, S-100	The tumor cells contain many organelles but only exceptionally melanosomes and melanin granules. The connective tissue was loose, poor in fibers, and sparsely vascularized		Secondary tumors Metastatic tumors Malignant melanoma
Adenocarcinoma of nonpigmented epithelium	Shows tubules and gland-like structure of pleomorphic epithelial cells, surrounded by hyalinized stroma	(+) for vimentin, EMA, S-100, and NSE	Shows tumor cells, desmosomes, areas of thick multilamellar basement membrane surrounding tumor cells and occasional intracytoplasmic intermediate filaments		Secondary tumors Metastatic tumors Malignant melanoma

(continued)

Table 50.2 (continued)

	Histology	Immunohistochemistry	Electron microscopy	Molecular diagnosis	Differential diagnosis
Adenoma of pigmented epithelium	Consists of pigmented cells, arranged in lobules, nodules, or sheets. Multiple vacuoles can be seen	(+) for CK, vimentin, and S-100	The tumor cells are rich in organelles, melanosomes, and mature melanin granules. A few single axons and fine bundles of unmyelinated nerve fibers can be seen		Secondary tumors Metastatic tumors Malignant melanoma
Adenocarcinoma of pigmented epithelium	Consist of tumor cells with abundant cytoplasm, hyperchromatic nuclei, and prominent nucleoli	(+) for CK, CAM 5.2, NSE, and vimentin	Shows poorly developed junctional complexes in the form of zonula occludens between tumor cells and multilaminar basement membrane partially surrounding individual cells		Secondary tumors Metastatic tumors Malignant melanoma
Schwannoma	Shows spindle-shaped tumor cells arranged as Antoni A and Antoni B patterns. Verocay bodies can be seen	(+) for type IV collagen, S-100, Leu 7, and GFAP	Consists of tumor cells with elongated and delicate processes and perineural capsular cells with smooth muscle differentiation		Astrocytoma Meningioma Ependymoma
Neurofibroma	Displays a solitary nodular mass or a diffuse thickened type with intertwining bundles of multiple-type cells and spread axons	(+) for NF, S-100, and EMA	Shows endoneural fibroblast, axon excess basement membrane, and perineurally neuromatous units of Schwann cells		Schwannoma

Leiomyoma	Classified as two types: mesectodermal type shows amelanotic, spindle-shaped cells with eosinophilic cytoplasm and long oval nuclei; mesodermal type shows interlacing bundles of spindle cells with eosinophilic cytoplasm and oval nuclei	(+) for muscle-specific antigen, smooth muscle actin, vimentin	Shows smooth muscle cells with investing basement membrane, plasmalemmal vesicles, intracytoplasmic filaments. The perikaryon contains parallel stacks of rough-surfaced endoplasmic reticulum reminiscent of Nissl substance		Malignant melanoma Amelanotic spindle cells nevus
Leiomyosarcoma	Consists of spindle cells with large round to oval hyperchromatic nuclei, abundant eosinophilic cytoplasm with indistinct borders, and slender cellular processes blending into a fibrillary background	(+) for muscle-specific antigen, synaptophysin, S-100, and NSE	Shows spindle cells, thin filaments with fusiform densities, pinocytotic vesicles, plasmalemmal densities, basement membranes, and underdeveloped desmosomes		Malignant melanoma
Rhabdomyosarcoma	Consists mainly of undifferentiated mesenchymal cells and scattered clusters of large polyhedral cells with an abundance of deeply eosinophilic cytoplasm or strap-like masses of cytoplasm	(+) for muscle-specific actin and myosin	Contains rhabdomyoblasts with incomplete basement membranes and fibrocytoid cells with considerable rough-surfaced endoplasmic reticulum		

(continued)

Table 50.2 (continued)

	Histology	Immunohistochemistry	Electron microscopy	Molecular diagnosis	Differential diagnosis
Hemangioma	Consists of a densely cellular infiltrate with numerous capillary channels	(+) for CD31, GLUT1, FLI-1	Disclose two or layers of smooth muscle cells surrounding the endothelial cells		Xanthogranuloma Angiosarcoma
Hemangiopericytoma	Consists of tightly packed, spindle cells with oval to round nuclei and poorly outlined eosinophilic cytoplasm. Focally, the tumor cells display slightly vesicular nuclei and more sharply outlined clear cytoplasm	(+) for actin and vimentin	Shows perivascular oval or spindle cells with few organelles, early smooth muscle, oval nuclei, spotty basement membrane, and pseudoluments surrounding extravasated erythrocytes		Xanthogranuloma Lymphangioma Hemangioma
Secondary and metastatic tumors	Tumors from the iris, choroid, retina can extend to the ciliary body. Tumors from lung, breast, renal and all others can metastasize to the ciliary body but are rare. They reveal neoplastic cells with numerous mitotic figures and suggest the origin of the primary tumors	Shows immunohistochemical features of the primary tumors	In women, breast carcinoma contains intracytoplasmic lumens, enriched by cytoplasmic filaments. In men, lung cancer is a common tumor to metastasize to the ciliary body, showing undifferentiated cells with or without core inclusions		Malignant melanoma Adenoma or adenocarcinoma of ciliary epithelium

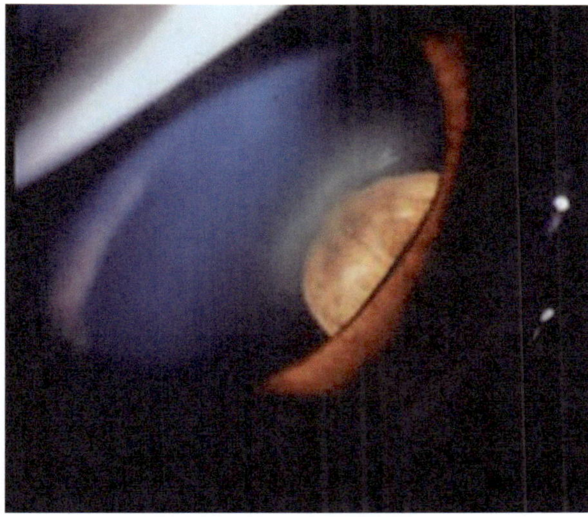

Fig. 50.1 Adenoma of nonpigmented ciliary epithelium. Gonioscopic examination shows a tan lobular tumor in the ciliary body

Pathology

The pathologic features in this group of tumors, including immunohistochemical findings, are shown in Table 50.2. Examples of adenoma (Fig. 50.2) and mesectodermal leiomyoma (Fig. 50.3) are shown.

Differential Diagnosis

The main differential diagnosis is melanoma. All of the entities in this category of tumors are in the differential diagnosis. The clinical and histologic differential diagnosis includes metastases.

Prophylaxis

There is no known prophylaxis for this group of tumors.

Therapy

Therapy for these tumors ranges from observation to iridocyclectomy to enucleation in cases of large tumors/medulloepithelioma.

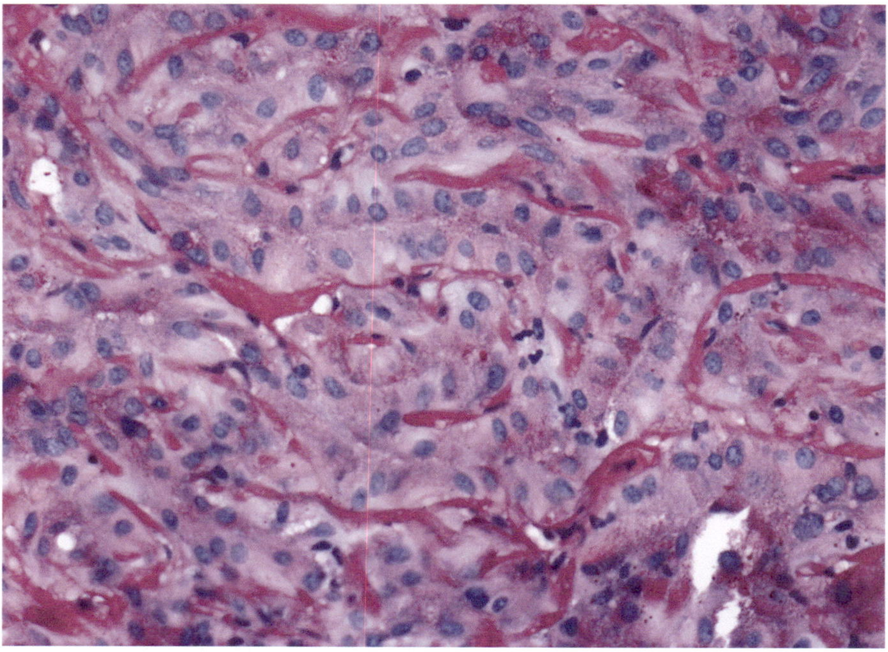

Fig. 50.2 Adenoma of nonpigmented ciliary epithelium. There are strands of nonpigmented epithelium and basement-membrane-like material present (periodic acid-Shiff, ×100)

Prognosis

The prognosis for this group of tumors is very good. The eye may be salvaged in most instances. There is a low risk of metastases of non-melanocytic malignant ciliary body tumors.

Epidemiology

Medulloepithelioma is found in children. Leiomyoma (mesectodermal leiomyoma) is found usually in young women. Other tumors in this category are found at any age equally in both sexes.

Cross-References

Ciliary epithelium adenoma, adenocarcinoma, medulloepithelioma (diktyoma), surgical techniques

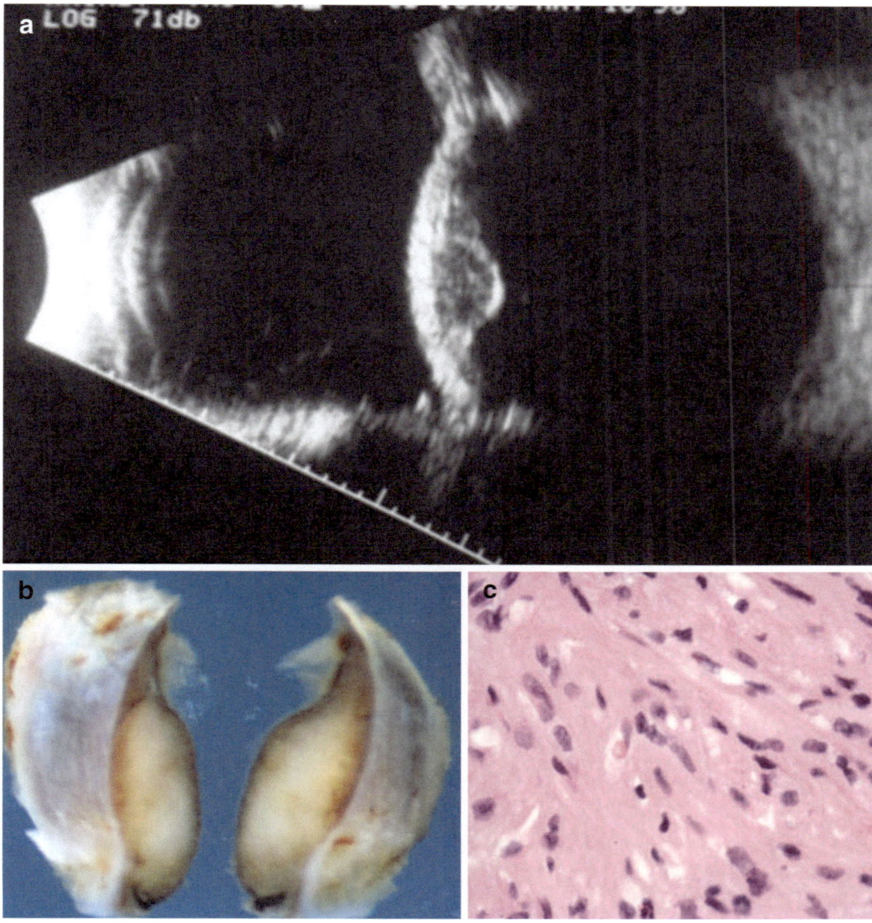

Fig. 50.3 Mesectodermal leiomyosarcoma. (**a**) B-scan shows ciliary body tumor. (**b**) Gross examination of resected tumor shows smooth surface. (**c**) The tumor is composed of amelanotic, spindle-shaped cells with eosinophilic cytoplasm and blunt-ended, cigar-shaped nuclei (hematoxylin and eosin, ×100)

Further Reading

Gieser SC, Hufnagel TJ, Jaros PA et al (1988) Hemangiopericytoma of the ciliary body. Arch Ophthalmol 106(9):1269–1272

Laver NM, Hidayat AA, Croxatto JO (1999) Pleomorphic adenocarcinomas of the ciliary epithelium. Immunohistochemical and ultrastructural features of 12 cases. Ophthalmology 106(1):103–110

Rao NA (1997) Biopsy pathology of the eye and ocular adnexa, 1st edn. Chapman & Hall, London, pp 215–225

Wilson ME, McClatchey SK, Zimmerman LE (1990) Rhabdomyosarcoma of the ciliary body. Ophthalmology 97(11):1484–1488

Uveal Lymphoma

51

Jim Sargent and Hans E. Grossniklaus

Synonyms

Reactive lymphoid hyperplasia; uveal lymphoid neoplasia; uveal lymphoid infiltrate; lymphoid tumor of the uvea.

Definition

Uveal lymphomas are either primary neoplasms of the uveal tract or secondary tumors in patients with disseminated disease. Primary uveal lymphomas are typically low-grade B cell neoplasms.

Etiology

No risk factors or causes for uveal lymphoma have been identified.

J. Sargent, M.D. (✉)
Emory Eye Center,
Atlanta, GA, USA
e-mail: j.sargent@emory.edu

H.E. Grossniklaus, M.D.
Emory University School of Medicine, Emory Eye Center,
Department of Ophthalmology,
Atlanta, GA, USA
e-mail: ophtheg@emory.edu

H.E. Grossniklaus (ed.), *Pocket Guide to Ocular Oncology and Pathology*,
DOI 10.1007/978-3-642-29782-3_51,

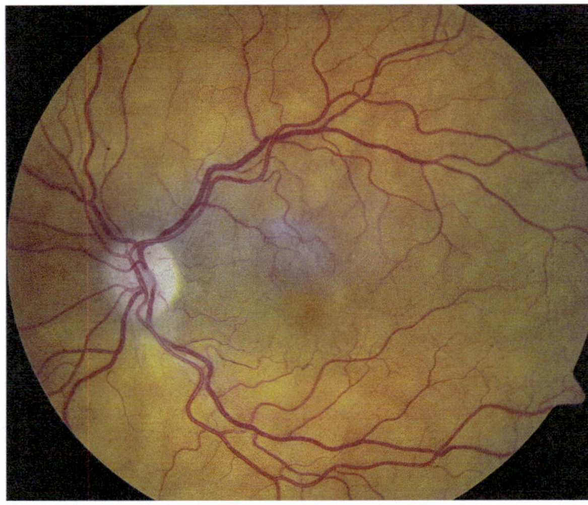

Fig. 51.1 Fundus photograph showing diffuse choroidal infiltration and shallow serous retinal detachment

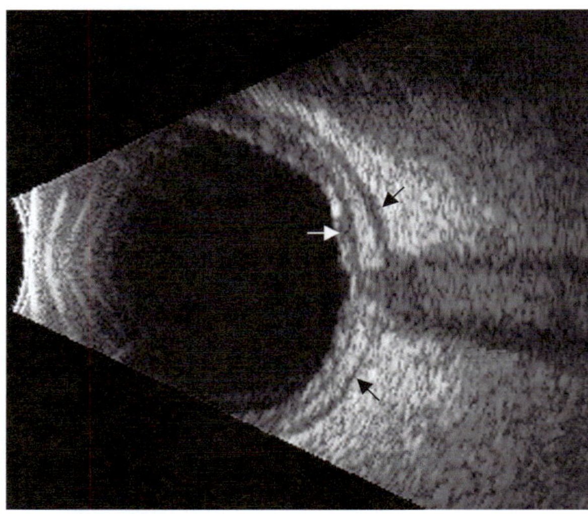

Fig. 51.2 A B-scan shows (*black arrows*) choroidal thickening, (*white arrow*) epibulbar nodules near the optic nerve, and a "whale tail" sign of the optic nerve

Clinical Presentation

Primary choroidal lymphoma is usually unilateral and is more common in men than women. Symptoms include painless blurred vision and metamorphopsia. Early signs include multifocal yellow-pink choroidal nodules on fundus examination. Later, a diffuse thickening of the uveal tract may become apparent. This is often associated with serous retinal detachments and fluorescein angiographic leakage (Fig. 51.1). The vitreous remains clear. Ultrasound findings include diffuse choroidal infiltrate with low internal reflectivity without choroidal or scleral excavation. Nodules around the optic nerve may be seen creating a "whale tale" sign (Fig. 51.2).

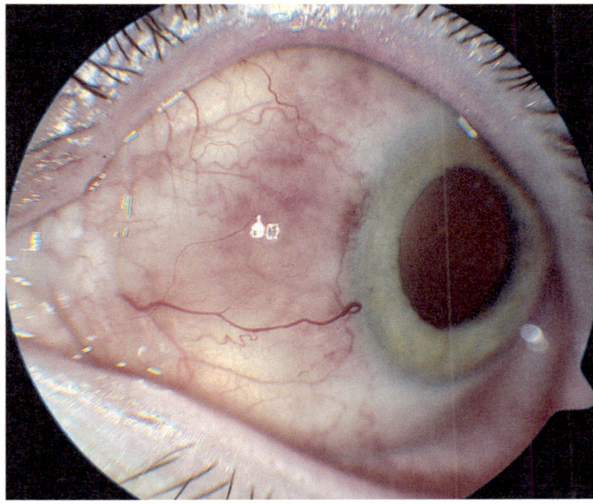

Fig. 51.3 Episcleral conjunctival nodule in a patient with a choroidal lymphoid proliferation

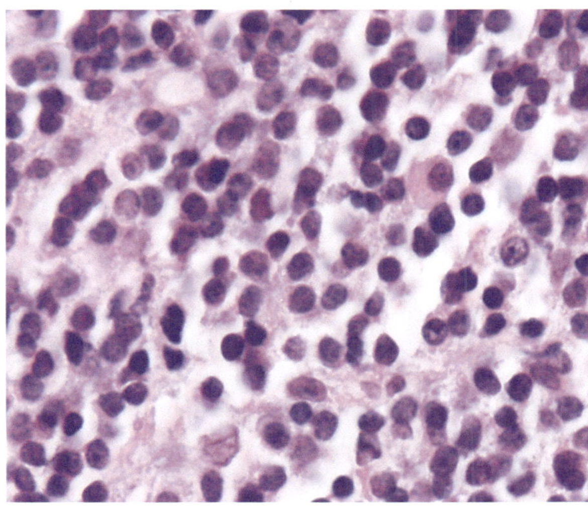

Fig. 51.4 The nodule is composed of sheets of small, round lymphocytes with occasional larger lymphocytes with open chromatin (hematoxylin and eosin, 100×)

In addition, episcleral conjunctival nodules can be seen (Fig. 51.3). Secondary choroidal lymphoma may be bilateral and associated with known systemic lymphoma.

Pathology

A biopsy may show diffuse infiltration of the substantia propria of the conjunctiva with lymphocytes (Fig. 51.4). These will be predominately B lymphocytes (Fig. 51.5) with or without kappa and lambda restriction. If there is clonality identified, the lesion represents a low-grade B cell lymphoma, in particular, a marginal zone B cell lymphoma.

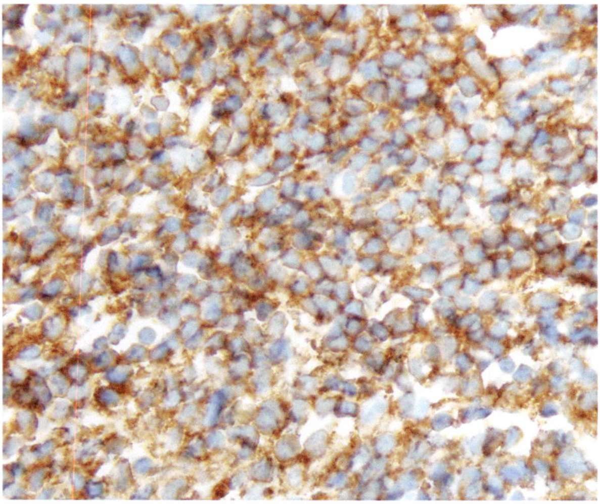

Fig. 51.5 Immunohistochemical stains are positive for CD20, indicating that most of the lymphocytes are B lymphocytes (peroxidase antiperoxidase, 100×)

Diagnostics

Diagnosis is made by clinical presentation with or without biopsy of an episcleral nodule. If systemic disease is suspected, evaluation by a medical oncologist and systemic work-up is indicated.

Differential Diagnosis

The clinical differential diagnosis includes melanoma, metastatic carcinoma, choroidal involvement from systemic lymphoma, and inflammatory conditions such as multifocal choroiditis, punctate inner choroiditis, Vogt-Koyanagi-Harada disease, birdshot retinochoroidopathy, acute multifocal posterior placoid pigment epitheliopathy, retinal detachment, and uveal effusion.

Prophylaxis

There is no prophylactic treatment for uveal lymphoid proliferation.

Therapy

Treatment includes high-dose systemic corticosteroids and low-dose external radiation therapy.

Prognosis

Primary choroidal lymphoma follows a protracted course. Without treatment, the lymphoma can cause glaucoma and serous retinal detachments. Systemic dissemination is rare. Treatment with radiotherapy and systemic corticosteroids usually induces complete tumor regression. Final visual acuity after treatment is unpredictable. Prognosis for secondary uveal lymphoma due to systemic dissemination depends on the subtype of systemic lymphoma.

Epidemiology

Primary uveal lymphoma most often occurs unilaterally and is more common in men than in women. It usually presents in the sixth and seventh decade.

Cross-Reference

Uveal metastatic tumors

Further Reading

Cockerham GC, Hidayat AA, Bijwaard KE, Sheng ZM (2000) Re-evaluation of "reactive lymphoid hyperplasia of the uvea": an immunohistochemical and molecular analysis of 10 cases. Ophthalmology 107:151–158

Coupland S, Damato B (2008) Understanding intraocular lymphomas. Clin Experiment Ophthalmol 36:564–578

Desroches G, Abrams G, Gass D (1983) Reactive lymphoid hyperplasia of the uvea: a case with ultrasonographic and computed tomographic studies. Arch Ophthalmol 101:725–728

Grossniklaus HE, Martin DF, Avery R, Shields JA, Shields CL, Kuo IC, Green RL, Rao N (1998) Uveal lymphoid infiltration: report of four cases and clinicopathologic review. Ophthalmology 105:1265–1273

Uveal Osseous Tumors

52

Jeffrey M. Goshe, Arun D. Singh, and Matthew Emanuel

Synonyms

Choroidal osteoma, Osseous choristoma, primary intraocular uveal osteoma, sclero-choroidal calcification

Definition

Choroidal osteoma is a benign primary tumor characterized by choristomatous presence of bony trabeculae and associated cellular elements within the choroid.

Etiology

The etiology is not completely understood, although inflammatory, genetic, metabolic, and hormonal factors have been suggested.

J.M. Goshe, M.D.
Cole Eye Institute, Cleveland Clinic Foundation,
9500 Euclid Avenue, Cleveland, OH 44195, USA

A.D. Singh, M.D. (✉)
Department of Ophthalmic Oncology,
Cole Eye Institute, Cleveland Clinic Foundation,
9500 Euclid Ave, Desk i-329,
Cleveland, OH 44195, USA
e-mail: singha@ccf.org

M. Emanuel, M.D.
Department of Ophthalmology,
Emory University School of Medicine,
Atlanta, GA, USA

H.E. Grossniklaus (ed.), *Pocket Guide to Ocular Oncology and Pathology*,
DOI 10.1007/978-3-642-29782-3_52,

Clinical Presentation

Approximately 75% of cases are unilateral. The majority of patients are asymptomatic at the time of diagnosis, although complaints of visual loss, metamorphopsia, and visual field defects are not uncommon. The typical appearance is that of a yellow-white, minimally elevated (<2.5 mm) choroidal mass with variable overlying RPE change (Figs. 52.1 and 52.2). The margins are characteristically wavy and well-demarcated. Lesions commonly occur in close proximity to the optic nerve and may extend to involve the macula. Overlying vascular tufts may be confused with secondary choroidal neovascularization (CNV) as suggested by exudation, hemorrhage, or adjacent subretinal fluid.

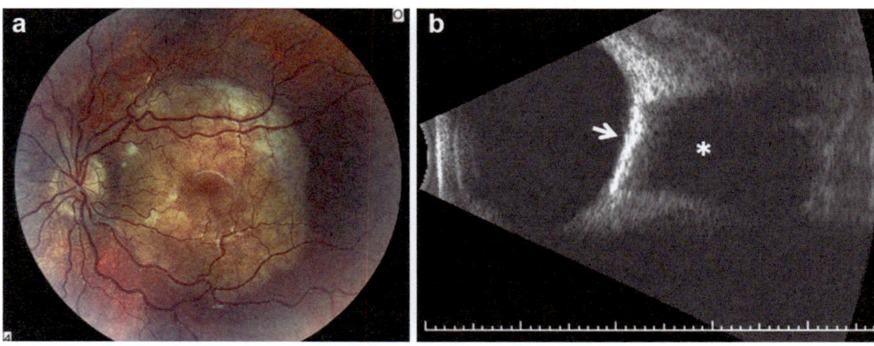

Fig. 52.1 Fundus photograph of the left eye. Note the yellow-white choroidal lesion with well-demarcated borders (**a**). B-scan ultrasonography demonstrates high reflectivity (*arrow*) at the level of the choroid and acoustic shadowing (*) suggestive of calcium deposition with posterior shadowing (**b**)

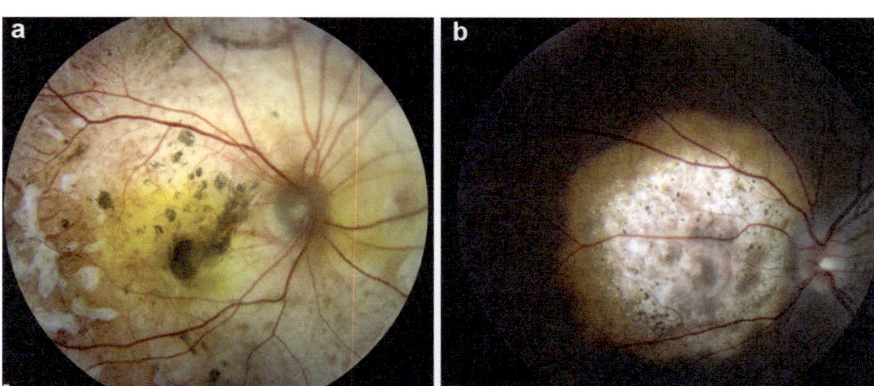

Fig. 52.2 Fundus photograph of the right and left eye of a 20-year-old female with bilateral choroidal osteomas. Note the extensive peripapillary and macular involvement with RPE changes over the lesion in the right eye (**a**) and a smaller lesion nasal to the optic disc in the left eye (**b**)

Diagnostics

The most useful ancillary study is ultrasonography, which demonstrates high reflectivity of the anterior face of the lesion (Fig 52.1b) with posterior shadowing. Fluorescein angiography shows patchy early hyperfluorescence and late diffuse staining and may assist in distinguishing fine overlying vascular tufts from CNV. ICG shows early hypofluorescence and late staining of the lesion. Computed tomography may reveal subtle choroidal calcification in the affected eye or reveal subclinical calcification in the ophthalmoscopically "normal" fellow eye. Optical coherence tomography may reveal irregular platelike high-signal intensity areas within the tumor and posterior tracks of high reflectivity.

Differential Diagnosis

Differential diagnosis includes amelanotic choroidal melanoma, choroidal metastasis, choroidal hemangioma, primary choroidal lymphoma, posterior scleritis, and sclerochoroidal calcification. Melanoma and lymphoma can be distinguished by their lower reflectivity on ultrasonography. Metastatic lesions may have a similar appearance but are typically multiple and discovered in patients with a known primary tumor. Choroidal hemangioma with overlying calcified RPE shows early diffuse hyperfluorescence on fluorescein angiography in contrast to the patchy hyperfluorescence seen with choroidal osteoma. Posterior scleritis is suggested by clinical history (e.g., pain, erythema, concurrent autoimmune disease) and usually demonstrates retrobulbar edema on ultrasonography. Sclerochoroidal calcification is the abnormal deposition of calcium in the sclera and, often, the adjacent choroid in an elderly individual. Although it appears to have increased prevalence in patients with disorders of calcium, phosphorus, or magnesium homeostasis (including congenital disorders such as Bartter syndrome and Gitelman syndrome), it has since been reported that most patients with sclerochoroidal calcification have no demonstrable metabolic abnormality. Calcification in these patients is generally believed to be secondary to a benign age-related degenerative process. The typical appearance is that of bilateral, multiple, round, yellow-white nodules with ill-defined margins clustered in the mid-periphery (Fig. 52.3). The lesions may be flat or minimally elevated and are often associated with overlying RPE atrophy. In the vast majority of patients, the ocular manifestations are stable and have no effect on visual function. The overall prognosis is excellent.

Prophylaxis

None

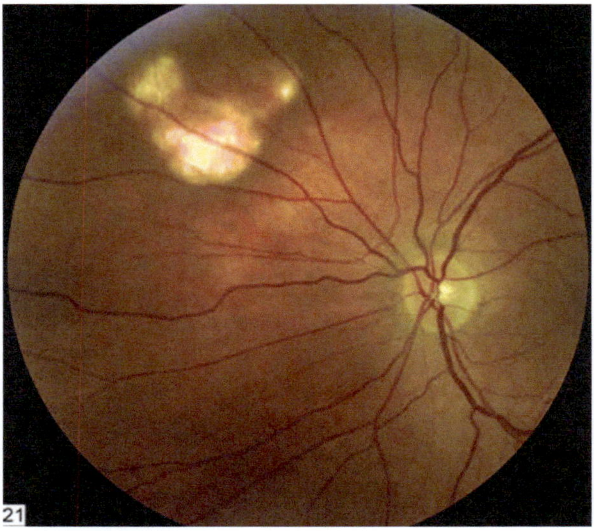

Fig. 52.3 Sclerochoroidal calcification in the superior nasal mid-periphery of the left eye

Therapy

There is no primary treatment for choroidal osteoma. Therapy is aimed at management of local complications, the most common of which is CNV (up to 50% of patients at 10 years). When indicated, treatment may consist of laser photocoagulation, photodynamic therapy, or antiangiogenic pharmacotherapy. Laser photocoagulation may be of limited benefit in these patients due to its poor uptake in a hypopigmented mass. Photodynamic therapy has the advantage of targeting the choroidal vasculature while sparing the overlying retina. Antiangiogenic (anti-VEGF) therapy, albeit novel, may offer comparable success with a good safety profile.

Prognosis

Due to the high rate of CNV, associated RPE degeneration, and the tendency of lesions to involve the macula, visual acuity is ultimately worse than 20/200 in most eyes after extended follow-up.

Epidemiology

Patients are predominantly young females (9:1 F/M ratio) with a mean age of 21.

Cross-References

Choroidal melanoma, Choroidal metastasis, Choroidal hemangioma, Primary choroidal lymphoma

Further Reading

Honavar SG, Shields CL, Demirci H, Shields JA (2001) Sclerochoroidal calcification: clinical manifestations and systemic associations. Arch Ophthalmol 119:833–840
Kadrmas EF, Weiter JJ (1997) Choroidal osteoma. Int Ophthalmol Clin 37:171–182
Schachat AP, Robertson DM, Mieler WF et al (1992) Sclerochoroidal calcification. Arch Ophthalmol 110:196–199
Shields CL, Shields JA, Augsburger JJ (1988) Choroidal osteoma. Surv Ophthalmol 33:17–27
Singh AD (2007) Clinical ophthalmic oncology. Saunders-Elsevier, Philadelphia, pp 305–310

Peripheral Nerve Sheath Tumors of Uveal Tract

53

Qing Zhang, Chris Bergstrom, and Hans E. Grossniklaus

Synonyms

Uveal schwannoma, Neurilemoma, Neurinoma, Neurofibroma.

Definition

Peripheral nerve sheath tumors describe a category of slow-growing tumors that mainly affect the head, neck, and extremities. These tumors arise in the sheath of peripheral nerves and can be subclassified as schwannoma or neurofibroma. Schwannoma is a tumor composed of a pure proliferation of Schwann cells, and neurofibroma is a tumor composed of a proliferation of Schwann cells, endoneural fibroblasts, and axons. Malignant peripheral nerve sheath tumors include malignant schwannoma, neurofibrosarcoma, perineural fibrosarcoma, and neurogenic sarcoma. Rarely, these tumors arise from ciliary nerves in the uvea or sclera and present as an intraocular mass.

Q. Zhang, M.D. (✉) • C. Bergstrom, M.D.
Department of Ophthalmology,
Emory University School of Medicine,
Atlanta, GA, USA
e-mail: qzhang7@emory.edu; cbergs2@emory.edu

H.E. Grossniklaus, M.D.
Emory University School of Medicine, Emory Eye Center,
Department of Ophthalmology,
Atlanta, GA, USA
e-mail: ophtheg@emory.edu

H.E. Grossniklaus (ed.), *Pocket Guide to Ocular Oncology and Pathology*,
DOI 10.1007/978-3-642-29782-3_53, © Springer-Verlag Berlin Heidelberg 2013

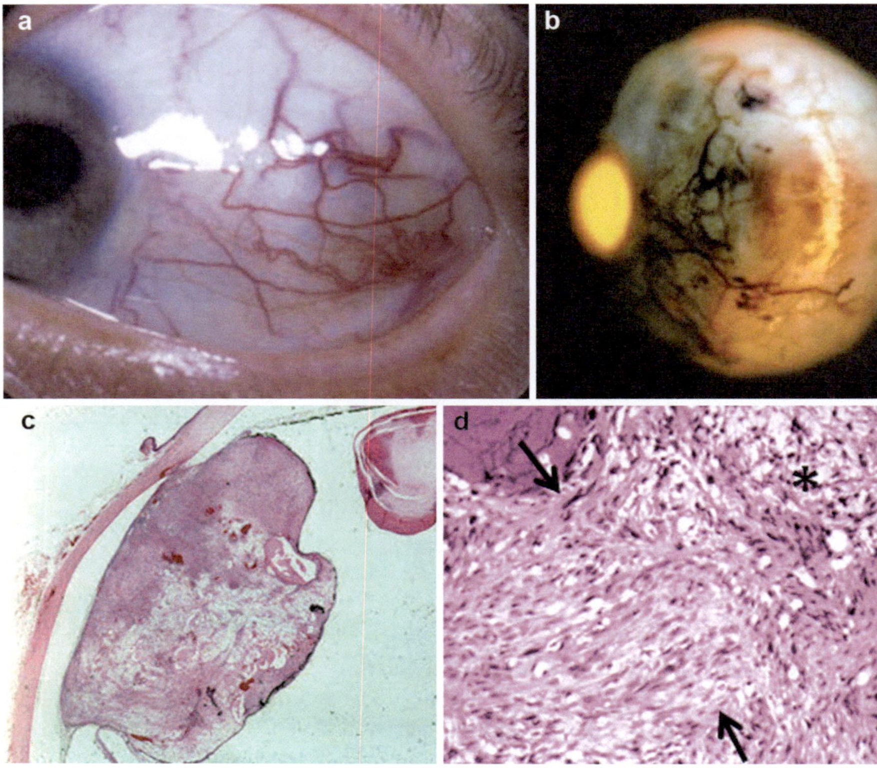

Fig. 53.1 (**a**) Clinical appearance with sentinel vessels over ciliary body. (**b**) Transillumination shows that the ciliary body mass transmits and does not block light. (**c**) There is an amelanotic tumor in the ciliary body. (**d**) The tumor is composed of compact fascicles between *arrows* (Antoni A pattern) and loosely cohesive (*) cells (Antoni B pattern) (**c**, hematoxylin and eosin, 2×; **d**, hematoxylin and eosin, 100×)

Etiology

These tumors are usually isolated with 10% of cases associated with a systemic disorder such as neurofibromatosis.

Clinical Presentation

Uveal schwannoma and neurofibroma typically presents as an amelanotic mass in the ciliary body or choroid (Fig. 53.1). A diffuse presentation throughout the uveal tract has been described.

Diagnostics

Diagnosis is made histologically, either by a fine-needle aspiration biopsy (FNAB), resection, or enucleation. It is not possible to differentiate uveal schwannoma or neurofibroma from melanoma on clinical exam or with ancillary testing. The presence of systemic finding of NF1 can help support the diagnosis of a nerve sheath tumor.

Pathology

Histologically, a uveal schwannoma appears as an elevated, circumscribed thickening of the uvea. It is composed of interwoven bundles of nonpigmented spindle-shaped cells. The cells have slender vesicular nuclei without prominent nucleoli. Antoni A pattern is where cells are arranged in a fascicular pattern with palisading nuclei. Antoni B pattern is characterized by a mucoid stroma. Verocay bodies may develop which are clusters of cells in areas of the tumor that resemble sensory corpuscles. Uveal neurofibroma is featured as spindle-shaped cells arranged in ribbons and cords in a matrix of myxoid tissue and contains axons.

Differential Diagnosis

The differential diagnosis includes uveal melanoma, metastatic tumors, and uveal lymphoma.

Prophylaxis

None

Therapy

Small anterior tumors may be diagnosed after resection. Others are diagnosed following enucleation for presumed melanoma. Since they can be mistaken for melanoma, it is likely that some are treated with brachytherapy.

Prognosis

Uveal schwannoma and neurofibroma are mostly benign tumors without metastatic potential; however, the ocular prognosis is guarded since they can show slow progressive growth and fill the entire globe.

Epidemiology

These tumors can occur sporadically or in association with neurofibromatosis type 1.

Cross-Reference

Phakomatoses

Further Reading

Dabbs DJ (2006) Diagnostic immunohistochemistry, 2nd edn. Churchill Livingstone, Philadelphia, pp 785–786

Jakobiec FA (1978) Ocular and adnexal tumors, vol 679, 1st edn. Aesculapius, Birmingham, 679, pp. 413–419. William H (1996) Spencer. Ophthalmic pathology, 4th edn. Saunders, Philadelphia, pp 2641–2662

Shields JA, Shields CL (1992) Intraocular tumors: a text and atlas, 1st edn. Saunders, Philadelphia, pp 285–295

Singh AD, Damato BE, Pe'er J, Murphree AL, Perry JD (eds) (2007) Clinical ophthalmic oncology. Saunders-Elsevier, Philadelphia

Uveal Metastatic Tumors

54

Jeffrey Yau Huei Chung, Arun D. Singh, Chris Bergstrom, and Hans E. Grossniklaus

Synonyms

Uveal metastases, choroidal metastasis

Definition

Spread of tumor from a distant location through blood or lymph channels to the iris, ciliary body, or the choroid of the eye. The choroid is the most common location of uveal metastasis, followed by iris and ciliary body. Up to half of patients present with bilateral metastasis.

J.Y.H. Chung, M.D.
Cole Eye Institute, Cleveland Clinic Foundation
9500 Euclid Avenue i-32, Cleveland, OH 44120, USA

A.D. Singh, M.D. (✉)
Department of Ophthalmic Oncology,
Cole Eye Institute, Cleveland Clinic Foundation
9500 Euclid Ave, Desk i-329, Cleveland, OH 44120, USA
e-mail: singha@ccf.org

C. Bergstrom, M.D.
Department of Ophthalmology, Emory University School of Medicine,
Atlanta, GA, USA
e-mail: cbergs2@emory.edu

H.E. Grossniklaus, M.D.
Emory University School of Medicine,
Emory Eye Center,
Department of Ophthalmology,
Atlanta, GA, USA
e-mail: ophtheg@emory.edu

H.E. Grossniklaus (ed.), *Pocket Guide to Ocular Oncology and Pathology*,
DOI 10.1007/978-3-642-29782-3_54, © Springer-Verlag Berlin Heidelberg 2013

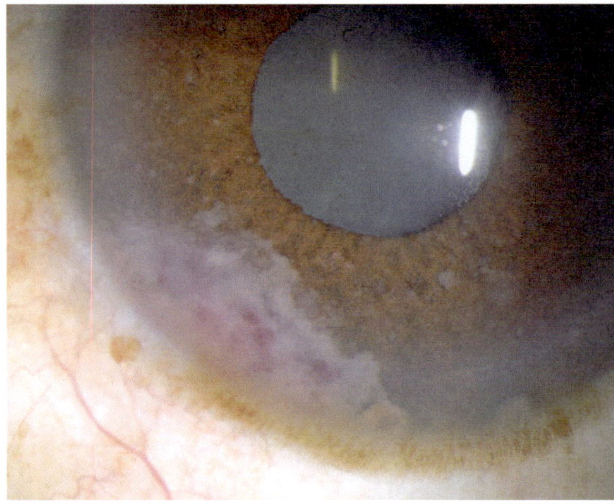

Fig. 54.1 Iris metastasis from renal cell carcinoma that initially presented with a hyphema

Etiology

The most common primary tumor sources are breast (47%), lung (21%), gastrointestinal tract (4%), kidney, skin, and prostate (2%). Breast cancer is the major source of metastasis in females, while lung cancer makes up 40% of source in males. Breast cancer commonly presents with bilateral metastasis. Other tumors that can metastasize to uvea include uterus, thyroid, pancreas, bladder, ovary, bile duct, testes, bone, and adrenal gland tumors.

Clinical Presentation

Presenting symptoms include blurred vision, scotoma, metamorphopsia, photopsia, floaters, and pain, or it may be asymptomatic. The majority of patients have decreased vision of 20/30 or worse caused mostly by exudative retinal detachment, progressive hypermetropia, or tumor growth in the visual axis. Iris metastases appear as a single yellow or white nodule at mid-iris, commonly in the inferior quadrant (Fig. 54.1). Glaucoma, irregular pupil, anterior segment inflammation, pseudohypopyon, and hyphema are commonly associated with iris and ciliary body metastases. Ciliary body metastases may be more difficult to detect. Choroidal metastases often present as a creamy dome or plateau-shaped subretinal mass commonly associated with exudative subretinal fluid. It is most commonly found posterior to the equator (92%) and in the lateral quadrants (Fig. 54.2).

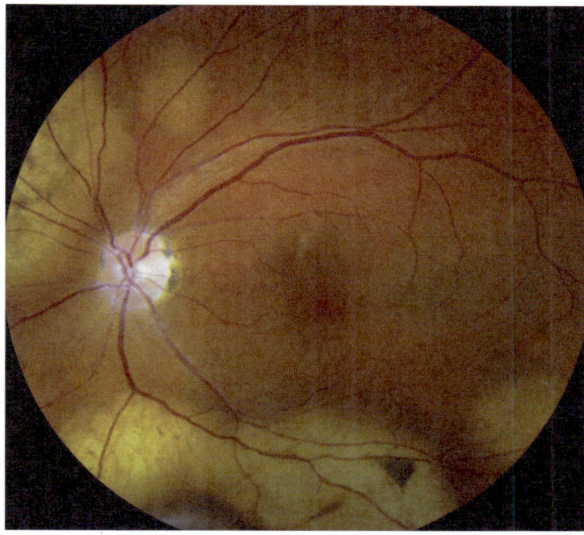

Fig. 54.2 Choroidal metastases from breast carcinoma presenting as multiple creamy dome-shaped subretinal masses

Diagnostics

Past medical history of malignancy and funduscopic exam are frequently all that is necessary to make the diagnosis of a metastatic choroidal tumor. Fluorescein angiogram shows blockage of choroidal flush, early hypofluorescence, and late leakage. Ultrasound may show moderate to high amplitude of internal reflectivity. MRI shows a lower T1 signal intensity than choroidal melanoma. As an initial step, a full systemic evaluation by oncologist is undertaken to detect a primary tumor, if unknown, and to identify other metastatic sites. Choroidal biopsy with immunostaining may be required to establish the diagnosis and find the location of the primary site.

Pathology

Most metastatic choroidal lesions are adenocarcinoma. Cytology and immunohistochemical staining features depend on the source of the primary tumor. A fine-needle aspiration biopsy, either transvitreally or transclerally, may be performed to obtain cells for a cytologic diagnosis (Figs. 54.3 and 54.4).

Differential Diagnosis

Amelanotic melanoma or nevus, lymphoma, choroidal hemangioma, choroidal osteoma, choroidal neovascularization, and posterior scleritis.

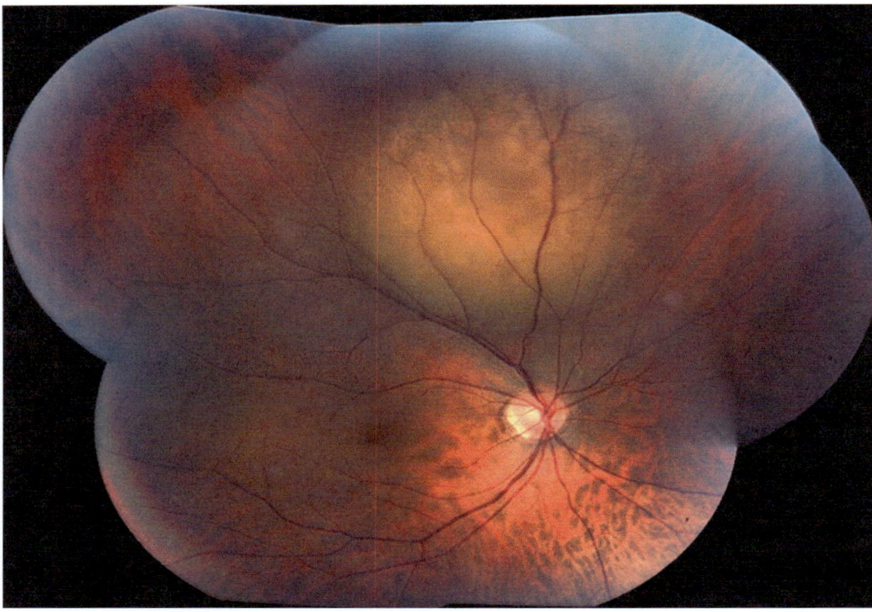

Fig. 54.3 Patient with metastatic breast carcinoma with single yellow choroidal mass

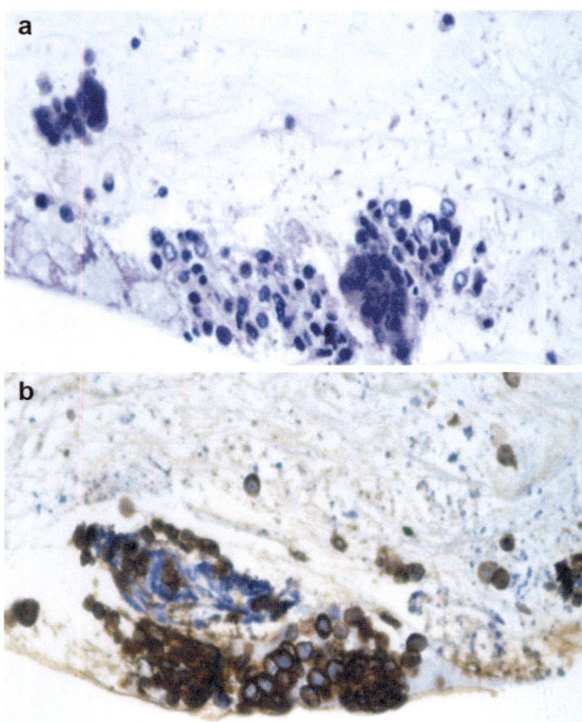

Fig. 54.4 A fine-needle aspiration biopsy (*FNAB*) was performed from the choroidal mass shown in Fig. 54.3. (**a**) There are clumps of cells with vesiculated pleomorphic nuclei and prominent nucleoli. (**b**) Immunohistochemical stains are positive for cytokeratins in the tumor cells, consistent with metastatic breast carcinoma (**a**, hematoxylin and eosin, 100×; **b**, peroxidase antiperoxidase, 100×)

Prophylaxis

Systemic treatment of known primary malignancy.

Therapy

Systemic chemotherapy or hormonal therapy is considered if there is evidence of metastasis elsewhere. If the metastasis is confined to the globe, then local therapy such as external beam radiation, plaque radiation, transpupillary thermotherapy, photodynamic therapy, and combination treatment may be used. External beam radiation treatment is given daily for 3–4 weeks for total dose of about 44 Gy. Complications include dry eye, cataract, and radiation retinopathy/neuropathy. Chemotherapy is reported to have a 65% response rate.

Prognosis

Uveal metastases occur relatively late in carcinoma. Between 70% and 86% of the patients have systemic metastasis elsewhere including lung, bone, liver, and CNS. Mean survival rate is 7–18 months from the time of uveal metastasis.

Epidemiology

Uveal metastasis is the most common uveal malignancy. In patients with carcinoma, the prevalence is 2–9%. Between 5% and 33% of patients with uveal metastasis as primary presentation have no history of cancer.

Cross-References

Choroidal melanoma, choroidal hemangioma, choroidal nevus, choroidal osteoma, surgical techniques

Further Reading

Bornfeld N (2007) Uveal metastatic tumors. In: Singh AD, Damato BE, Pe'er J, Murphree AL, Perry JD (eds) Clinical ophthalmic oncology. Saunders-Elsevier, Philadelphia, pp 322–327

Kanthan G, Jayamohan J, Yip D et al (2007) Management of metastatic carcinoma of the uveal tract: an evidence-based analysis. Clin Experiment Ophthalmol 35:553–565

Shields CL, Shields JA, Gross NE et al (1997) Survey of 520 eyes with uveal metastasis. Ophthalmology 104:1265–1276

Soysal HG (2007) Metastatic tumors of the uvea in 38 eyes. Can J Ophthalmol 42:832–835

Uveal Vascular Tumors 55

Mary E. Aronow, Arun D. Singh, and Chris Bergstrom

Synonyms

Circumscribed choroidal hemangioma, Localized choroidal hemangioma, Diffuse choroidal hemangioma

Definition

Uveal vascular tumors are benign, hamartomatous disorders classified as hemangiomas that occur in two distinct forms: circumscribed and diffuse.

Circumscribed Choroidal Hemangioma

Synonyms

Localized choroidal hemangioma

M.E. Aronow, M.D.
Department of Ophthalmic Oncology, Cole Eye Institute,
Cleveland Clinic Foundation, Cleveland, OH, USA

A.D. Singh, M.D. (✉)
Department of Ophthalmic Oncology,
Cole Eye Institute, Cleveland Clinic Foundation,
9500 Euclid Ave, Desk i-329, Cleveland, OH 44195, USA
e-mail: singha@ccf.org

C. Bergstrom, M.D.
Department of Ophthalmology,
Emory University School of Medicine,
Atlanta, GA, USA
e-mail: cbergs2@emory.edu

H.E. Grossniklaus (ed.), *Pocket Guide to Ocular Oncology and Pathology*,
DOI 10.1007/978-3-642-29782-3_55, © Springer-Verlag Berlin Heidelberg 2013

Definition

Circumscribed choroidal hemangiomas are benign vascular hamartomas that are likely congenital.

Etiology

These tumors typically occur sporadically in the absence of systemic disease.

Clinical Presentation

Although commonly asymptomatic, circumscribed choroidal hemangiomas can be associated with exudative retinal detachment resulting in reduced visual function, metamorphopsia, and photopsias.

Diagnostics

On ophthalmoscopic examination, a circumscribed choroidal hemangioma appears as an orange choroidal mass with indistinct margins that blend with the surrounding choroid (Fig. 55.1). They are frequently located in the macular region of the posterior pole and are not usually thicker than 6 mm. Although these tumors are highly vascular, dilated and tortuous feeder vessels are not typically observed. Surrounding subretinal fluid with exudative retinal detachment involving the macula is common in symptomatic cases (Fig. 55.2). Retinal hard exudates are minimal or absent. B-scan ultrasound shows a dome-shaped choroidal mass with smooth contours (Fig. 55.3a), and A-scan reveals high internal reflectivity (Fig. 55.3a). Fluorescein angiography demonstrates a lacy vascular network with early hyperfluorescence and variable leak-

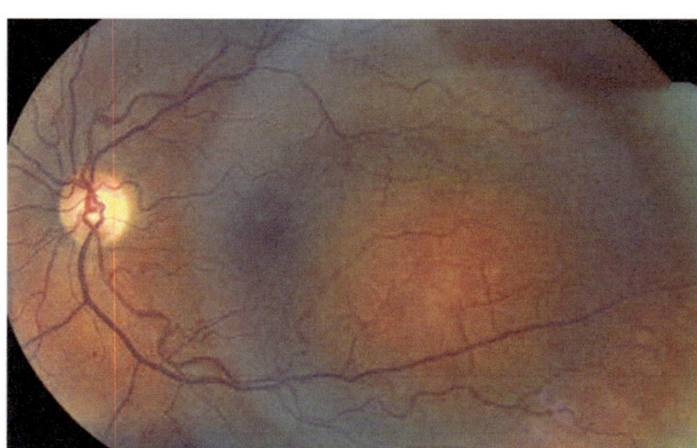

Fig. 55.1 Fundus photograph of a left eye with an asymptomatic circumscribed choroidal hemangioma

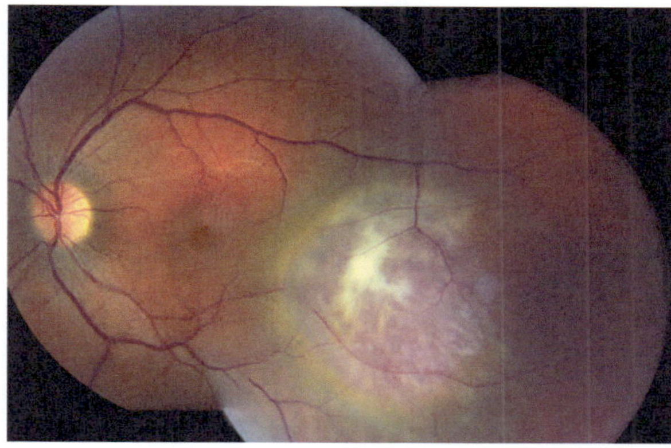

Fig. 55.2 Fundus photograph of a left eye with a symptomatic circumscribed choroidal hemangioma. Note the subretinal exudate and fluid involving the macula

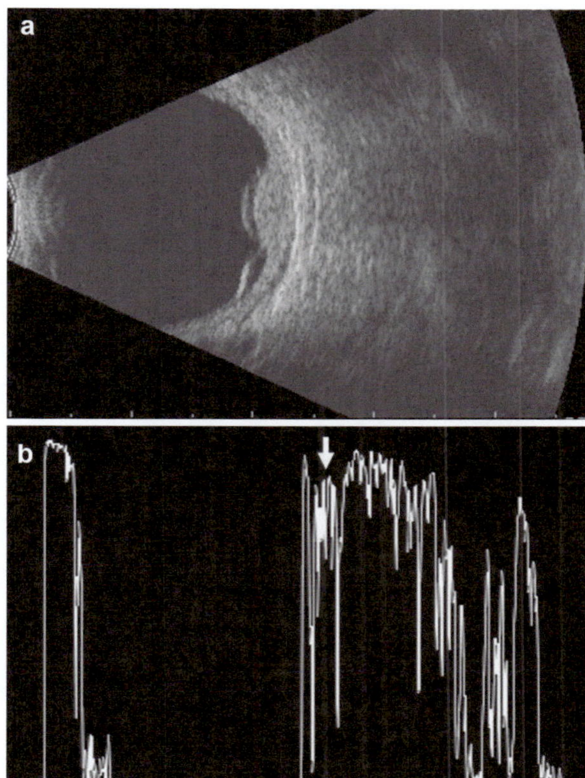

Fig. 55.3 B-scan ultrasound showing a smooth-contoured, dome-shaped choroidal mass (**a**). Diagnostic A-scan demonstrates high internal reflectivity (**b**)

age in late views (Fig. 55.4a). Indocyanine green angiography reveals intrinsic vasculature with a characteristic "dye washout" late in the study. Optical coherence tomography is helpful in evaluating secondary changes in the overlying retina (Fig. 55.4b).

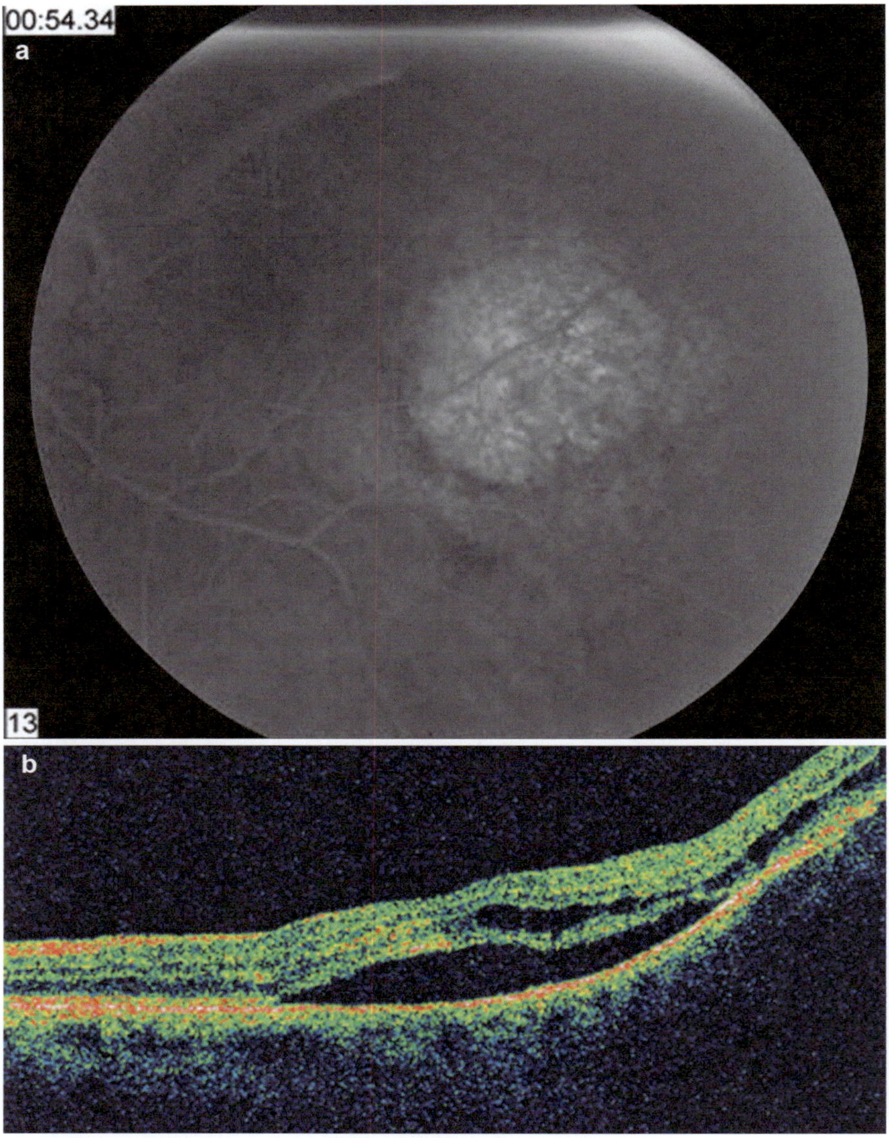

Fig. 55.4 Fluorescein angiography demonstrates a lacy vascular network with early hyperfluorescence (**a**). OCT of the same tumor showing retinal tilt with intraretinal and subretinal fluid (**b**)

Pathology

Hemangiomas of the choroid are classified histopathologically by the prevailing types of vessels within the tumor: capillary, cavernous, or mixed. The capillary type is composed of small vessels separated by loose connective tissue. The cavernous type is composed of larger vessels separated by little connective tissue.

Differential Diagnosis

Differential diagnosis includes: melanoma of the choroid, osteoma of the choroid, metastatic eye disease, granuloma of the choroid, posterior scleritis, or atypical central serous chorioretinopathy.

Prophylaxis

None

Therapy

Observation is warranted for asymptomatic cases. When vision loss occurs, therapy is aimed at inducing tumor atrophy with resolution of subretinal fluid and foveal distortion. Treatment options include photodynamic therapy, laser photocoagulation, transpupillary thermotherapy, and radiotherapy.

Prognosis

Long-term visual prognosis is poor secondary to vision loss induced by subretinal fluid, cystoid macular edema, foveal distortion, and treatment side effects.

Epidemiology

The incidence is unknown. These tumors typically present between the second and fourth decades of life. Nearly all cases reported have occurred in Caucasians, and there is no sex predilection.

Diffuse Choroidal Hemangioma

Synonyms

Choroidal hemangioma

Definition

Diffuse choroidal hemangiomas are benign vascular hamartomas that typically occur as part of neuro-oculocutaneous hemangiomatosis or Sturge-Weber syndrome.

Etiology

Diffuse choroidal hemangiomas are usually evident at birth and typically occur as part of neuro-oculocutaneous hemangiomatosis (Sturge-Weber syndrome).

Clinical Presentation

Diffuse choroidal hemangiomas may be asymptomatic. As with circumscribed hemangiomas, there may be associated exudative retinal detachment that often does not become manifest until adolescence. Symptoms include: reduced visual acuity, metamorphopsia, and photopsias. Leptomeningeal hemangiomatosis can lead to a seizure disorder in Sturge-Weber syndrome.

Diagnostics

Diffuse choroidal hemangiomas are typically unilateral and ipsilateral to the characteristic nevus flammeus or port-wine stain, seen in association with Sturge-Weber syndrome (Fig. 55.5). Clinically, these tumors appear as a red-orange, diffuse choroidal thickening (Fig. 55.6). The funduscopic appearance is described as a "tomato catsup" fundus. Focal regions of excessively thickened choroid within the diffuse hemangioma may simulate circumscribed hemangioma. There may be associated exudative retinal detachment (Fig. 55.5 inset). Glaucoma occurs in up to 70% of cases ipsilateral to the port-wine stain. Anisometropia with a hyperopic shift in the involved eye is common. B-scan ultrasound demonstrates a diffusely thickened choroid (Fig. 55.7a). A-scan ultrasound shows high internal reflectivity (Fig. 55.7b).

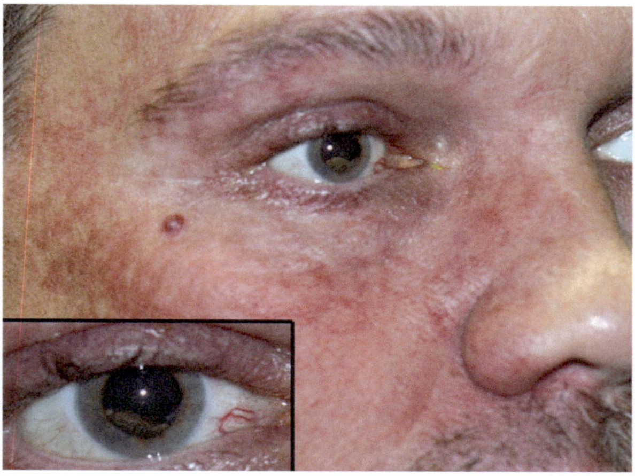

Fig. 55.5 Cutaneous hemangioma distribution typical of Sturge-Weber syndrome. Note the exudative retinal detachment in the right eye visible through the dilated pupil (*inset*)

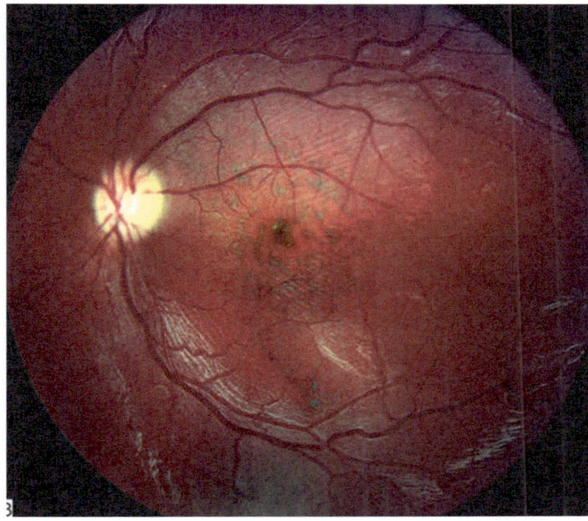

Fig. 55.6 Fundus photograph showing diffuse choroidal thickening with RPE changes due to chronic subretinal fluid

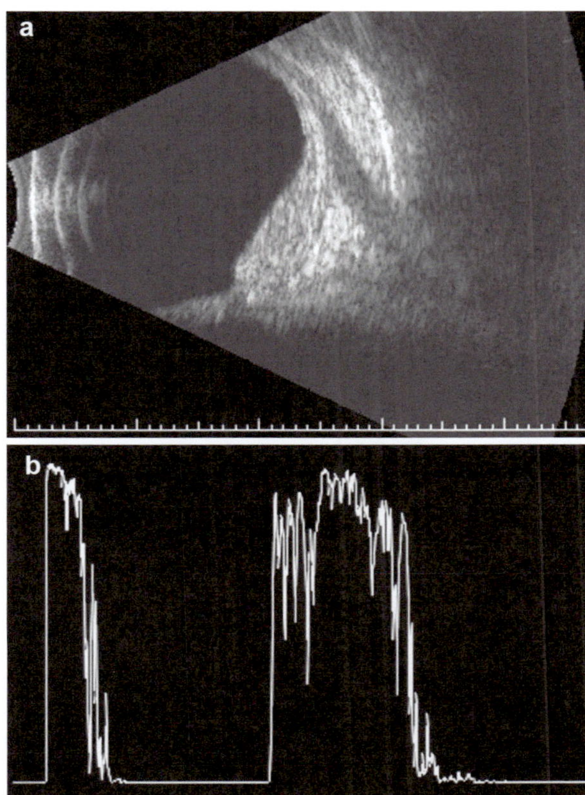

Fig. 55.7 B-scan ultrasonograph showing a diffusely thickened choroid mass (**a**) with high internal reflectivity on diagnostic A-scan (**b**)

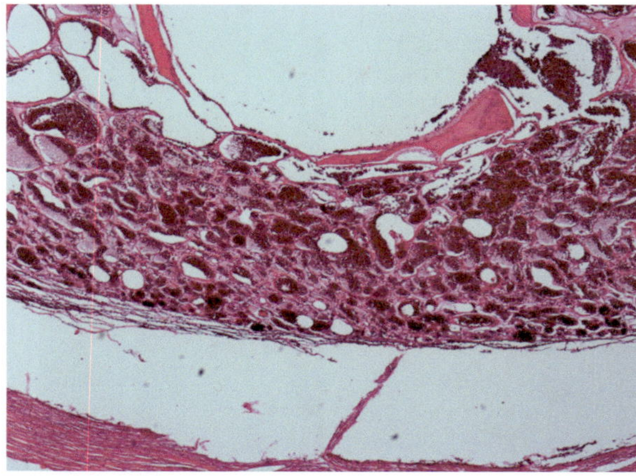

Fig. 55.8 A choroidal hemangioma contains dilated, thin-walled vascular channels that are congested with erythrocytes (hematoxylin and eosin, 25×)

Pathology

See circumscribed choroidal hemangioma. These tumors are composed collections of diffusely dilated thin-walled choroidal vascular channels which are congested with erythrocytes (Fig. 55.8).

Differential Diagnosis

In the setting of Sturge-Weber syndrome with typical cutaneous features, the diagnosis of diffuse choroidal hemangioma is straightforward.

Prophylaxis

None

Therapy

Observation is appropriate for asymptomatic cases. When visual loss occurs, therapy is aimed at inducing tumor atrophy and resolution of exudative retinal detachment and foveal distortion. Low-dose lens sparing radiotherapy and photodynamic therapy are currently the preferred methods of treatment. Recently, the use of oral propranolol has been shown to decrease exudation associated with these tumors. Diffuse choroidal hemangiomas are associated with variable visual loss secondary to exudative retinal detachment. Vision loss can also be caused by congenital glaucoma, which is also associated with Sturge-Weber syndrome.

Prognosis

The visual prognosis for patients with diffuse choroidal hemangioma is guarded.

Epidemiology

Approximately half of patients with Sturge-Weber syndrome have a diffuse choroidal hemangioma.

Cross-References

Choroidal melanoma, choroidal osteoma, choroidal metastasis

Further Reading

Schilling H, Sauerwein W, Lommatzsch A (1997) Long term results after low dose ocular irradiation for choroidal hemangioma. Br J Ophthalmol 81:267–273
Shields C, Honavar S, Shields J et al (2001) Circumscribed choroidal hemangioma: clinical manifestations and factors predictive of visual outcome in 200 consecutive cases. Ophthalmology 108:2237–2248
Singh A, Kaiser P (2007) Uveal vascular tumors. In: Singh A (ed) Clinical ophthalmic oncology, 1st edn. Saunders-Elsevier, Philadelphia, pp 289–299
Sullivan T, Clarke M, Morin J (1992) The ocular manifestations of the Sturge-Weber syndrome. J Pediatr Ophthalmol Strab 29:349–356
Witschel H, Font R (1976) Hemangioma of the choroid. A clinicopathologic study of 71 cases and a review of the literature. Surv Ophthalmol 20:415–431

Part VI

Uveal Tumors: Nevus and Melanoma

Uveal Tract Melanocytoma

56

Martina C. Herwig and Hans E. Grossniklaus

Synonyms

Magnocellular nevus

Definition

Melanocytomas of the uveal tract can affect the iris, ciliary body, and choroid. They are characterized by a benign nature and pigmented appearance with typical histological features and the ability for invasion of local tissues.

M.C. Herwig, M.D. (✉)
Department of Ophthalmology, University of Bonn,
Bonn, Germany

Department of Ophthalmology,
Emory University School of Medicine,
Atlanta, GA, USA
e-mail: martina.herwig@ukb.uni-bonn.de

H.E. Grossniklaus, M.D.
Emory University School of Medicine, Emory Eye Center,
Department of Ophthalmology,
Atlanta, GA, USA
e-mail: ophtheg@emory.edu

H.E. Grossniklaus (ed.), *Pocket Guide to Ocular Oncology and Pathology*,
DOI 10.1007/978-3-642-29782-3_56,

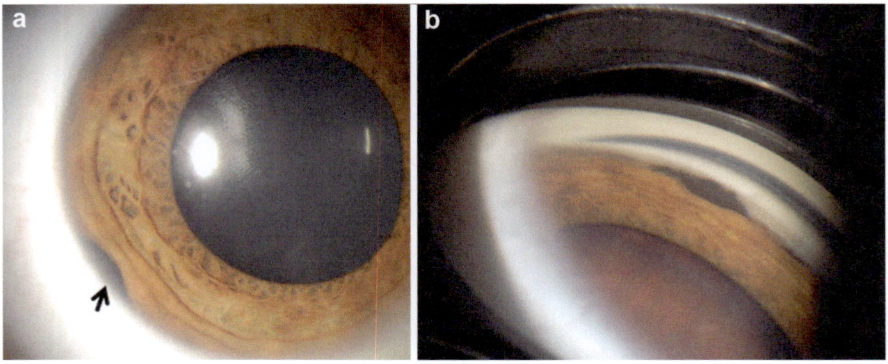

Fig. 56.1 Clinical picture of a dark-brown melanocytoma (*arrow*) involving the angle of the eye (**a**). Gonioscopic image of the same patient (**b**)

Etiology

Melanocytomas are a variant of melanocytic nevi and are thought to develop from proliferating melanocytes of the uvea.

Clinical Presentation

In uveal melanocytomas, necrosis and pigment dispersion may occur leading to discohesiveness of the tumor cells followed by seeding into the angle and secondary glaucoma.

The usual age of presentation for iris melanocytoma is the third or fourth decade of life. These tumors are nodular and deeply pigmented and have a predilection for involving the angle of the eye (Fig. 56.1). They lack intrinsic vascularity. Patients with iris melanocytoma are typically asymptomatic, and the lesion is discovered on routine examination or gonioscopy. Ciliary body melanocytoma are nodular and have a black appearance. They tend to extend into the anterior chamber and may present with extraocular extension mimicking a malignant tumor. Choroidal melanocytoma typically is dome-shaped and darkly pigmented. It can be indistinguishable from choroidal melanoma on ophthalmoscopy, angiography, and ultrasonography.

Diagnostics

In contrast to melanocytoma of the optic disc, the diagnosis of uveal melanocytoma is rarely made on clinical appearance because of the difficulty to distinguish it from malignant melanoma.

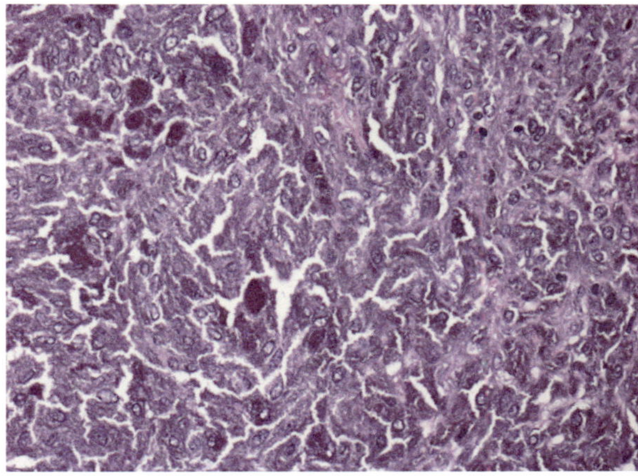

Fig. 56.2 Histopathology reveals predominantly necrotic tumor cells as well as polyhedral melanocytoma cells with small nuclei (hematoxylin and eosin, bleached, 100×)

Serial ultrasonography reveals a stable tumor although slow growth can occur. Fine-needle aspiration biopsy shows typical histologic features.

Pathology/Histology

Histology unequivocally confirms the diagnosis as it reveals a tumor composed of uniform deeply pigmented cells with melanosomes. After bleaching (Fig. 56.2), round or slightly polyhedral plump cells with abundant cytoplasm and small uniform nuclei with inconspicuous nucleoli (type I cells) as well as spindle-shaped, sparsely pigmented cells (type II cells) become visible. Scattered melanomacrophages can be observed. Mitotic figures are uncommon. Ciliary body melanocytomas may exhibit cystoid spaces.

Differential Diagnosis

Melanocytoma of the iris: malignant melanoma

Melanocytoma of the ciliary body: malignant melanoma, carcinoma, adenoma or adenocarcinoma of the pigmented ciliary body epithelium, medulloepithelioma, or hyperplasia of the pigmented ciliary epithelium (secondary to trauma or surgery)

Melanocytoma of the choroid: choroidal melanoma and congenital hypertrophy of the retinal pigment epithelium

Prophylaxis

None

Therapy

Melanocytomas are benign tumors that do not require treatment, except for secondary complications such as glaucoma. Since enlarging melanocytomas can be indistinguishable from melanoma using noninvasive studies, some are inevitably treated with surgery.

Prognosis

Melanocytomas are benign pigmented tumors with a good prognosis. Malignant transformation has been documented but is extremely uncommon.

Epidemiology

Unlike melanocytoma of the optic disc, most uveal tract melanocytomas occur in whites.

Cross-References

Melanocytoma optic nerve head, choroidal melanoma, iris melanoma, ciliary body melanoma

Further Reading

Baker-Griffith AE, McDonald PR, Green WR (1976) Malignant melanoma arising in a choroidal magnocellular nevus (melanocytoma). Can J Ophthalmol 11:140–146
Brownstein S, Dorey MW, Mathew B, Little JM, Lindley JI (2002) Melanocytoma of the choroid: atypical presentation and review of literature. Can J Ophthalmol 37:247–252
Green WR (1996a) Uveal tract. In: Spender WH (ed) Ophthalmic pathology: an atlas and textbook, 4th edn. WB Saunders Company, Philadelphia, pp 1608–1611
Green WR (1996b) Uveal tract. In: Spender WH (ed) Ophthalmic pathology: an atlas and textbook, 4th edn. WB Saunders Company, Philadelphia, pp 1679–1682
Green WR (1996c) Uveal tract. In: Spender WH (ed) Ophthalmic pathology: an atlas and textbook, 4th edn. WB Saunders Company, Philadelphia, pp 1699–1700
Juarez CP, Tso MO (1980) An ultrastructural study of melanocytomas (magnocellular nevi) of the optic disk and uvea. Am J Ophthalmol 90:48–62
Robertson DM, Campbell RJ, Salomao DR (2002) Mushroom-shaped choroidal melanocytoma mimicking malignant melanoma. Arch Ophthalmol 120:82–85

Uveal Tract Choroidal Melanoma

57

Claudia Perez-Straziota, Chris Bergstrom,
and Hans E. Grossniklaus

Synonyms

Uveal melanoma, Ocular melanoma

Definition

Choroidal melanoma is a proliferation of malignant neoplastic cells that primarily arises from the choroid of the eye. It is the most common primary intraocular malignant tumor. Choroidal melanoma can lead to vision loss or even death.

Etiology

The etiology of choroidal melanoma remains unknown. Among host factors, white race has the strongest association. Choroidal melanoma is rare in nonwhite races. Environmental factors such as sunlight and chemical exposure have been

C. Perez-Straziota, M.D. • C. Bergstrom, M.D.
Department of Ophthalmology,
Emory University School of Medicine,
Atlanta, GA, USA
e-mail: cbergs2@emory.edu

H.E. Grossniklaus, M.D.
Emory University School of Medicine,
Emory Eye Center,
Department of Ophthalmology,
Atlanta, GA, USA
e-mail: ophtheg@emory.edu

H.E. Grossniklaus (ed.), *Pocket Guide to Ocular Oncology and Pathology*,
DOI 10.1007/978-3-642-29782-3_57,

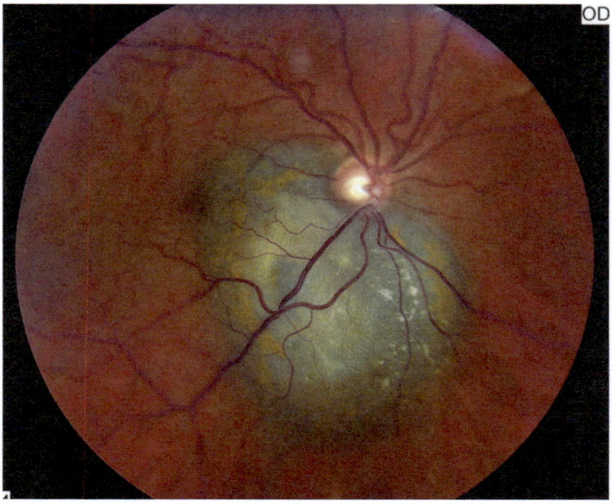

Fig. 57.1 A juxtapapillary dome-shaped choroidal melanoma with lipofuscin

investigated; however, none have been clearly implicated in the etiology of choroidal melanoma.

Clinical Presentation

Choroidal melanoma is most often diagnosed during a dilated fundus examination in a patient with a complaint of decreased visual acuity or blurred vision. Other common presenting symptoms include floaters, flashing lights, or visual field defects. Occasionally, choroidal melanoma is found during a routine dilated fundus examination in an asymptomatic patient.

Diagnostics

The diagnosis of choroidal melanoma is clinical, and the gold standard in making the diagnosis is the funduscopic examination. Combined with ultrasonography, the diagnostic accuracy exceeds 99% for medium- and large-sized tumors. Pigmentation can vary from amelanotic to deeply pigmented. RPE changes over the lesion or the presence of lipofuscin (orange pigment) are common (Fig. 57.1). Most choroidal melanomas are localized, dome-shaped tumors arising from the choroid. The characteristic collar-button configuration occurs when the tumor breaks through Bruch's membrane (Fig. 57.2). Subretinal fluid, exudative detachments, and rarely subretinal hemorrhage, choroidal hemorrhage, or vitreous hemorrhage can also be seen with choroidal melanoma. The most important ancillary study in the diagnosis of choroidal melanoma is ultrasound. On B-scan, the tumors are most often internally homogeneous. Diagnostic

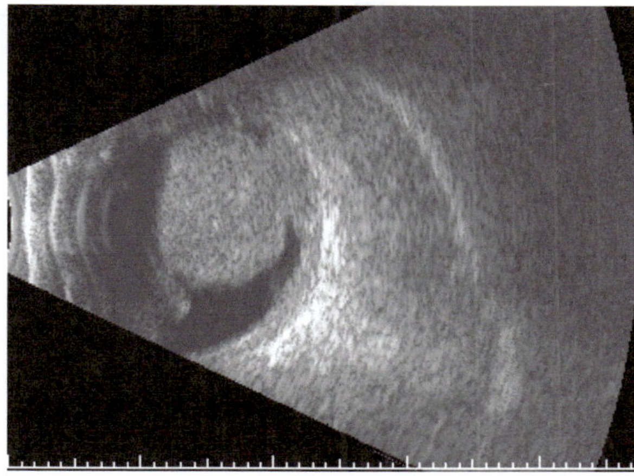

Fig. 57.2 B-scan ultrasound of a large choroidal melanoma with a collar-button configuration

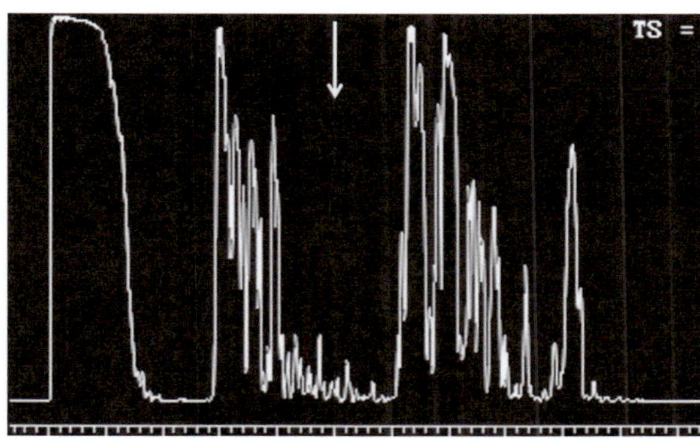

Fig. 57.3 A scan of the same tumor in Fig. 57.2 demonstrating low to medium internal reflectivity (*arrow*)

A-scan demonstrates characteristic low to medium internal reflectivity (Fig. 57.3). Fluorescein angiography may demonstrate an intrinsic tumor circulation (secondary circulation) in larger tumors. Rarely is biopsy required for diagnostic purposes.

Pathology

Spindle cell nevus: low nuclear-to-cytoplasmic ratios. No nucleoli or mitosis observed.

Spindle cell melanoma: higher nuclear-to-cytoplasmic ratios. Granular chromatin and large nuclei. Present mitotic figures and nucleoli but sparse.

Epithelioid melanoma: poorest prognosis. Cells have abundant eosinophilic cytoplasm and enlarged oval nuclei, therefore they resemble epithelial cells. Marked pleomorphism; nuclei with dense chromatin and prominent nucleoli.

Mixed-cell type: mixture of spindle and epithelioid cells (Figs. 57.4 and 57.5).

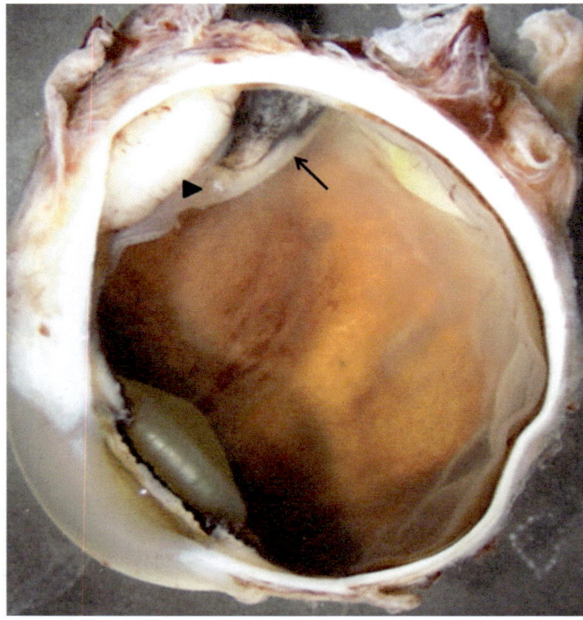

Fig. 57.4 This enucleated eye contains a choroidal melanoma that straddles the equator. A portion of the tumor is melanotic (*arrow*) and a portion is amelanotic (*arrowhead*)

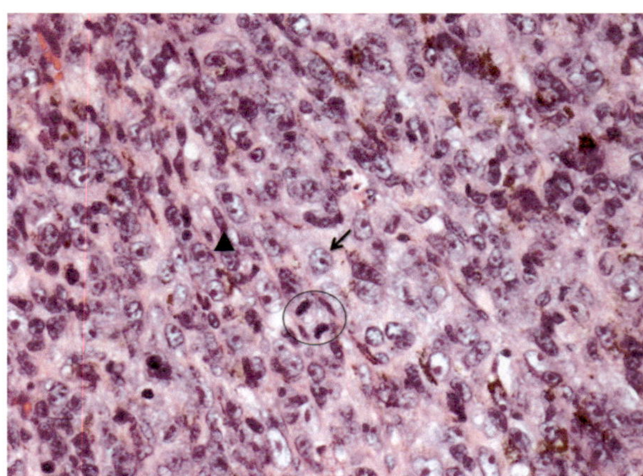

Fig. 57.5 The melanoma contains spindle (*arrowhead*) and epithelioid cells (*arrow*), making it mixed-cell type. A mitotic figure is observed (within *circle*) (hematoxylin and eosin, 100×)

Immunohistochemistry

Immunohistochemical stains that are usually positive in uveal melanoma include S100, HMB45, melan A, and microphthalmia transcription factor (MITF).

Electron Microscopy

The electron microscopic features of uveal melanoma include high nuclear-to-cytoplasm ratio, irregular nuclear chromatin, and intracytoplasmic melanin and melanin precursor granules.

Differential Diagnosis

Choroidal nevus, choroidal hemorrhage, disciform lesions, choroidal hemangioma, melanocytoma, choroidal osteoma, congenital hypertrophy of the retinal pigment epithelium, choroidal metastasis, posterior nodular scleritis

Prophylaxis

There is no known prophylaxis for choroidal melanoma.

Therapy

Brachytherapy using COMS dosing, proton beam radiotherapy, enucleation, thermotherapy, stereotactic radiotherapy, and surgical resection and observation are alternatives based on the size of the tumor, condition of the eye, institutional capabilities, and patient preference.

Prognosis

Tumor-related mortality rates from uveal melanoma approach 50% in some studies. Important clinical characteristics of uveal melanoma that portend a poorer prognosis include increased tumor thickness, larger basal diameter, advanced patient age, ciliary body location, extrascleral extension, subretinal fluid, and intraocular hemorrhage. It has been recently shown that for each millimeter of thickness, the metastatic risk increases by 5%. Cytogenetic testing on tumor specimens obtained from enucleated eyes or FNAB is superior in predicting metastatic risk when compared to high-risk clinical characteristics. Monosomy 3 and class 2 gene expression profiling have both correlated with a high risk of developing metastatic disease.

Epidemiology

Choroidal melanoma is an uncommon disease, with incidence ranging from 4 to 6 cases per million population. The rate is slightly higher in males than females. The incidence and mortality rates have been stable over the past several decades.

Cross-References

Ciliary body melanoma, choroid nevus, surgical techniques

Further Reading

Shetlar DJ, Chevez-Barros P, Dubovy S, Rosa Jr. RH, Syed N, Wilsen MW, Pelton RW, and Pe'er J. Publisehd by the American Academy of Ophthalmology, San Francisco, CA, USA

Dennis M, Robertson MD (2003) Changing concepts in the management of choroidal melanoma. Am J Ophthalmol 136(1):161–170

Oosterhuis JA (1995) Transpupillary thermotherapy in choroidal melanomas. Arch Ophthalmol 113:315–324

Oosterhuis JA et al (1998) Transpupillary thermotherapy results in 50 patients with choroidal melanoma. Arch Ophthalmol 116:157–162

Shields CL et al (2009) Metastasis of uveal melanoma millimeter-by-millimeter in 8033 consecutive eyes. Arch Ophthalmol 127(8):989–998

The Collaborative Ocular Melanoma Study Group (1997) Factors predictive of growth and treatment of small choroidal melanoma. COMS report no. 5. Arch Ophthalmol 115:1537–1544

The Collaborative Ocular Melanoma Study Group (1999) Mortality in patients with small choroidal melanoma. COMS report no. 4. Arch Ophthalmol 115:886–893

The Collaborative Ocular Melanoma Study Group (2001) Randomized trial of iodine 125 brachytherapy for choroidal melanoma III: initial mortality rates. COMS report no. 18. Arch Ophthalmol 119:969–982

Wilson DJ et al (2002) Choroidal melanoma treated with cryotherapy. Arch Ophthalmol 120:393–395

Choroidal Nevus

58

Arun D. Singh and Alexandre A.C.M. Ventura

Synonyms

None

Definition

A choroidal nevus is a benign melanocytic tumor of neural crest origin. According to the Collaborative Ocular Melanoma Study (COMS) criteria, a choroidal nevus is classified as a melanocytic choroidal lesion that is ≤5 mm in the largest basal dimension and is ≤1 mm in height.

Etiology

There is no known etiology for choroidal nevi.

Clinical Presentation

Choroidal nevi do not usually cause any symptoms, and most are diagnosed by routine ophthalmoscopy. A nevus in the macula can cause visual loss from photoreceptor atrophy, serous detachment, and choroidal neovascularization. Subretinal

A.D. Singh (✉)
Department of Ophthalmic Oncology, Cole Eye Institute, Cleveland Clinic Foundation,
9500 Euclid Ave, Desk i-329, Cleveland, OH 44195, USA
e-mail: singha@ccf.org

A.A.C.M. Ventura
Cole Eye Institute, Cleveland Clinic Foundation,
Cleveland, OH, USA

H.E. Grossniklaus (ed.), *Pocket Guide to Ocular Oncology and Pathology*,
DOI 10.1007/978-3-642-29782-3_58,

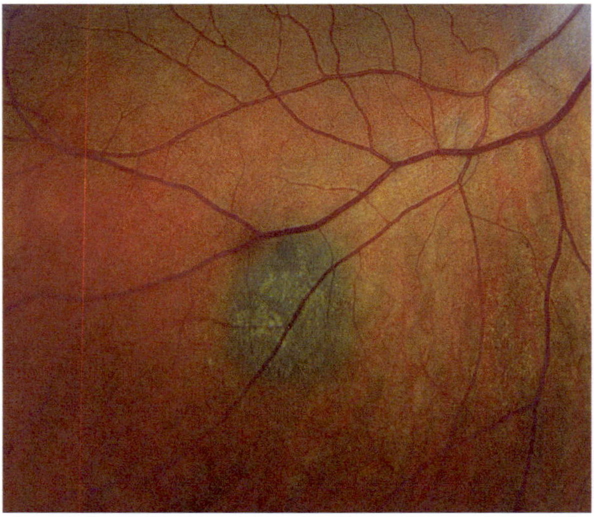

Fig. 58.1 This small choroidal nevus exhibits overlying drusen

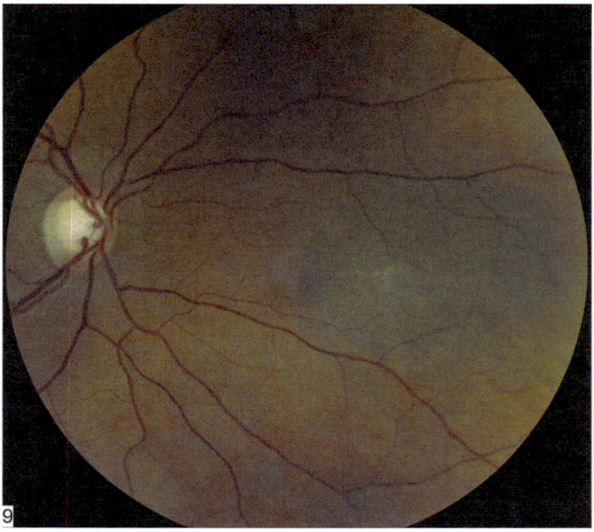

Fig. 58.2 This larger gray to black flat choroidal nevus has somewhat ill-defined borders

fluid in association with a nevus may induce symptoms of metamorphopsia or photopsia. Choroidal nevi appear as a slate-gray to brown lesions with minimal thickness, and the margins may be well defined or ill defined. These nevi range in size from small (Fig. 58.1) to large (Fig. 58.2). These lesions, especially large nevi, should be followed for the possible development of melanoma. The clinical features suspicious of melanoma are: symptoms, tumor size (basal diameter > 12 mm; height > 2 mm) and proximity to the optic nerve <2 mm, intrinsic vascularity on ICG,

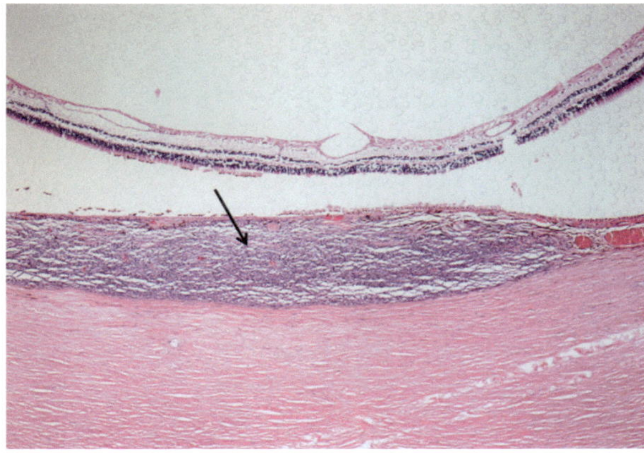

Fig. 58.3 A choroidal nevus (*arrow*) is composed of a cellular proliferation between Bruch's membrane and the sclera (hematoxylin and eosin, 10×)

presence of orange pigmentation, subretinal fluid, rapid growth, ultrasonographic hollowness, and absence of a halo. A recent long-term follow-up study showed that about 30% of choroidal nevi showed slight enlargement without clinical evidence of transformation into melanoma, and the frequency of enlargement was inversely related to patient age.

Diagnostics

Detailed dilated fundus exam with photographic documentation is utilized for documenting the appearance of the lesion. A and B ultrasonography scans are used to measure thickness and internal reflectivity. Fluorescein angiography (FA) and ocular coherence tomography (OCT) over the lesion may be performed but are not necessary to make the diagnosis of choroidal nevus.

Pathology

Four types of choroidal cells have been described: plump polyhedral, slender spindle, plump fusiform dendritic, and balloon cells. These cells contain bland nuclear chromatin (Figs. 58.3 and 58.4). In the modified Callender's classification of uveal melanoma, tumors composed entirely of spindle A cells are regarded as nevi.

Differential Diagnosis

The differential diagnosis includes choroidal melanoma, RPE hyperplasia, congenital hypertrophy of the RPE, melanocytoma, suprachoroidal hemorrhage, atypical disciform scar associated with AMD, and choroidal hemangioma with RPE hyperpigmentation.

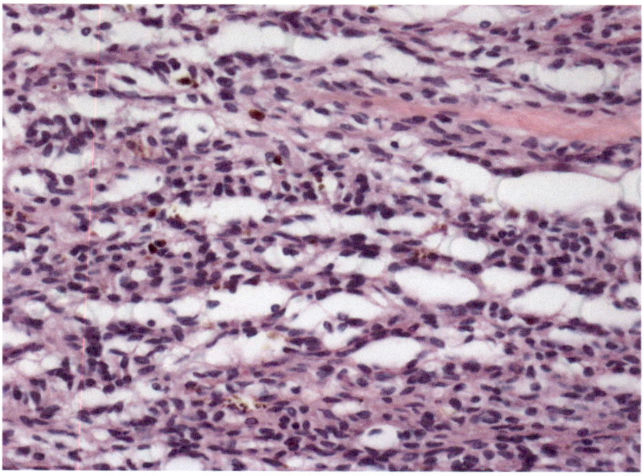

Fig. 58.4 Closer inspection of the choroidal nevus shown in Fig. 58.3 shows that it is composed of spindle-shaped cells with bland nuclei (hematoxylin and eosin, 100×)

Prophylaxis

There is no prophylaxis for this lesion.

Therapy

Generally, no treatment is necessary. Lesions are followed by serial photography and ultrasonography. In cases of subretinal fluid causing decreased vision, light laser photocoagulation may be applied.

Prognosis

The prognosis for choroidal nevi is excellent.

Epidemiology

Choroidal nevi may occur in 7% of the population. The risk of malignant transformation is 1 in 8,845 (1 in 269,565 for 15–19 years of age and 1 in 3,664 for those 80–84 years of age).

Cross-References

Choroidal melanoma, ultrasound techniques

Further Reading

Ophthalmic pathology and intraocular tumors. American Academy of ophthalmology basic and clinical science course. 2006–2007. pp 156–157

Jakobiec FA, Silbert G (1981) Are most iris 'melanomas' really nevi? A clinicopathologic study of 189 lesions. Arch Ophthalmol 99:2117–2132

Shields JA, Karan DS, Perry HD, Donosa LA (1985) Epithelioid cell nevus of the iris. Arch Ophthalmol 1–3:235–237

Singh AD (2007) Clinical ophthalmic oncology. WB Saunders Company, Philadelphia, pp 185–186

Ciliary Body Melanoma

59

Harry H. Brown and Chris Bergstrom

Synonyms

Ciliary body melanoma, Ring melanoma

Definition

Ciliary body melanoma is a malignant tumor that arises in the ciliary body. It may be circumscribed or annular (ring).

Etiology

No definite causes for ciliary body melanoma have been identified; risk factors include ocular melanocytosis and xeroderma pigmentosum. An association with sunlight exposure is controversial.

H.H. Brown, M.D. (✉)
Department of Pathology, University of Arkansas School of Medicine,
Harvey and Bernice Jones Eye Institute, University of Arkansas for Medical Sciences,
Little Rock, AR, USA
e-mail: brownharryh@uams.edu

C. Bergstrom, M.D.
Department of Ophthalmology, Emory University School of Medicine,
Atlanta, GA, USA
e-mail: cbergs2@emory.edu

H.E. Grossniklaus (ed.), *Pocket Guide to Ocular Oncology and Pathology*,
DOI 10.1007/978-3-642-29782-3_59, © Springer-Verlag Berlin Heidelberg 2013

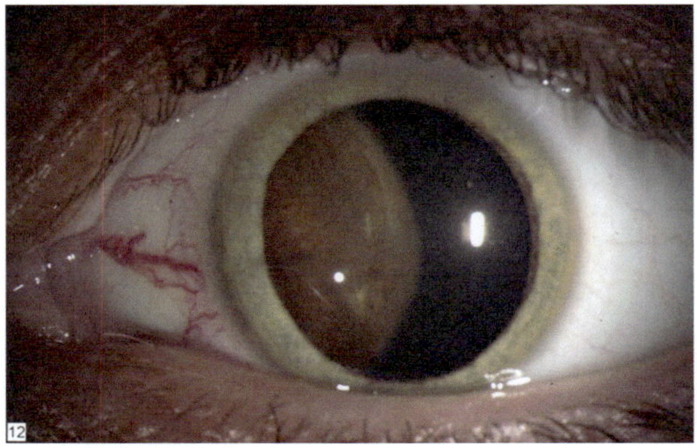

Fig. 59.1 Large ciliary body melanoma. Note the prominent sentinel vessels

Clinical Presentation

Malignant melanoma of the ciliary body is often delayed in recognition by the patient and the clinician due to the absence of symptoms and the location of the ciliary body, posterior to the iris and peripheral to the lens. Tumors that involve the anterior face of the ciliary body may be visible on biomicroscopy and gonioscopy, and if angle structures are affected may result in elevated intraocular pressure. Tumors that encroach on the lens may cause visual difficulties due to cataract and/or lens displacement. Extrascleral extension along emissarial channels may be visible as acquired pigmentation of the sclera. A prominent episcleral "sentinel" vessel may also be a clue as to the presence of a ciliary body melanoma (Fig. 59.1).

Diagnostics

The clinical diagnosis is suggested by the signs mentioned above. Visualization of the ciliary body requires a widely dilated pupil or the use of a Goldmann 3-mirror lens at the time of biomicroscopy. Ultrasound biomicroscopy may be helpful in confirming and delineating the presence of a mass lesion. Melanomas of the ciliary body may grow in a diffuse circumferential pattern rather than an elevated circumscribed mass; such tumors are termed ring melanoma. Melanomas of the ciliary body and choroid may be treated presumptively, that is, without pathological tissue confirmation of the diagnosis.

Pathology

Pathological specimens demonstrate proliferation of uveal melanocytes, enlarging the ciliary body proper. Tumor cells may spread anteriorly to involve the iris and anterior chamber angle or posteriorly into the choroid (Fig. 59.2). Histological examination shows some combination of two types of melanocytes: spindle cells with elongated nuclei and inconspicuous nucleoli, and epithelioid cells with rounded nuclei and prominent nucleoli (Fig. 59.3).

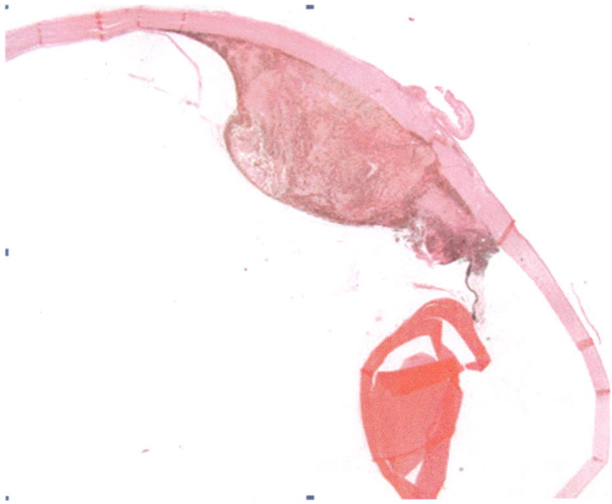

Fig. 59.2 Ciliary body melanoma with invasion of the iris and anterior chamber angle anteriorly and the peripheral choroid posteriorly (hematoxylin and eosin, 10×)

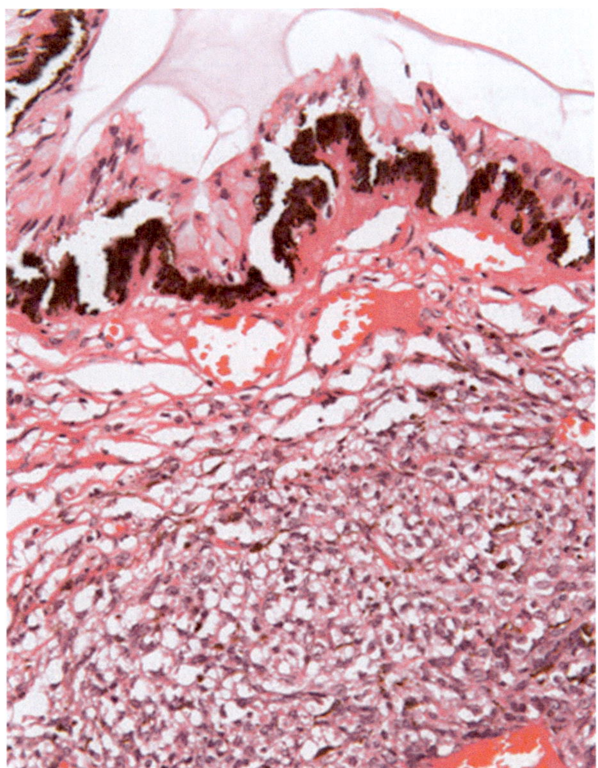

Fig. 59.3 Predominantly epithelioid cell-type ciliary body melanoma. Note the normal overlying pigmented and nonpigmented ciliary epithelium (hematoxylin and eosin, 100×)

Differential Diagnosis

The differential diagnosis includes benign melanocytic proliferations (nevus, melanocytoma), tumors of stromal lineage (leiomyoma, schwannoma), and tumors of ciliary epithelium (adenoma, adenocarcinoma, medulloepithelioma).

Prophylaxis

There is no prophylactic treatment for ciliary body melanoma.

Therapy

Treatment consists of either radiation or surgical extirpation. Radiation usually delivered using brachytherapy using COMS doses or proton beam irradiation. Surgical treatment is either local resection (iridocyclectomy) or enucleation. The treatment options are based on size and extent of the tumor as well as patient preference.

Prognosis

Prognostic factors include tumor basal diameter, cell type, and chromosomal aberration: larger tumors and especially ring configuration, epithelioid cell type, class 2 gene expression profile, and monosomy 3 are all unfavorable findings.

Epidemiology

Occurrence in Caucasians predominates, but other ethnicities may rarely be afflicted; males are slightly more predisposed than females. Melanomas are rare in children and increase in incidence with increasing age, reaching a peak in the sixth to seventh decades.

Cross-References

Choroidal melanoma, surgical techniques

Further Reading

Demirci H, Shields CL, Shields JA et al (2002) Ring melanoma of the ciliary body: report on twenty-three patients. Retina 22:698–706

Laver NV, McLaughlin ME, Duker JS (2010) Ocular melanoma. Arch Pathol Lab Med 134:1778–1784

Simpson ER (2004) Ciliary body melanoma: a special challenge. Can J Ophthalmol 39:365–371

Singh AD, Turell ME, Topham AK (2011) Uveal melanoma: trends in incidence, treatment, and survival. Ophthalmology 118:1881–1885

Ciliary Body Nevus

60

Hans E. Grossniklaus

Synonyms

Melanocytic nevus, melanocytoma (special form of nevus)

Definition

A ciliary body nevus is a proliferation of nevocellular nevus cells within the stroma of the ciliary body.

Etiology

Ciliary body nevi are due to full thickness stromal growth of nevus cells. There may be an increased incidence of ciliary body nevi in ocular and oculodermal melanocytosis (see Chapters 59 and 75). There also might be an increased incidence in patients with dysplastic nevus syndrome.

H.E. Grossniklaus, M.D.
Emory University School of Medicine, Emory Eye Center,
Department of Ophthalmology,
Atlanta, GA, USA
e-mail: ophtheg@emory.edu

H.E. Grossniklaus (ed.), *Pocket Guide to Ocular Oncology and Pathology*,
DOI 10.1007/978-3-642-29782-3_60,

Clinical Presentation

Ciliary body nevi are asymptomatic and are often an incidental finding in examination of an eye-bank eye or surgically enucleated eye. A ciliary body melanocytoma may present as a darkly pigmented ciliary body mass seen on examination of the pars plana/ora serrata area in dilated fundus examination. Transillumination will block light.

Diagnosis

Diagnosis is clinically made by serial observation without evidence of growth. A trans-scleral or anterior chamber fine-needle aspiration biopsy may be performed which will yield nevus cells.

Pathology

The nevus is composed of spindle, fusiform, plump polyhedral, or balloon nevus cells. A melanocytoma is composed of heavily pigmented plump polyhedral cells and may extend into the angle (Figs. 60.1, 60.2, and 60.3). It may be histologically difficult to distinguish between melanoma cells and melanocytoma cells in some instances.

Differential Diagnosis

The differential diagnosis includes melanoma, melanocytoma, suprachoroidal hemorrhage, leiomyoma, peripheral nerve sheath tumor, tumor of ciliary epithelium (adenoma, adenocarcinoma), and metastatic carcinoma.

Prophylaxis

There is no known prophylaxis for ciliary body nevus.

Therapy

The treatment of choice is observation. It is possible that a melanoma may arise in a nevus. The nevus should be followed by ultrasound examination and clinical examination, including examination of the irido-corneal angle, iris, anterior chamber, and a dilated fundus examination. Signs of growth are worrisome for melanoma (see Chap. 59). At that time, radioactive plaque brachytherapy, iridocyclectomy/eye wall resection, or enucleation, depending on the patient's health, condition of the eye and fellow eye may be elected.

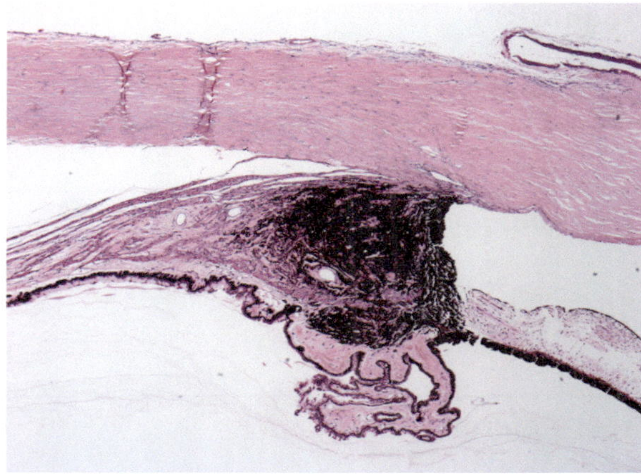

Fig. 60.1 This nevus (melanocytoma) was incidentally found in an eye-bank eye as a heavily pigmented lesion in the ciliary body (hematoxylin and eosin, 10×)

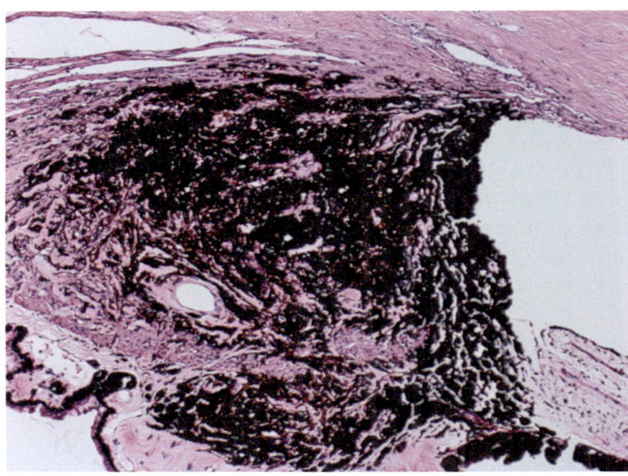

Fig. 60.2 The ciliary body melanocytoma extends into the angle, where it would have been able to be visualized gonioscopically (hematoxylin and eosin, 25×)

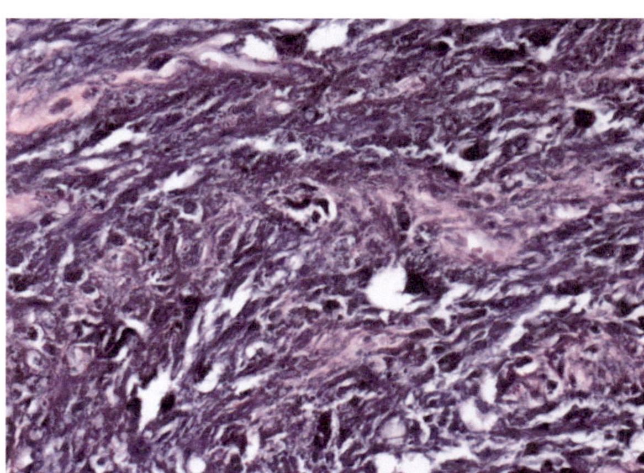

Fig. 60.3 The ciliary body melanocytoma is composed of polyhedral melanocytes with bland nuclei (bleached, hematoxylin and eosin, 100×)

Prognosis

The prognosis for nevus is excellent for both vision, preservation of the eye and life. If the nevus progresses to melanoma, the prognosis is guarded.

Epidemiology

The frequency of ciliary body nevus appears to be similar in men and women and may increase with age.

Cross-References

Ciliary body melanoma, phakomatoses

Further Reading

Shetlar DG, Chevez-barrios P, Dubovy S, Rosa RH, Syed N, Wilson MW, Pelton RW, Pe'er J. Ophthalmic Pathology and Intraocular Tumors. Section 4, Basic and Clinical Science Text, American Academy of Ophthalmology, 2007–2008, p 187

Green WR (1996) The uveal tract. In: Spencer WH (ed) Ophthalmic pathology: an atlas and textbook, 4th edn. Saunders, Philadelphia, pp 1699–1712

Singh AD (2007) Tumors of the uvea: benign melanocytic tumors. In: Singh AD, Damato BE, Pe'er J (eds) Clinical ophthalmic oncology. Saunders, Philadelphia, pp 187–190

Iris Melanoma

61

Jill R. Wells and Hans E. Grossniklaus

Synonyms

There are no synonyms for iris melanoma.

Definition

Iris melanoma is a malignant melanocytic uveal tumor of the iris.

Etiology

The etiology is unknown, although there is some weak evidence of sun exposure as a risk factor.

Clinical Presentation

This tumor may occur as a circumscribed (Fig. 61.1), diffuse, or tapioca-like lesion on the iris. A diffuse iris melanoma can be a result of primary infiltration of

J.R. Wells, M.D. (✉)
Department of Ophthalmology, Emory University School of Medicine,
Atlanta, GA, USA
e-mail: Jwells4@emory.edu

H.E. Grossniklaus, M.D.
Emory University School of Medicine,
Emory Eye Center,
Department of Ophthalmology,
Atlanta, GA, USA
e-mail: ophtheg@emory.edu

H.E. Grossniklaus (ed.), *Pocket Guide to Ocular Oncology and Pathology*,
DOI 10.1007/978-3-642-29782-3_61,

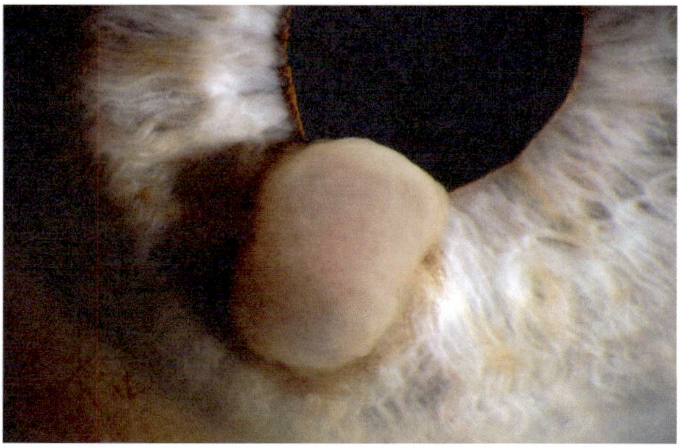

Fig. 61.1 This iris melanoma exhibited growth over a several month period

the iris stroma or seeding of tumor cells from a circumscribed iris or ciliary body melanoma. Nodular-shaped iris melanoma with variable pigmentation tends to arise in the inferior half of the iris. In lightly pigmented or amelanotic tumors, blood vessels are often visible. Involvement of the lesion in the angle may be a ciliary body melanoma extending into the iris or iris melanoma extending into the ciliary body. Topical antiglaucoma drugs such as Xalatan may cause iris pigmentation changes and make following a pigmented iris lesion challenging. It is not recommended to do a glaucoma shunt procedure in an eye with a possible iris melanoma. Signs suggesting malignancy include extensive size greater than 3-mm ectropion iridis, prominent vascularity, presence of symptoms, hyphema, sectoral cataract, secondary glaucoma, diffuse heterochromia, tapioca appearance, seeding of the peripheral angle structures, extrascleral extension, and documented progressive growth.

Diagnostics

Iris melanomas may invade the ciliary body, so it is important to perform gonioscopy and UBM (Fig. 61.2) on these lesions prior to treatment. If the diagnosis is still in question, a biopsy may be performed. A metastatic work-up is necessary, and patients need long-term follow-up.

Pathology

The tumor is composed of surface sheets, clusters and/or stromal sheets, and clusters of melanoma cells. There may be nevus cells also present and, in general, iris melanomas are cytologically more bland than ciliary body/choroidal melanomas. The stromal tumor proliferation disrupts the normal iris architecture (Fig. 61.3). Tumor cells on the surface may be loosely coherent (Fig. 61.4) and seed the angle. The modified Callender classification is used for the cytologic classification of uveal melanomas: spindle cell melanoma, epithelioid melanoma, and mixed-cell type (mixture of spindle and epithelioid cells). This classification may not be applicable

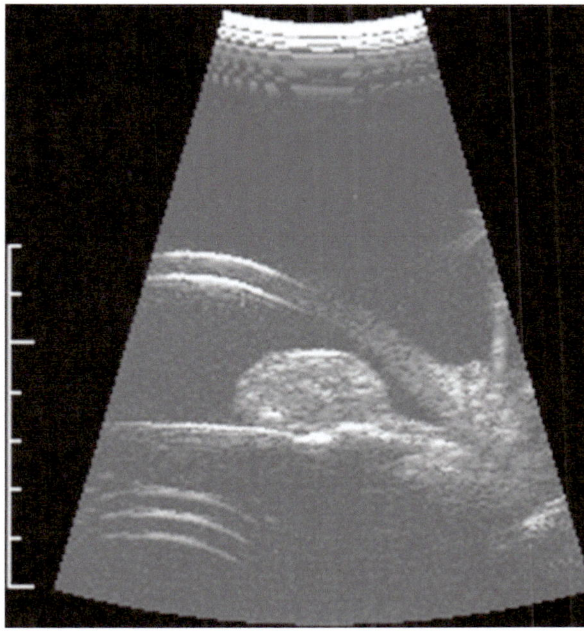

Fig. 61.2 A B-scan ultrasound demonstrates the nodular nature of the melanoma

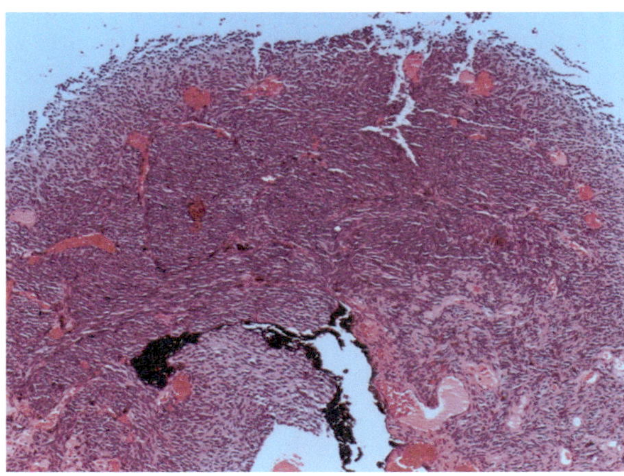

Fig. 61.3 The tumor is very cellular, although the nuclear features of many of the cells are bland (hematoxylin and eosin, 25×)

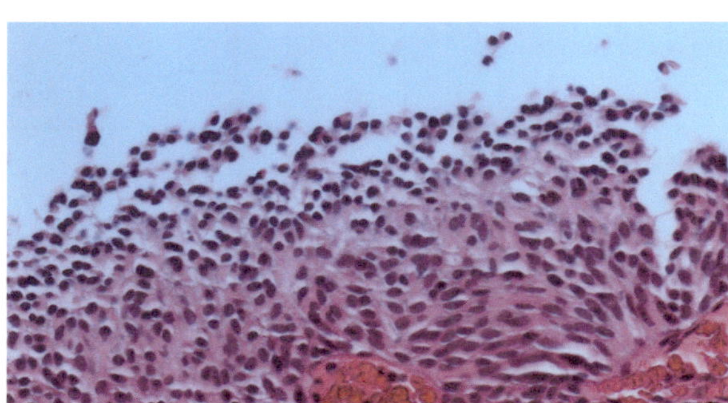

Fig. 61.4 Note the loosely cohesive nature of the tumor cells on the surface of the tumor (hematoxylin and eosin, 100×)

to iris melanomas in terms of prognostic significance, because iris melanomas have a relatively benign course.

Differential Diagnosis

The differential diagnosis includes iris nevus, primary iris cyst (pigment epithelial and stromal), essential iris atrophy, iris foreign body, peripheral anterior synechia, metastatic carcinoma to iris, aphakic iris cyst, pigment epithelial hyperplasia, juvenile xanthogranuloma, medulloepithelioma, and retained lens material simulating iris nodule.

Prophylaxis

There is no known prophylaxis for iris melanoma.

Therapy

Plaque brachytherapy with COMS dosing is now commonly used to treat iris melanoma. The dimension of the plaque is usually 4 mm greater than the largest basal diameter of the melanoma. The plaque should cover any ciliary body extension of the tumors. Any ciliary body involvement may be determined by preoperative ultrasound and demonstrated intraoperatively by transillumination. An amniotic membrane may be placed on the surface of the cornea to help with patient comfort, and a tarsorrhaphy may be performed at the time of placement. Another option is complete excision including an iridectomy. If the ciliary body is involved, an iridocyclectomy may be performed. Excision may result in cystoid macular edema; tumor cells may shed during removal, therefore close clinical follow-up with examination of the iridocorneal angle and anterior segment ultrasound examination is recommended.

Prognosis

The prognosis for survival for patients with iris melanoma is very good. It is much better than ciliary body/choroidal melanoma. The risk of metastasis is low (3–5% at 10 years).

Epidemiology

The annual incidence of iris melanoma is approximately 1/100,000. The average age of onset is 40–50 years. It should be remembered, however, that iris melanoma can occur in children.

Cross-References

Iris nevus, iris melanoma diffuse, iris melanoma tapioca, surgical techniques

Further Reading

Shetlar DJ, Chevez-Barrios P, Dubovy S, Rosa Jr RH, Syed N, Wilson MW, Pelton RW, and Pe'er J. Published by the American Academy of Ophthalmology, San Francisco, CA, USA, p 217–221

Demirci H, Shields CL, Shields JA et al (2002) Diffuse iris melanoma: a report of 25 cases. Ophthalmology 109:1553–1560

Onken MD, Worley LA, Harbour JW (2010) Association between gene expression profile, proliferation and metastasis in uveal melanoma. Curr Eye Res 35(9):857–863

Singh AD (2007) Clinical ophthalmic oncology. WB Saunders Company, Philadelphia, p 205

Iris Melanoma: Diffuse

62

Hans E. Grossniklaus

Synonyms

This tumor may also be termed diffuse seeding of iris melanoma

Definition

An extensive iris melanoma with involvement of the entire iris, usually with multiple pigmented lesions and/or heterochromia

Etiology

This tumor may arise in preexisting nevi.

Clinical Presentation

The patient will have diffuse pigmentation of the iris, usually consisting of multiple pigmented lesions, causing minimal thickening of the iris (Fig. 62.1). There will usually be raised intraocular pressure in the involved eye, many times causing unilateral glaucoma. Gonioscopic examination will show pigment in the angle.

H.E. Grossniklaus, M.D.
Emory University School of Medicine, Emory Eye Center,
Department of Ophthalmology,
Atlanta, GA, USA
e-mail: ophtheg@emory.edu

H.E. Grossniklaus (ed.), *Pocket Guide to Ocular Oncology and Pathology*,
DOI 10.1007/978-3-642-29782-3_62,

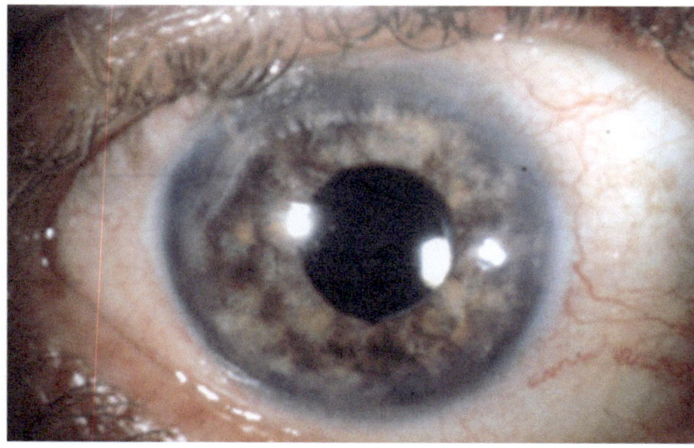

Fig. 62.1 Diffuse iris melanoma, clinical appearance. There are multiple pigmented areas in the iris of this patient with heterochromia and unilateral glaucoma Photo courtesy of Nasreen Syed MD and Lee Alward MD

Ultrasound biomicroscopy should be performed to measure the thickness of the iris and examine for extension into the face of the ciliary body.

Diagnosis

There should be a high clinical index of suspicion in cases of possible diffuse iris melanoma, as the clinical appearance and pathology may be inconspicuous. Care should be taken to examine the angle, perform careful ultrasound examination, and examine the iris surface and corneal endothelium by specular microscopy. A biopsy should be performed in suspicious cases. There are a variety of biopsy techniques including fine-needle aspiration biopsy (FNAB), punch biopsy, and using a vitrectomy cutter.

Pathology

The pathology shows a diffuse melanocytic infiltration of the iris and loosely cohesive melanoma cells in the iris surface (Fig. 62.2) which may be inconspicuous.

Differential Diagnosis

The differential diagnosis includes a diffuse nevus, melanosis oculi, and pigment dispersion syndrome. Iridocorneal endothelial syndrome may be also misdiagnosed in these patients and vice versa.

Prophylaxis

There is no known prophylaxis for diffuse iris melanoma.

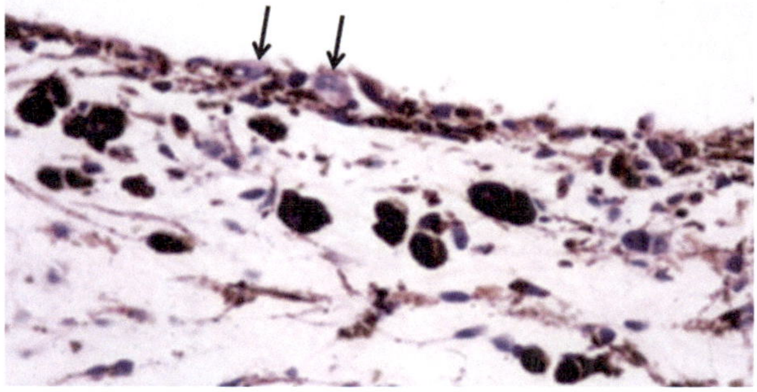

Fig. 62.2 Diffuse iris melanoma, pathology. There are pigmented macrophages in the iris stroma, a prominent anterior border layer, and several amelanotic cells with atypical cytology features on the surface of the anterior border layer (*arrows*). The diagnosis may be difficult due to limited cellularity and somewhat bland appearance of the melanoma cells (hematoxylin and eosin, 100×)

Therapy

Once the diagnosis is established, there are several therapeutic options. One option is observation, as there is a low risk of metastatic spread. Other options include enucleation and radiation plaque brachytherapy. If the eye has poor vision due to secondary glaucoma, enucleation is recommended. If there is good vision, you can consider submitting cells for molecular profiling. If there is low risk of metastasis, observation and plaque brachytherapy covering the entire cornea (Fig. 62.3) are options. If there is high risk of metastasis, plaque brachytherapy and enucleation are options. The treatments are highly individualized and depend on an extensive discussion with the patient.

Prognosis

The prognosis for life is good, as iris melanoma in general is associated with a favorable prognosis for life. The prognosis for vision is limited, as this tumor usually results in secondary glaucoma and plaque brachytherapy may cause a cataract or possibly neovascularization of the iris.

Epidemiology

Men and women appear to be equally affected by this tumor.

Cross Reference

Iris melanoma, ultrasound techniques, surgical techniques

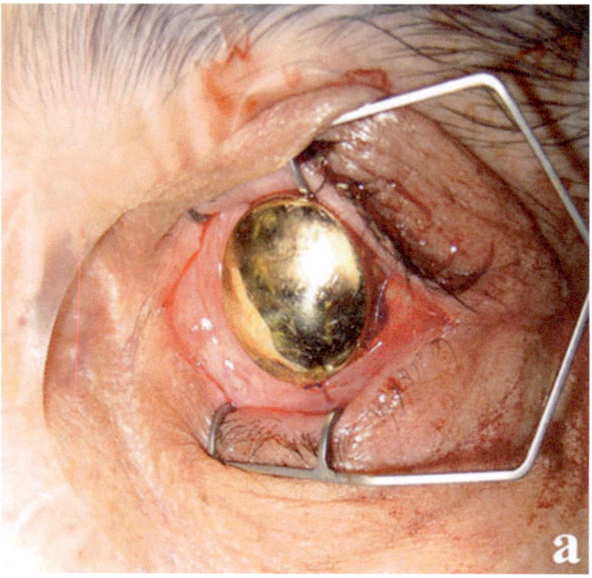

Fig. 62.3 A plaque covering the entire iris is sewn onto the ocular surface with interrupted 6.0 nylon sutures

Further Reading

Demirci H, Shields CL, Shields JA, Eagle RC Jr, Honavar SG (2002) Diffuse iris melanoma: report of 25 cases. Ophthalmology 109:1553–1560

Grossniklaus H (1992) Fine needle aspiration biopsy of the iris. Arch Ophthalmol 110:969–976

Pe'er J, Blumenthal EZ, Frenkel S (2007) Punch biopsy of iris lesions: a novel technique for obtaining histologic samples. Br J Ophthalmol 91:660–662

Petousis V, Finger PT, Milman T (2011a) Anterior segment tumor biopsy using aspiration cutter technique: clinical experience. Am J Ophthalmol 152:771–775

Petousis V, Finger PT, Milman T (2011b) Multifocal iris melanoma treated with total anterior segment palladium-103 plaque radiation therapy. Graefes Arch Clin Exp Ophthalmol 249:937–940

Shields CL, Shields MV, Viloria V, Pearstein H, Say EA, Shields JA (2011) Iridocorneal endothelial syndrome masquerading as iris melanoma in 71 cases. Arch Ophthalmol 129:1023–1029

Skalicky SE, Giblin M, Conway RM (2007) Diffuse iris melanoma: report of a case with review of the literature. Clin Ophthalmol 1:339–342

Iris Melanoma: Tapioca

63

Harry H. Brown

Synonyms

Malignant melanoma, Iris

Etiology

No risk factors or causes for tapioca melanoma of the iris have been identified; risk factors for iris melanoma include fair skin and lightly pigmented irides (blue gray). Association with degree of sunlight exposure has been proposed but not universally accepted. Conditions predisposing to iris melanoma include ocular melanocytosis and possibly neurofibromatosis type 1.

Clinical Presentation

The term "tapioca" refers to the clinical/biomicroscopical appearance of multiple confluent yellow-white nodules on the anterior surface of an iris tumor, reminiscent of tapioca pudding. It may be localized, circumferential, or diffuse (Fig. 63.1). The tumor is usually slow growing, and individual surface nodules may dissociate from the tumor mass and be deposited elsewhere, often in the inferior anterior chamber angle.

H.H. Brown, M.D.
Department of Pathology, Harvey and Bernice Jones Eye Institute,
Universitiy of Arkansas School of Medicine,
Little Rock, AR, USA
e-mail: brownharryh@uams.edu

H.E. Grossniklaus (ed.), *Pocket Guide to Ocular Oncology and Pathology*,
DOI 10.1007/978-3-642-29782-3_63,

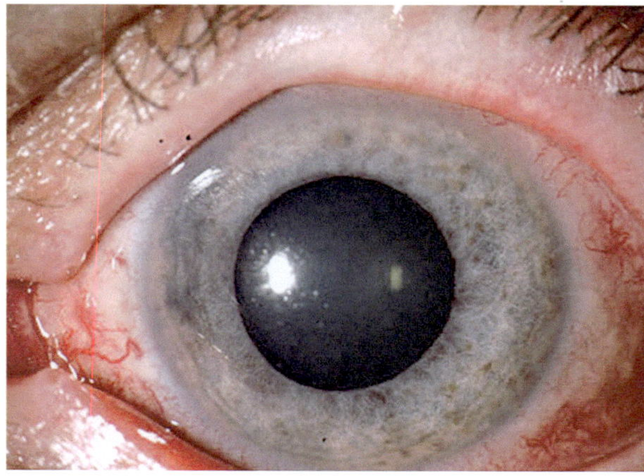

Fig. 63.1 Tapioca melanoma appears as small, inconspicuous nodules on the anterior iris surface (Courtesy of Ralph C. Eagle Jr., MD)

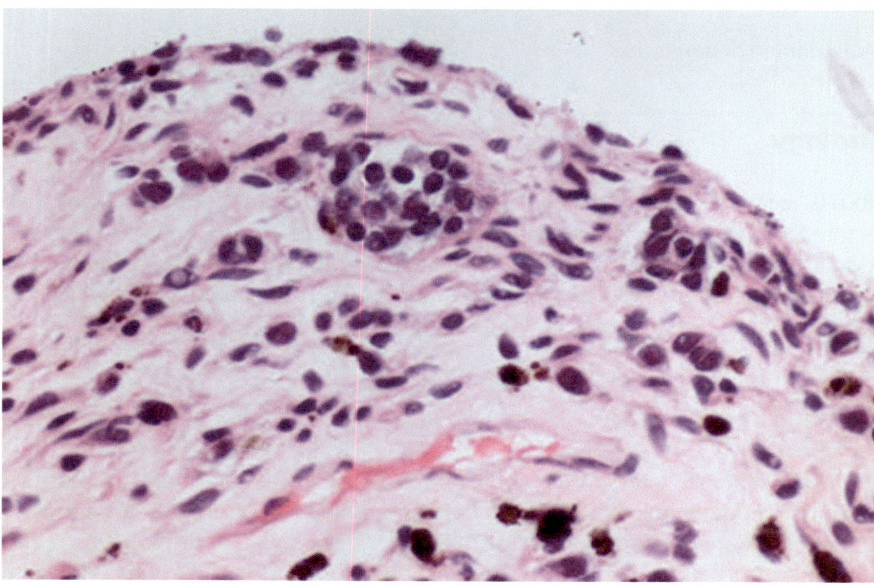

Fig. 63.2 The melanoma forms small, inconspicuous islands of cells near the iris surface (hematoxylin and eosin, 100×)

Diagnosis

Diagnosis is made by clinical appearance, ultrasonography, and biopsy or resection of the iris mass. The tumor on histological examination is usually an inconspicuous low-grade melanocytic proliferation, often lacking visible cytoplasmic melanin pigment (Fig. 63.2). Epithelioid and mixed cell types are less common but possible.

Immunohistochemical stains may be helpful in confirming the melanocytic nature of the tumor cells; a panel of markers (S100, HMB-45, Melan-A positive) should be employed due to possible variability in staining patterns.

Differential Diagnosis

The clinical differential diagnosis includes iris nevus, hemangioma, nonmelanocytic spindle cell tumors (leiomyoma, peripheral nerve sheath tumors), inflammatory nodules (juvenile xanthogranuloma, sarcoid, infectious granulomas), and metastatic tumors to the iris (typically carcinomas).

Prophylaxis

There is no prophylactic treatment for tapioca melanoma of the iris.

Therapy

Treatment is based on observed tumor growth and may include sector iridectomy if localized or iridocyclectomy if angle involvement is observed. Plaque radiotherapy is a treatment option, particularly for unresectable lesions. Enucleation may be required if more extensive disease is present. Detached tumor nodules may be aspirated from the anterior chamber.

Prognosis

As with most iris melanomas, tapioca melanoma has an excellent prognosis with a very low incidence of metastatic disease (3–5%). If amenable to local resection, visual prognosis is good.

Epidemiology

Tapioca melanoma usually affects younger patients than other uveal melanoma, with an average age around 30. No sex predisposition is apparent. All reported cases have been unilateral and in Caucasians.

Cross-References

Iris melanoma, iris melanoma: diffuse, surgical techniques

Further Reading

Henderson E, Margo CE (2008) Iris melanoma. Arch Pathol Lab Med 132:268–272
Pick ZS, Wilson GA (2009) Tapioca melanoma of the iris. Clin Exp Optom 2:154–156
Viestenz A, Conway RM, Küchle M (2004) Tapioca melanoma of the iris mimicking a vascular tumour: a clinicopathological correlation. Clin Experiment Ophthalmol 32:327–330
Zakka KA, Foos RY, Sulit H (1979) Metastatic tapioca iris melanoma. Br J Ophthalmol 63:744–749

Iris Nevus

64

Jill R. Wells and Hans E. Grossniklaus

Synonyms

Nevocellular nevus

Definition

An iris nevus is a local proliferation of benign melanocytic cells that generally appears as a pigmented (although some may be amelanotic) lesion of the iris stroma with some distortion of the iris architecture.

Etiology

There is no known etiology for this lesion.

J.R. Wells, M.D. (✉)
Department of Ophthalmology,
Emory University School of Medicine,
Atlanta, GA, USA
e-mail: jwells4@emory.edu

H.E. Grossniklaus, M.D.
Emory University School of Medicine,
Emory Eye Center,
Department of Ophthalmology,
Atlanta, GA, USA
e-mail: ophtheg@emory.edu

H.E. Grossniklaus (ed.), *Pocket Guide to Ocular Oncology and Pathology*,
DOI 10.1007/978-3-642-29782-3_64, © Springer-Verlag Berlin Heidelberg 2013

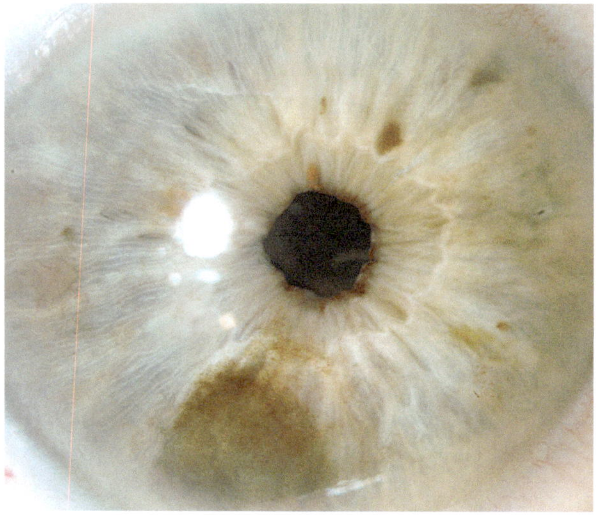

Fig. 64.1 This inferior iris nevus is moderately pigmented. It does not extend to the pupillary margin

Clinical Presentation

Iris nevus typically appears solitary and circumscribed and is located in the lower half of the iris (Fig. 64.1). Pupillary changes including corectopia, irregularity of the margin, and ectropion iridis may occur in nevi and do not necessarily imply malignancy (Fig. 64.2). There may be extension of the nevus into the trabecular meshwork. A nevus may shed pigment which appears smooth on gonioscopy compared to irregular nodules seen with tumor seeding from iris melanoma.

An iris nevus must be differentiated from iris melanoma, although the only way to definitely differentiate is the histopathologic evaluation. Worrisome clinical features are outlined in *Iris Melanoma*.

Diagnostics

A detailed anterior segment exam with gonioscopy is necessary to evaluate for tumor vascularity, pigment dispersion, and hyphema (features of iris melanoma).

Intraocular pressure should be obtained as increased pressure may be a sign of tumor seeding. Photographic documentation at the first examination is helpful for documenting growth in future examination. High-frequency ultrasound biomicroscopy provides tumor size measurements, detects any ciliary body involvement, and differentiates a solid from a cystic mass.

Pathology

There are a variety of types of iris nevus, including melanocytoma (plump polyhedral cell nevus), spindle cell nevus with surface plaque, spindle cell nevus with

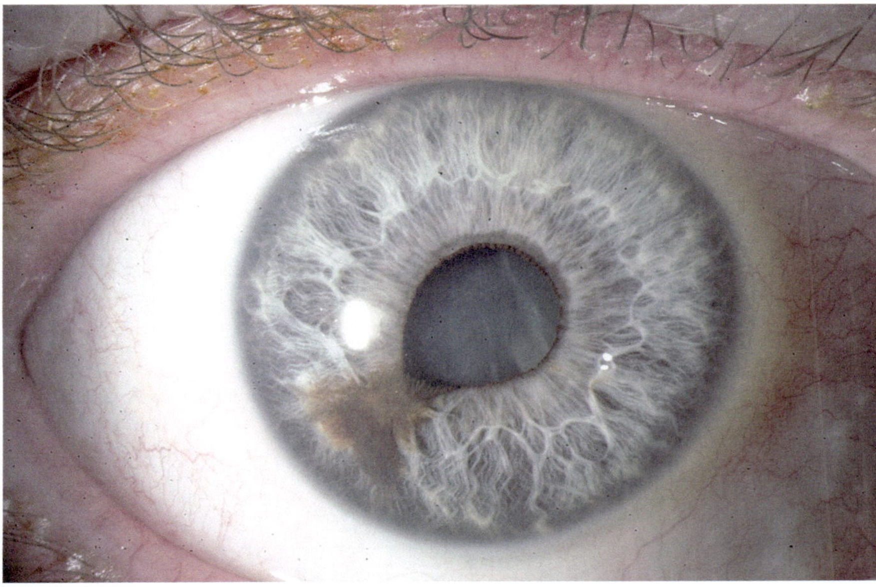

Fig. 64.2 This iris nevus causes distortion of the stromal crypt and valley architecture. It extends to the pupil causing ectropion uveae

stromal component, and epithelioid cell nevus. The nevus cells contain bland nuclear chromatin and may contain intranuclear pseudoinclusions (invaginations of cytoplasm).

Differential Diagnosis

The differential diagnosis of iris nevus includes melanoma, primary iris cyst (pigment epithelial and stromal), essential iris atrophy, iris foreign body, peripheral anterior synechia, metastatic carcinoma to iris, aphakic iris cyst, pigment epithelial hyperplasia, juvenile xanthogranuloma, medulloepithelioma, and retained lens material simulating iris nodule.

Prophylaxis

There is no known prophylaxis for iris nevus.

Therapy

Serial photographic documentation and ultrasonography are recommended.

Prognosis

The prognosis for iris nevus is excellent, as only a small minority will give rise to iris melanoma.

Epidemiology

Approximately 4–6% of the population have iris nevi. The incidence of iris freckle (prominent anterior border layer melanocytes) can be seen in up to 60% of the population.

Cross-References

Iris melanoma, ultrasound techniques

Further Reading

Shetlar DJ, Chevez-barrios P, Dubovy S, Rosa Jr. RH, Syed N, Wilson MW, Pelton RW, and Pe'er J. (2006–2007) American Academy of Ophthalmology Ophthalmic pathology and intraocular tumors. In: Basic and clinical science course. San Francisco, CA, USA, p 156–157

Jakobiec FA, Silbert G (1981) Are most iris 'melanomas' really nevi? A clinicopathologic study of 189 lesions. Arch Ophthalmol 99:2117–2132

Shields JA, Karan DS, Perry HD, Donosa LA (1985) Epithelioid cell nevus of the iris. Arch Ophthalmol 1–3:235–237

Singh AD (2007) Clinical ophthalmic oncology. WB Saunders Company, Philadelphia, pp 185–186

Uveal Melanoma: Epidemiology

65

Felicia Fountain and Hans E. Grossniklaus

Overview

Uveal melanoma is a malignant neoplasm of melanocyte origin arising from the iris, ciliary body, or choroid of the eye. Melanomas arising from the ciliary body/choroid are the most common primary intraocular malignancies in adults.

Epidemiology/Incidence

Among all melanomas reported in the United States, approximately 5% arise from the ocular and adnexal structures (85% of which originate in the uveal tract). The age-adjusted incidence historically in the US has ranged 6–7 cases per million. An age-adjusted incidence of 5.1 reported in recent study by Singh et al. using the SEER program database for analysis with a statistically higher incidence found in males compared to females. The aforementioned study also showed that the incidence of uveal melanoma has been relatively stable over the study period 1973–2008. European studies have reported incidences of 5.3–7.4 per million. Virgili et al. reported a trend of increasing incidence with latitude in Europe but

F. Fountain, M.D. (✉)
Department of Ophthalmology,
Emory University School of Medicine,
Atlanta, GA, USA
e-mail: felicia.c.fountain@emory.edu

H.E. Grossniklaus, M.D.
Emory University School of Medicine,
Emory Eye Center,
Department of Ophthalmology,
Atlanta, GA, USA
e-mail: ophtheg@emory.edu

H.E. Grossniklaus (ed.), *Pocket Guide to Ocular Oncology and Pathology*,
DOI 10.1007/978-3-642-29782-3_65,

overall stable incidence for years 1983–1994. Isager et al. reported an incidence of 0.78/100,000 in men and 0.65/100,000 person-years in women in Denmark for years 1943–1997. The incidence was noted to be stable over that time period. The median age at diagnosis is approximately 55 years with most being affected in their 50s or early 60s in contrast to the median age of diagnosis in cutaneous melanoma of 45 years. Uveal melanoma overwhelmingly occurs in fair-skinned Caucasians who have eight times the risk of African-Americans and three times the risk of Asians. In a recent study by Singh et al. evaluating 4,070 cases of uveal melanoma between 1973 and 2008, 97.8% occurred in whites with a white to black ratio of 196:1. Despite the high prevalence of disease in fair-skinned individuals, the causative role of UV exposure is controversial as there has been no increase in incidence of uveal melanoma over the last 40 years compared to cutaneous melanoma and no higher incidence found in the most light-exposed areas of the eye. Other risk factors of uveal melanoma may include (1) ocular or oculodermal melanocytosis (Nevus of Ota), (2) genetic predisposition (dysplastic nevus syndrome), and (3) cigarette smoking.

Survival/Prognosis

Despite advancements in treatment modalities, the overall survival rate of uveal melanoma has not changed over the last 30 years. Singh et al. reported a 5-year survival rate ~81.6% between 1973 and 2008, despite transition in treatment from enucleation to radiation therapy. In 2003, Singh and Topham published survival rates of 77–84% between 1973 and 1997. Survival rates diminish with metastatic disease. The Collaborative Ocular Melanoma Study (COMS) reported cumulative rates of metastasis of 25% and 34% at 5 and 10 years, respectively. Most common sites of metastasis are liver (90%), lung (24%), and bone (16%). Those with metastasis confined to extrahepatic sites have longer survival rates of 19–28 months than patients with hepatic metastases. The median survival for hepatic metastasis is approximately 6 months: estimated 15–20% survival at 1 year and 10% at 2 years regardless of treatment.

The most reliable prognostic tumor morphology feature appears to be LTD (largest tumor diameter). Mclean et al. reported a 10-year mortality based on LTD which is a better parameter than tumor thickness in contrast to cutaneous melanoma. The 10-year mortalities for patients with <11, 11–15, and >15 mm LTDs are 20%, 40%, and 60%, respectively. Other prognostic features are as follows:

- Age (older age with worse prognosis).
- Location: 10–15% rate of metastasis for iris melanoma versus 40–50% for choroidal/posterior uveal melanoma; worse prognosis with anterior tumor location (ciliary body) and juxtapapillary tumors.
- Gender (worse in males).
- Tumor histology: 5-year survival rates of approximately 88% in pure spindle cell versus 60% for epithelioid or mixed; worse prognosis also with numerous mitotic figures/scleral invasion/complete vascular loops/mean of ten largest nuclei.
- Worse with tumor regrowth after globe-conserving treatment.

- Genetics: worse prognosis with monosomy 3 or trisomy 8 chromosomal abnormalities and gene expression profiling of Class I and II. Recent series of 500 patients with uveal melanoma with monosomy 3 abnormality showed significantly worse 3-year prognosis compared to partial monosomy 3 and disomy 3. Monosomy 3 chromosomal abnormality showed association with larger tumor size at diagnosis, and epithelioid cell type in the previously mentioned series (5). Class I represents tumors with disomy 3 and other advantageous chromosomal aberrations such as gain of 6p. Class II (monosomy 3) has deleterious aberrations like gain 8p and/or isochromosome 8p conferring high metastatic potential.

Proposed Serum Markers

- Vascular endothelial growth factor (VEGF) overexpression in uveal melanoma; has been associated with increased metastatic potential; increased levels proposed to occur in presence of micrometastasis and parallel extent of liver disease.
- The tyrosinase enzyme is involved in melanin production; serum mRNA levels of this enzyme have been shown to be increased in primary uveal melanoma and correlate with tumor dimensions.
- Insulin-like growth factor 1 (IGF-1) expression is associated with a worse prognosis; binding to its receptor triggers important steps in metastasis such as cell proliferation/prevention of apoptosis/integrin adhesion and invasion of basement membranes; levels fall with presence of metastatic disease. Molecular markers are currently under investigation and have a limited role in tumor surveillance at this point.

Surveillance

To date, there is no universally accepted method of surveillance for metastatic disease.

The COMS used chest x-ray and liver function tests for screening biannually for at least 5 years (LFTs have high specificity but low sensitivity for detecting metastasis). Other modalities employed for detection of metastatic disease include abdominal ultrasound, PET/CT, and abdominal CT. Recently published literature review on surveillance testing for metastasis from primary uveal melanoma concluded that to date there is no compelling evidence in the peer-reviewed literature of survival benefit to routine screening of patients who underwent definitive treatment for their disease.

Further Reading

All-Ericsson C, Girnita L, Seregard S, Bartolazzi A, Jager MJ, Larsson O (2002) Insulin-like growth factor-1 receptor in uveal melanoma: a predictor for metastatic disease and a potential therapeutic target. Invest Ophthalmol Vis Sci 43(1):1–8

Augsburger James J, Correa Zelia M, Shaikh Adeel H (2009) Effectiveness of treatments for metastatic uveal melanoma. Ophthalmology 148(1):119–127
Bakalian S, Marshall JC, Logan P et al (2008) Molecular pathways mediating liver metastasis in patients with uveal melanoma. Clin Cancer Res 14(4):951–956
Bedician AY (2006) Metastatic uveal melanoma therapy: current options. Int Ophthalmol Clin 46(1):151–166
Filali M, Missotten G, Maat W et al (2010) Regulation of VEGF-A in uveal melanoma. Invest Ophthalmol Vis Sci 51(5):2329–2337
Frenkel S, Barak V, Zioto O, Pe'er J (2011) Novel biomarkers for detecting uveal melanoma metastases. In: Proceedings of the spring meeting of Ocular Oncology Group, Copenhagen, 2011
Isager P et al (2005) Uveal and conjunctival malignant melanoma in Denmark, 1943–1997: incidence and validation study. Ophthalmic Epidemiol 12(4):223–232
Mclean IW, Foster DW, Zimmerman LE (1982) Uveal melanoma: localization, size, cell type and enucleation as risk factors in metastasis. Hum Pathol 13:123–132
Onken MD, Worley LA, Harbour JW (2010) Association between gene expression profile, proliferation and metastasis in uveal melanoma. Curr Eye Res 35(9):857–863
Papastefenou VP, Cohen VM (2011) Uveal melanoma. J Skin Cancer 2011. doi: 10.1155/2011/573974, 573974
Pinzani P, Mazzini C, Salvianti F et al (2010) Tyrosinase mRNA levels in the blood of uveal melanoma patients: correlation with the number of circulating tumor cells and tumor progression. Melanoma Res 20(4):303–310
Sheidow TG, Hooper PL, Crukley C, Young J, Heathcote JG (2000) Expression of vascular endothelial growth factor in uveal melanoma and its correlation with metastasis. Br J Ophthalmol 84(7):750–756
Shields CL, Ganguly A, Bianciotto CG, Turaka K, Tavallali A, Shields JA (2011) Prognosis of uveal melanoma in 500 cases using genetic testing of fine-needle aspiration biopsy specimens. Ophthalmology 118(2):396–401
Singh AD, Topham A (2003) Survival rates with uveal melanoma in the United States: 1973–1997. Ophthalmology 110:962–965
Singh AD, Turell ME, Topham AK (2011) Uveal melanoma: trends in incidence, treatment, and survival. Ophthalmology 118(9):1881–1885
Virgili G et al (2007) Incidence of uveal melanoma in Europe. Ophthalmology 114(12): 2309–2315
Woll E et al (1999) Uveal melanoma: natural history and treatment options for metastatic disease. Melanoma Res 9:575–581

Uveal Melanoma: Brachytherapy

66

Aimee V. Chappelow, Arun D. Singh, and Chris Bergstrom

Synonyms

Plaque radiotherapy.

Definition

Brachytherapy is a radiation-based treatment for small- to medium-sized ciliary body and choroidal melanoma (<16-mm basal diameter) that employs a metal plaque implanted with radioactive isotope (I-125, Ru-106, or other) sutured to the episclera for a precalculated duration, and offers similar 12-year tumor-specific mortality rates as treatment by enucleation.

Indication

Treatment of small- to medium-sized ciliary body and choroidal melanoma (>2.5 mm in height, <16 mm in basal diameter, <10 mm in apical height).

A.V. Chappelow, M.D.
Cole Eye Institute, Cleveland Clinic,
Cleveland, OH, USA

A.D. Singh, M.D. (✉)
Department of Ophthalmic Oncology,
Cole Eye Institute, Cleveland Clinic Foundation,
9500 Euclid Ave, Desk i-329,
Cleveland, OH 44195, USA
e-mail: singha@ccf.org

C. Bergstrom, M.D.
Department of Ophthalmology,
Emory University School of Medicine, Atlanta, GA, USA
e-mail: cbergs2@emory.edu

H.E. Grossniklaus (ed.), *Pocket Guide to Ocular Oncology and Pathology*,
DOI 10.1007/978-3-642-29782-3_66, © Springer-Verlag Berlin Heidelberg 2013

Contraindication

Large ciliary body and choroidal melanoma (>16 mm in basal diameter).

Background

Traditionally, uveal melanoma was treated by enucleation. However, in 1978, Zimmerman, McLean, and Foster observed a transient rise in posttherapeutic mortality and hypothesized that enucleation accelerated the systemic dissemination of tumor. Though data now supports early micrometastases at the time of enucleation as a more probable explanation, this proposition provided the impetus for a quarter century of research on alternative treatment options for uveal melanoma. Among these, brachytherapy has emerged as the most widely used alternative to enucleation for the treatment of uveal melanoma.

Techniques and Principles

A bowl-shaped heavy metal plaque implanted with a radioactive isotope is sized to exceed tumor margins (determined by ophthalmoscopy, ultrasonography, and transillumination) by 2 mm (Fig. 66.1). It is then sutured to episclera (Fig. 66.2) underlying the tumor base for a period of 2–7 days (Fig. 66.3). Duration of therapy is determined by radiation dosimetry with a goal of delivering 80–100 Gy to the tumor apex. Depending on the dose distribution of the isotope, the tumor base receives up to nine times as much radiation as the apex. Plaques have been custom designed to treat choroidal melanoma at various locations in the eye while minimizing radiation dosage to the macula, optic nerve, and lens. Juxtapapillary and macular choroidal melanomas can be treated with notched plaques, and ciliary body and iris melanomas can be treated with curvilinear plaques.

Preoperative Evaluation

Though most patients with choroidal melanoma <16-mm basal diameter do not present with detectable systemic metastases, preoperative evaluation should include a complete physical exam, a complete blood count, serum liver function studies, and a CT scan of chest, abdomen, and pelvis.

Outcome

Between 1986 and 1994, the Collaborative Ocular Melanoma Study (COMS) screened 6,078 patients with choroidal melanoma at 43 clinical centers. A total of 1,317 patients with tumors between 2.5 and 10 mm in apical height and no more

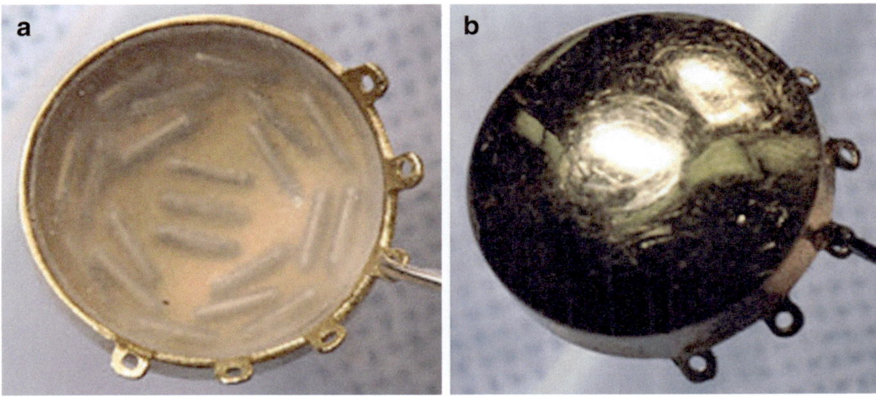

Fig. 66.1 (**a**) shows the concave surface of an Iodine-125 plaque. Note the Iodine-125 seeds loaded in the gold disc. (**b**) shows the smooth convex surface of the plaque being held at a suture eyelet by a forcep

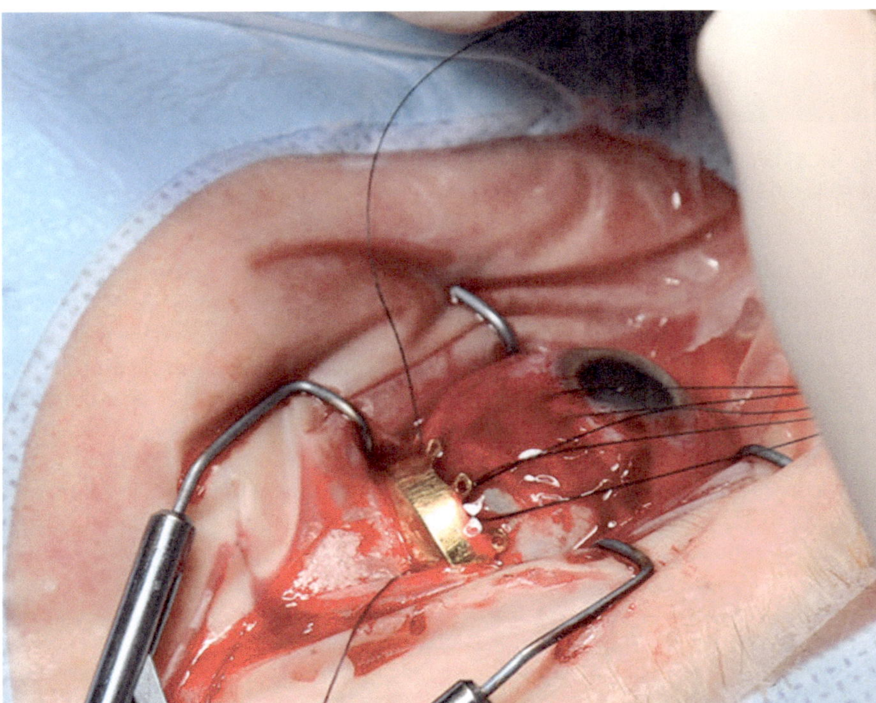

Fig. 66.2 Intraoperative photo of radioactive plaque being sutured to the sclera

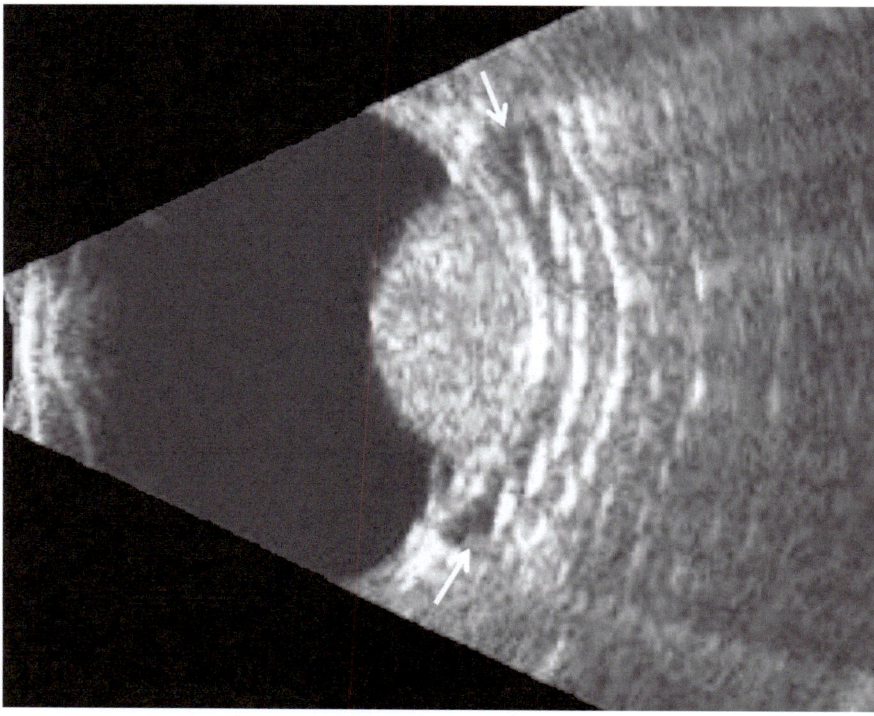

Fig. 66.3 Intraopertive B-scan ultrasound image of an appropriately placed radioactive plaque covering the tumor. *Arrows* demarcate the plaque edges

than 16 mm in basal diameter (classified as medium-sized) were randomized to receive either Iodine-125 (I-125) brachytherapy or enucleation. The 5-, 10-, and 12-year rates of death with histopathologically confirmed melanoma metastasis were similar for I-125 brachytherapy (10 %, 18 %, and 21%) and enucleation (11 %, 17 %, and 17%). As a result of the COMS, I-125 has become the most common isotope used in brachytherapy in North America.

There have been no randomized trials comparing different isotopes due to the large sample size required to detect a difference in treatment outcome. Combination of brachytherapy and adjunctive transpupillary thermotherapy (TTT) has also been reported to produce favorable local tumor control rates.

Complications

Dose-dependent cataract, radiation-related optic neuropathy, radiation retinopathy, and sequelae (such as neovascular glaucoma and vitreous hemorrhage) occur in up to 50% of patients.

Cross-References

Thermotherapy, Collaborative Ocular Melanoma Study (COMS), ultrasonography techniques, surgical techniques

Further Reading

COMS Group (2006) The COMS randomized trial of iodine 125 brachytherapy for choroidal melanoma: V. Twelve-year mortality rates and prognostic factors: 3. COMS report No. 28. Arch Ophthalmol 124:1684–1693

Finger PT (1997) Microwave thermoradiotherapy for uveal melanoma: results of a 10-year study. Ophthalmology 104:1794–1803

Melia M, Moy CS, Reynolds SM et al (2006) Quality of life after iodine 125 brachytherapy vs enucleation for choroidal melanoma: 5-year results from the 5. Collaborative Ocular Melanoma Study: COMS QOLS Report No. 3. Arch Ophthalmol 124:226–238

Singh AD, Rennie IG, Kivela T, Seregard S, Grossniklaus H (2004) The Zimmerman-McLean-foster hypothesis: 25 years later. Br J Ophthalmol 88:962–967

Metastatic Uveal Melanoma to the Liver 67

Hans E. Grossniklaus

Overview

The sites of metastases of uveal melanoma include liver (93%), lung (24%), and bone (16%). Multiple sites are involved in 87% of cases. Current treatments for treating metastatic uveal melanoma are largely ineffective.

Screening

Molecular testing for high-grade (high metastatic potential) versus low-grade (low metastatic potential) uveal melanoma includes cytogenetics for monosomy 3, fluorescent in situ hybridization (FISH) for monosomy 3, gene expression profiling (Class IA, IB; Class II), genotyping (for GNAQ/GNA11, BAP1 mutations), and multiplex ligation-dependent probe amplification (MLPA) for monosomy 3. Serum tests to monitor for metastases include liver function tests (alkaline phosphatase, AST, ALT, GGT, bilirubin).

Biomarkers are under investigation—osteopontin, melanoma inhibitory activity (MIA), and vascular endothelial growth factor (VEGF). Circulating melanoma cells under investigation regarding tumor progression are also being investigated. Imaging to monitor for metastases includes chest and abdominal CT, liver ultrasound, MRI, and PET/CT. Controversies include no standard method of follow-up, no definitive evidence that any surveillance method leads to increased survival, and genotyping and detection of metastases early may enable enrollment into clinical trial.

H.E. Grossniklaus, M.D.
Emory University School of Medicine, Emory Eye Center,
Department of Ophthalmology,
Atlanta, GA, USA
e-mail: ophtheg@emory.edu

H.E. Grossniklaus (ed.), *Pocket Guide to Ocular Oncology and Pathology*,
DOI 10.1007/978-3-642-29782-3_67,

Table 67.1 Clinical trials for metastatic uveal melanoma

Uveal melanoma clinical trials.gov				
Trial	Sponsor	Location	Requirements	Agent(s)
NCT01034787	Alberta Health Sciences	Alberta, Toronto	Unresectable or metastatic uveal melanoma	IV drug CP-675,206
NCT00929019	Radboud University	Nijmegen, Rotterdam	High-risk melanoma expressing gp100 and/or tyrosinase	Vaccine
NCT00506142	Talon Therapeutics	Los Angeles, Denver, Philadelphia, Houston	Metastatic uveal melanoma	Vincristine sulfate liposome injection
NCT01100528	Cleveland Clinic	Cleveland	Monosomy 3 melanoma <56 days from treating primary	Interferon alpha 2b sc dacarbazine iv
NCT01200342	MD Anderson Hospital	Houston	Metastatic uveal melanoma	Genasense iv Paclitaxel iv Carboplatin iv
NCT01252251	Memorial Sloan Kettering	New York	Metastatic uveal melanoma	Pasireotide im Everolimus po
NCT01143402	Memorial Sloan Kettering	New York, New Haven, Miami Beach, Boston, Philadelphia	Metastatic uveal melanoma	Temozolomide po AZD6244 po
NCT00738361	Ohio State	Columbus	Metastatic uveal melanoma	Paclitaxel nanoparticles iv
NCT00110123	European Organization for Research and Treatment of Cancer	Italy, Poland, Switzerland, UK	Metastatic uveal melanoma	Fotemustine isolated hepatic perfusion
NCT01217398	Institute Curie	Paris	Metastatic uveal melanoma	Bevacizumab iv Temozolomide po
NCT00471471	University of Pittsburgh	Pittsburgh	Unresectable or metastatic uveal melanoma	Vaccine
NCT00792545	NCI	Bethesda	Unresectable or metastatic uveal melanoma	Bevacizumab iv Dasatinib po
NCT00489944	San Diego Pacific Oncology and Hematology	San Diego	Large uveal melanoma >16×10mm	Cisplatin Sunitinib Tamoxifen
NCT00813423	University of New Jersey Medicine and Dentistry	New Brunswick, NJ	Failed chemotherapy for metastatic uveal melanoma	Hydroxychloroquine sunitinib
NCT01311466	Oslo University Hospital	Oslo	Metastatic uveal melanoma to liver	Liver transplant

Treatments for Metastatic Uveal Melanoma to Liver

There are a number of medical treatments (chemotherapy) used to treat metastatic uveal melanoma to the liver. These treatments are dependent on the treating cancer center and medical oncologist. The treatments consist of various combinations of the following agents: temozolomide, interferon alpha 2b, genasense, paclitaxel, carboplatin, paseriotide, everolimus, AZD6244, bevacizumab, dasatinib, sunitinib, tamoxifen, verapamil, and SAHA. Treatment protocols differ from center to center. Examples of experimental protocols are shown in Table 67.1. Current centers and protocols may be found at www.clinicaltrials.gov. Locoregional management may include surgical resection, drug eluting beads (DEBs), radiospheres, intrahepatic arterial infusion (IHA), hepatic arterial infusion (HAI), isolated hepatic perfusion (IHP), radiofrequency ablation (RFA), transarterial chemoembolization (TACE), transarterial immunoembolization (TAIE), and percutaneous hepatic perfusion (PHP). The efficacy and choice of treatment are dependent on time of diagnosis and number and volume of metastases as well as institutional availability and experience

Further Reading

Augsburger JJ, Correa ZM, Shaikh AH (2009) Effectiveness of treatments for metastatic uveal melanoma. Am J Ophthalmol 148:119–127

Augsburger JJ, Correa ZM, Trichopolous N (2011) Surveillance testing for metastases from primary uveal melanoma and effect on patient survival. Am J Ophthamol 152:5–9

Barak V, Frenkel S, Kalickman I (2007) Serum markers to detect metastatic uveal melanoma. Anticancer Res 27:1897–1900

Callejo SA, Antecka E, Blanco PL et al (2007) Identification of circulating malignant cells and its correlation with prognostic factors and treatment in uveal melanoma. A prospective longitudinal study. Eye 21:752–759

Callejo SA, Dopierala J, Coupland SE, Damato B (2011) Sudden growth of a choroidal melanoma and multiplex ligation-dependent probe amplification findings suggesting late transformation to monosomy 3 type. Arch Ophthalmol 129:958–960

Collaborative Ocular Melanoma Study Group (2001) Assessment of metastatic disease status at death in 435 patients with large choroidal melanoma in the Collaborative Ocular Melanoma Study (COMS): COMS report no. 15. Arch Ophthalmol 119:670–676

Diener West M, Reynolds SM, Agugliaro DG et al (2004) Screening for metastasis from choroidal melanoma: the Collaborative Ocular Melanoma Study Group Report 23. J Clin Oncol 22:2438–2444

Finger PT, Kurli M, Wesley P (2005) Whole body PET/CT for initial staging of choroidal melanoma. Br J Ophthalmol 89:1270–1274

Harbour JW, Onken MD, Roberson ED (2010) Frequent mutation of BAP1 in metastasizing uveal melanoma. Science 330:1410–1413

Haritoglu I, Wolf A, Maier T et al (2009) Osteopontin and "melanoma inhibitory activity": comparison of two serologic tumor markers in metastatic uveal melanoma patients. Ophthalmologica 223:239–243

Onken MD, Whorley LA, Harbour JA (2010) An accurate, clinically feasible, multi-gene expression assay for predicting metastases in uveal melanoma. J Mol Diagn 12:461–468

Pardo M, Garcia A, Antrobus R et al (2007) Biomarker discovery from uveal melanoma secrotomes: identification of gp 100 and cathepsin D in patient serum. J Proteome Res 6:2802–2811

Sato T (2010) Locoregional management of hepatic metastases from primary uveal melanoma. Semin Oncol 37:127–138

Van Raamsdonk CD, Bezrookove V, Green G et al (2009) Frequent somatic mutations of GNAQ in uveal melanoma and blue naevi. Nature 457:599–602

Proton Beam Radiotherapy

68

Victoria M.L. Cohen and Arun D. Singh

Synonyms

External beam radiation therapy, EBRT, Heavy charged particle irradiation

Definition

The use of heavy charged particle external beam radiotherapy for the treatment of intraocular tumors, most commonly uveal melanoma

Treatment

Proton beam radiotherapy is a radiotherapy that achieves a high rate of local tumor control. The proton beam exhibits low linear energy transfer (LET, minimal scatter of energy due to its mass) and exerts a Bragg peak effect (the deposition of most of its energy at the end of its range). The beam can be modulated to broaden the Bragg peak, hence tumors of varying thickness can be treated (Fig. 68.1). In addition, a custom designed collimator is used to conform the beam to a specific tumor volume. These properties limit radiation complications and improve tumor control rates. Proton beam is not recommended for tumors that occupy at least 30% of the eye or are associated with extrascleral extension or neovascular glaucoma.

V.M.L. Cohen (✉)
Ocular Oncology Service,
Moorfields Eye Hospital and St. Bartholomew's Hospital,
London, UK
e-mail: victoria.lendrum@googlemail.com

A.D. Singh, M.D.
Department of Ophthalmic Oncology, Cole Eye Institute, Cleveland Clinic Foundation,
9500 Euclid Ave, Desk i-329, Cleveland, OH 44195, USA

H.E. Grossniklaus (ed.), *Pocket Guide to Ocular Oncology and Pathology*,
DOI 10.1007/978-3-642-29782-3_68, © Springer-Verlag Berlin Heidelberg 2013

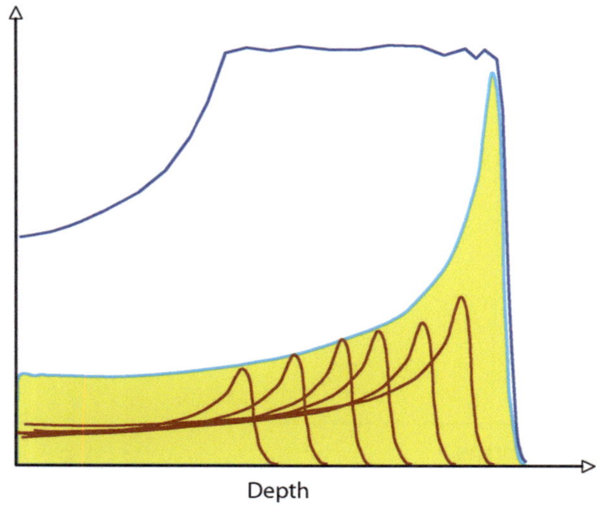

Fig. 68.1 This graph demonstrates modulation of the proton beam. The Bragg peak is moved backward and forward during the process of modulation, allowing treatment of tumors with differing thickness. Note the entry-level dose increases but remains lower than the dose received at the end of the proton beam range

Technique

Before proton beam therapy, the patient must undergo treatment planning. A- and B-scan ocular ultrasonography are used to measure the tumor dimensions. The tumor is surgically localized by standard techniques of transillumination and indirect ophthalmoscopy. Four radiopaque tantalum markers are sutured to the sclera at known distances from the tumor margins (Fig. 68.2). Iris tumors do not require surgical localization as the tumor margin can be identified using anatomical landmarks. A computerized three-dimensional model of the eye is created using the information from ocular ultrasonography, digital photography, and intraoperative measurements with radiographs showing the tantalum marker positions. A face-mask and bite block are molded to immobilize the patient during treatment (Fig. 68.3). Uveal melanoma is treated with a dose of 70 cobalt Gy equivalents (CGE), administered in four or five fractions over a week. Each treatment session lasts less than 1 min.

Indications

Proton beam radiotherapy is used for the treatment of uveal melanoma, especially medium- to large-sized tumors. This modality allows delivery of a homogeneous dose to the tumor while sparing the surrounding normal tissue. This makes it an attractive procedure for tumors that cannot be easily treated by plaque because of juxtapapillary or peripapillary location. Some centers use proton beam radiotherapy for the treatment of iris melanoma. It can also be used for the treatment of choroidal hemangiomas and retinoblastoma.

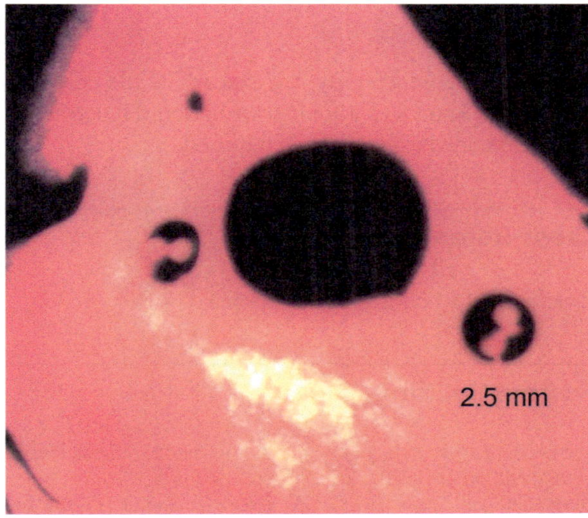

Fig. 68.2 Transillumination of the eye reveals a dark shadow from an intraocular tumor. Tantalum markers are sutured to the sclera at know distances from the tumor margin. These distances are recorded for the planning or simulation of proton beam treatment

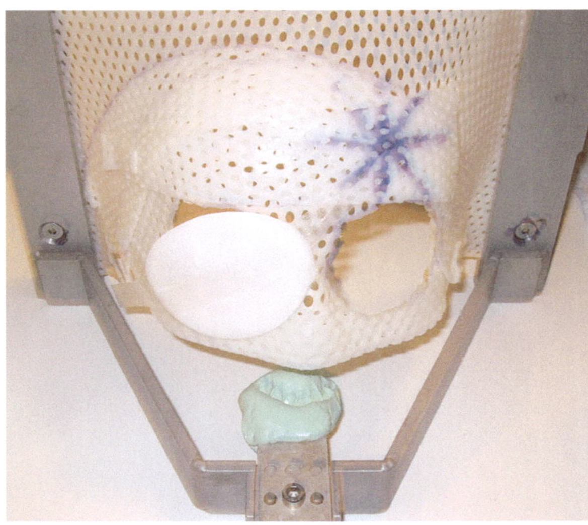

Fig. 68.3 The facemask and bite block are custom designed for each patient to prevent movement of the head when the proton beam is switched on

Complications

Early complications include eyelid erythema or ulceration and conjunctivitis. Late complications include eyelid damage, loss of the eyelashes, scarring or depigmentation, canalicular obstruction leading to epiphoria keratitis, conjunctival telangiectasia, and neovascular glaucoma. A large tumor diameter and the presence of a retinal detachment are significant risk factors for the development of rubeosis. Radiotherapy may result in radiation retinopathy, maculopathy, optic neuropathy, and ipsilateral cataract. The higher the dose received to the lens, the greater the risk of posterior subcapsular cataract formation.

Interactions

Concurrent chemotherapy can exacerbate the complications induced by radiotherapy, this is known as chemopotentiation. Hyperthermia increases radiosensitivity, therefore a lower total dose is required.

Cross-References

Brachytherapy, choroidal melanoma

Further Reading

Damato B (2000) Ocular tumours: diagnosis and treatment. Radiotherapy. Butterworth-Heinemann, Oxford, pp 213–222

Gragoudas ES, Lane AM (2005) Uveal melanoma: proton beam irradiation. Ophthalmol Clin North Am 18(1):111–118

Lane AM, Gragoudas ES (2007) Uveal malignant melanoma: management options – proton beam radiotherapy. In: Singh AD, Damato BE, Pe'er J, Murphree AL, Perry JD (eds) Clinical ophthalmic oncology. Elsevier-Saunders, Philadelphia, pp 248–253

Uveal Melanoma: Resection Technique 69

Evelyn X. Fu and Arun D. Singh

Synonyms

Choroidectomy, Endoresection

Definition

The surgical removal of tumor and choroid

Transscleral Choroidectomy

Indications

Bulky choroidal melanoma (thickness >8 mm) that cannot be adequately treated with brachytherapy or proton beam radiation. It is also used to treat local recurrence and remove irradiated tumor with significant exudative retinal detachment and neovascular glaucoma.

E.X. Fu, M.D.
Department of Ophthalmic Oncology,
Cole Eye Institute, Cleveland Clinic Foundation,
9500 Euclid Avenue,
Cleveland, OH 44195, USA

A.D. Singh, M.D. (✉)
Department of Ophthalmic Oncology,
Cole Eye Institute, Cleveland Clinic Foundation,
9500 Euclid Avenue, Desk i-329,
Cleveland, OH 44195, USA
e-mail: singha@ccf.org

H.E. Grossniklaus (ed.), *Pocket Guide to Ocular Oncology and Pathology*,
DOI 10.1007/978-3-642-29782-3_69,

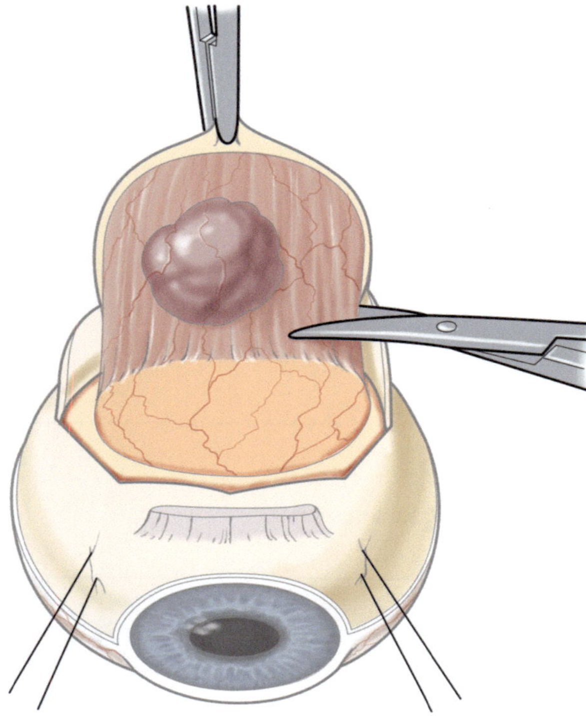

Fig. 69.1 Transscleral choroidectomy (Reproduced with permission from Damato (1999))

Contraindications

Patients with systemic diseases that preclude hypotensive anesthesia and tumors with basal diameter exceeding 16 mm, optic disc involvement, more than three clock hours of ciliary body or angle involvement, or extensive retinal invasion. Extraocular extension is not a contraindication if the tumor is otherwise resectable or treatable with adjunctive radiotherapy.

Techniques and Principles (Fig. 69.1)

Hypotensive anesthesia is induced to avoid intraocular hemorrhage. A 180–360° limbal peritomy is created, two scleral traction sutures are placed, and extraocular muscles overlying the tumor are disinserted to provide exposure. The tumor is localized by transpupillary transillumination. A polyhedral shaped lamellar flap with 90% scleral depth and at least 3-mm of margin is dissected with a no. 59 Beaver Blade. Vortex veins or long posterior ciliary arteries in the flap are cauterized. A triple row of penetrating diathermy is placed around the tumor to prevent intraocular bleeding. One to 1.5 mL of vitreous is removed via a limited pars plana vitrectomy

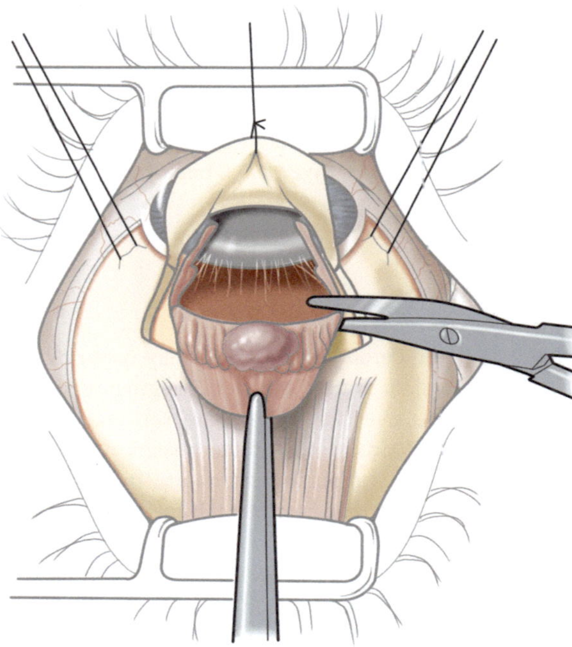

Fig. 69.2 Technique of iridocyclectomy (Reproduced with permission from Damato (1999))

to prevent retinal prolapse through the scleral window. Incisions with a diamond knife into the deep sclera are made 1–2 mm closer to the tumor margins in relation to the superficial flap to create a stepped wound edge and facilitate closure. Blunt-tipped scissors are used to excise the tumor with the deep scleral lamella. The retina usually separates spontaneously from the tumor but in cases with retina-tumor adhesion, the intraretinal part of the tumor may be left in situ and treated with adjunctive radiotherapy. The scleral window is closed with interrupted 8-0 nylon sutures using a fresh set of instruments to prevent possible seeding of tumor cells. The globe is reformed with balanced salt solution, the extraocular muscles are reinserted, and the conjunctiva is closed. If adjunctive brachytherapy is to be applied, a 25-mm ruthenium plaque delivering approximately 100 Gy to a depth of 1–2 mm is favored because of the limited range of beta irradiation, the convenience of a long half-life, and the thin shape of the implant. If the ciliary body is involved (Fig. 69.2), the anterior margin of the superficial scleral flap is placed at or near the limbus so that the deep scleral incision enters the anterior chamber. As much of the ciliary epithelium as possible is conserved by perforating the choroid posterior to the ora serrata and bluntly dissecting the ciliary epithelium from uvea before cutting the uveal tissue with scissors. Postoperatively, the patient is positioned with the surgical coloboma situated below the macula to prevent any subretinal blood from gravitating toward the macula. Residual subretinal fluid from the preoperative exudative retinal detachment generally resorbs within a few days despite the absence of the underlying retinal pigment epithelium and choroid.

Outcomes

Uveal melanomas ≥16 mm in height have better visual function and lower complications when treated with transscleral local resection than iodine-125 plaque brachytherapy. Tumors located nasally or are more than one disc diameter away from the optic disc or fovea have better visual outcome than tumors in the posterior pole.

Complications

Myocardial and cerebral infarctions may occur during profound hypotensive anesthesia. Incomplete tumor resection, rhegmatogenous retinal detachment, choroidal tears, and expulsive hemorrhage are serious ocular complications. Tumor recurrence may result from incomplete resection, microscopic subclinical deposits, or failure to detect extraocular extension. Intraoperative penetrating diathermy and adjunctive brachytherapy reduce the incidence of local recurrence. Retina break is complicated by proliferative vitreoretinopathy and must be repaired with total vitrectomy, endolaser retinopexy, and silicone oil tamponade immediately. Choroidal tear may occur if the tumor is pulled excessively during resection. The incidence of metastatic disease after local excision is not significantly different from that after enucleation or plaque radiotherapy.

Transretinal Endoresection

Indication

Reserved for selected cases of juxtapapillary tumors when visual loss as a result of optic neuropathy is inevitable with radiotherapy.

Contraindications

Tumor basal diameter exceeds 10 mm or involves more than 4–5 h of the optic disc margin.

Techniques and Principles (Fig. 69.3)

A pars plana vitrectomy is performed, and the tumor is accessed via a retinotomy at the apex of the lesion. In tumors involving the macula, a peripheral retinectomy is created, and the retina is folded away from the lesion. A 20-gauge vitrector is used to remove the growth, beginning at the apex to form a crater into which hemorrhage

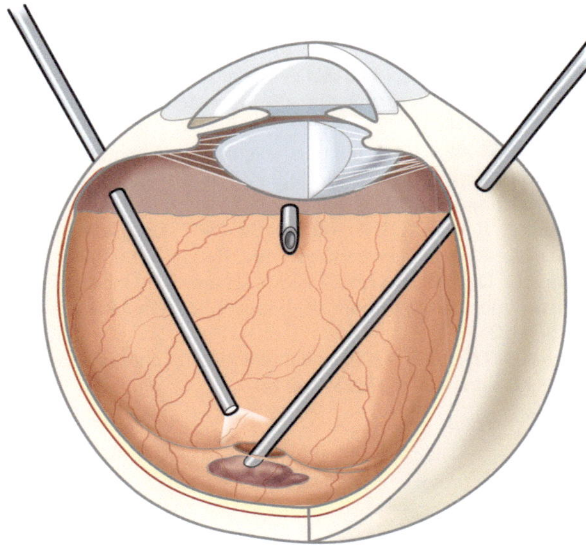

Fig. 69.3 Transretinal endoresection (Reproduced with permission from Damato (1999))

will pool. Intraoperative bleeding is controlled by temporarily elevating the intraocular pressure. Endodiathermy is applied to the tumor margins, and endolaser is administered to the exposed scleral bed to destroy any residual tumor. Fluid-air exchange and endolaser retinopexy are performed to reattach the retina. The eye is then filled with silicone oil for 12 weeks.

Outcomes

The eye can be successfully conserved in more than 90% of cases. The final vision depends on the tumor location.

Complications

The main concern regarding endoresection is tumor seeding. Widespread dissemination has only been reported in one patient whose local recurrence was not immediately detected and treated because of opaque media. Local recurrence is infrequent and can be further reduced with adjunctive brachytherapy and proton beam radiation.

Cross-References

Choroid melanoma, uveal peripheral nerve sheath tumor, surgical techniques

Further Reading

Bechrakis NE, Bornfeld N, Zoller I et al (2002) Iodine 125 plaque brachytherapy versus transscleral tumor resection in the treatment of large uveal melanomas. Ophthalmology 109:1855–1861

Damato B (1999) Ocular tumours: diagnosis and treatment. Butterworth Heinemann, Oxford

Damato B, Groenewald C, McGalliard J et al (1998) Endoresection of choroidal melanoma. Br J Ophthalmol 82:213–218

Karkhaneh R, Chams H, Amoli FA et al (2007) Long-term surgical outcome of posterior choroidal melanoma treated by endoresection. Retina 27:908–914

Puusaari I, Damato B, Kivela T (2007) Transscleral local resection versus iodine brachytherapy for uveal melanomas that are large because of tumour height. Graefes Arch Clin Exp Ophthalmol 245:522–533

Singh AD, Triozzi PL (2008) Endoresection for choroidal melanoma: palliative or curative intent? Br J Ophthalmol 92:1015–1016

Uveal Melanoma: Thermotherapy 70

Werner Wackernagel, Arun D. Singh, Chris Bergstrom, and Hans E. Grossniklaus

Synonyms

Transpupillary thermotherapy, Infrared thermotherapy, TTT

Definition

Thermotherapy is the destruction of intraocular tumors by heating tumor tissue to temperatures of 60–65°C, usually by means of an infrared diode laser (810 nm). Thermotherapy is a distinct independent therapeutic modality and different from photocoagulation, which induces coagulation of tumor tissue at temperatures above 65°C. It is also different from hyperthermia, which induces heating to less than 45°C and causing only limited disturbance of tumor cells. Thermotherapy induces irreversible cell damage, tumor necrosis, and vascular occlusion up to a depth of 3.9 mm.

W. Wackernagel, M.D.
Department of Ophthalmology and Optometry,
Medical University Graz, Auenbruggerplatz 4, 8036 Graz, Austria
e-mail: werner.wackernagel@medunigraz.at

A.D. Singh, M.D. (✉)
Department of Ophthalmic Oncology, Cole Eye Institute, Cleveland Clinic Foundation,
9500 Euclid Ave, Desk i-329, Cleveland, OH 44195, USA
e-mail: singha@ccf.org

C. Bergstrom, M.D.
Department of Ophthalmology, Emory University School of Medicine,
Atlanta, GA, USA
e-mail: cbergs2@emory.edu

H.E. Grossniklaus, M.D.
Emory University School of Medicine,
Emory Eye Center,
Department of Ophthalmology,
Atlanta, GA, USA
e-mail: ophtheg@emory.edu

H.E. Grossniklaus (ed.), *Pocket Guide to Ocular Oncology and Pathology*,
DOI 10.1007/978-3-642-29782-3_70, © Springer-Verlag Berlin Heidelberg 2013

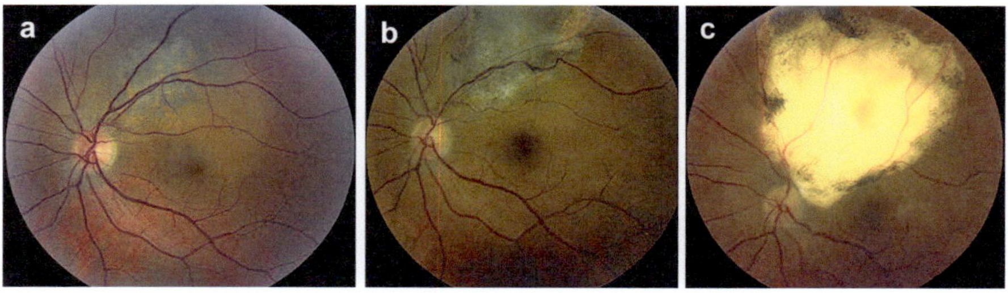

Fig. 70.1 Small choroidal melanoma treated with three sessions of TTT. (**a**) Shows the tumor prior to treatment. Note the *orange* pigment on the tumor surface and the subretinal fluid that extends under the fovea. (**b**) Is 3 months after the first treatment and (**c**) is 1 year after the third treatment

Indications

Thermotherapy is commonly used for the following indications:

(a) Small choroidal melanoma: TTT as a sole treatment may be used only for small melanomas, up to a height of about 3 mm (Fig. 70.1). However, because of the uncertainty about the efficacy of TTT as a sole treatment, it is currently being recommended for use in combination with brachytherapy, even for small melanomas.
(b) Medium-sized and large choroidal melanoma: For tumors higher than 3 mm, TTT is always used in combination with plaque brachytherapy. This technique (sandwich therapy) is used for tumors too high to be treated with plaque brachytherapy alone or to reduce radiation dose, thus minimizing radiation side effects.
(c) Juxtapapillary choroidal melanoma in combination with a notched radioactive plaque.
(d) TTT has successfully been used to treat tumor recurrence after radiotherapy and also to quicken tumor regression.
(e) Side effects after radiation, such as subretinal fluid and cystoid macular edema, have also been treated with TTT, using lower energy settings to treat exuding melanoma.

Contraindications

(a) TTT is contraindicated as a sole treatment for tumors thicker than 4 mm.
(b) Media opacities, such as lens opacifications or vitreous bleeding, not only hinder visibility of the tumor but also absorb part of the laser energy.
(c) Retinal detachment and subretinal fluid overlying the tumor also hamper correct alignment of the laser beam.
(d) Amelanotic melanoma: As absorption of laser energy depends much on tumor pigmentation, TTT is less effective in less pigmented tumors, though absorption may be increased by intravenous ICG (indocyanine green).

Techniques and Principles

The infrared laser can be attached to a slit lamp, the operation microscope, or an indirect ophthalmoscope. TTT is performed after full dilation of the pupil, and usually retro- or peribulbar anesthesia is given before treatment. The laser is set to a beam diameter of 2–3 mm, to an exposure time of 1 min, and to an energy of 300–600 mW. Energy settings are adjusted after each spot for the tumor to show a grayish color after 30–40 s. White coagulation effects on the tumor surface should be avoided, as this will reduce depth of penetration. The entire tumor surface and a safety margin of 1–2 mm are covered with overlapping spots.

Outcomes

TTT as a sole treatment for small melanomas also shows a high initial response rate of over 90%. However, long-term outcomes are less favorable with a recurrence rate of about 22% after 3 years and 33% after 10 years. Several cases of extrascleral recurrence after complete regression of the intraocular tumor emphasize the need for continuous follow-up with ultrasound exams for many years (Fig. 70.2). Visual

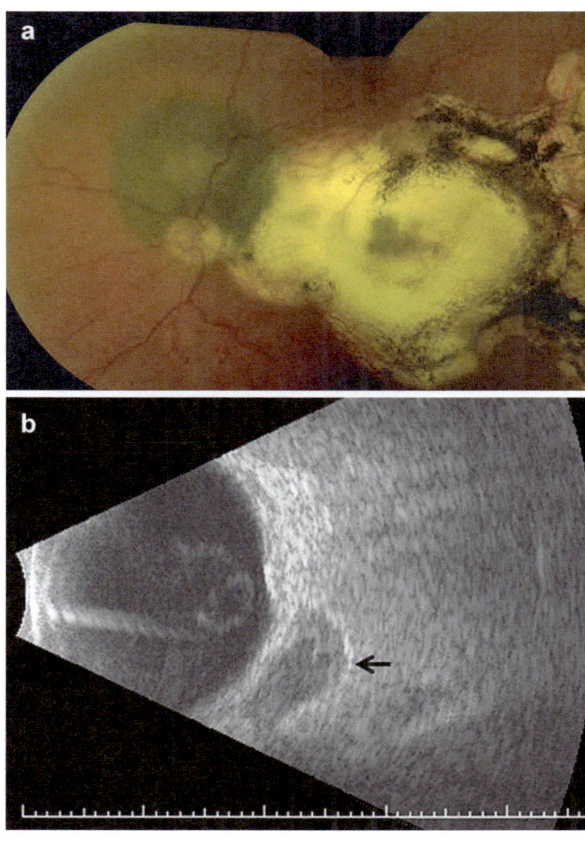

Fig. 70.2 Tumor recurrence following TTT. (**a**) Fundus photograph showing tumor recurrence superior to the optic disc at the nasal edge of a TTT scar. (**b**) A B-scan ultrasonography of the same patient demonstrating a nodular extrascleral extension along the base of the original tumor (*arrow*)

results after TTT are comparable with radiotherapy. TTT induces absolute scotoma in the treated area, and visual outcome depends much on tumor location.

Complications

Complications include transient retinal edema, subretinal fluid, and exudation. Severe complications such as retinal artery and vein occlusion, superficial bleeding, or retinal breaks are rare, however. Intense TTT might eventually result in the formation of epiretinal membranes, jeopardizing otherwise good visual outcome.

Pathology

The pathology of TTT treated uveal melanoma shows early hemorrhages and necrosis, followed by atrophy and fibrosis of the tumor. In cases of recurrent melanoma, the melanoma may be relatively flat within the choroids or cause a mound. Extraocular extension via an emissary canal may occur due to insulated tumor within the sclera (Fig. 70.3).

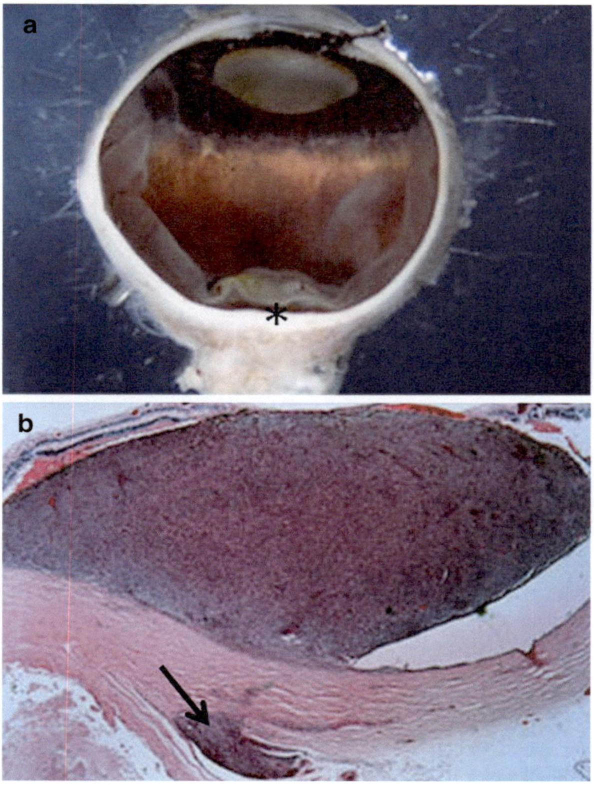

Fig. 70.3 (**a**) A recurrent choroidal tumor (*) after TTT is present in this enucleate eye. (**b**) The tumor exhibits extraocular extension via an emissary canal (*arrow*) (**b**: Hematoxylin and eosin, ×25)

Cross-References

Choroidal melanoma, brachytherapy, radiotherapy

Further Reading

Aaberg TM Jr, Bergstrom CS, Hickner ZJ, Lynn MJ (2008) Long-term results of primary transpupillary thermal therapy for the treatment of choroidal malignant melanoma. Br J Ophthalmol 92(6):741–746

Harbour JW, Meredith TA, Thompson PA (2003) Transpupillary thermotherapy versus plaque radiotherapy for suspected choroidal melanomas. Ophthalmology 110:2207–2214; discussion 2215

Journée-de Korver H, Midena E, Singh AD (2005) Infrared thermotherapy: from laboratory to clinic. Ophthalmol Clin North Am 18:99–110

Journée-de Korver H, Schalij-Delfos N, Imhof S (2007) Uveal malignant melanoma: management options – thermotherapy. In: Singh AD, Damato BE, Pe'er J, Murphree AL, Perry JD (eds) Clinical ophthalmic oncology. Saunders-Elsevier, Philadelphia, pp 232–240

Shields CL, Shields JA, Perez N (2002) Primary transpupillary thermotherapy for small choroidal melanoma in 256 consecutive cases: outcomes and limitations. Ophthalmology 109:225–234

Singh AD, Rundle PA, Berry-Brincat A, Parsons MA, Rennie IG (2004) Extrascleral extension of choroidal malignant melanoma following transpupillary thermotherapy. Eye 18:91–93

Singh AD, Kivelä T, Seregard S, Robertson D, Bena JF (2008) Primary transpupillary thermotherapy of "small" choroidal melanoma: is it safe? Br J Ophthalmol 92:727–728

Zaldivar RA, Aaberg TM, Sternberg P Jr, Waldron R, Grossniklaus HE (2003) Clinicopathologic findings in choroidal melanomas after failed transpupillary thermotherapy. Am J Ophthalmol 135(5):657–663

Part VII

Optic Nerve Tumors and Phakomatoses

Optic Nerve Glioma

71

Hans E. Grossniklaus

Synonyms

Juvenile pilocytic astrocytoma

Definition

A low-grade (grade 1) glioma involving the optic nerve

Etiology

Glioma may be associated with neurofibromatosis, with optic nerve glioma in 12–37% of patients with neurofibromatosis type 1.

Clinical Presentation

Optic nerve glioma (Fig. 71.1): Patients will have decreased vision and an afferent papillary defect in the affected eye. The optic disc may be swollen and contain dilated vessels; it also later appears pale and atrophic. There may be a loss of color vision. Other signs include axial proptosis and ophthalmoplegia. Visual fields may show a central scotoma or enlarged blind spot. Patients with NF1 will have other sequelae of neurofibromatosis.

H.E. Grossniklaus, M.D.
Emory University School of Medicine,
Emory Eye Center,
Department of Ophthalmology,
Atlanta, GA, USA
e-mail: ophtheg@emory.edu

H.E. Grossniklaus (ed.), *Pocket Guide to Ocular Oncology and Pathology*,
DOI 10.1007/978-3-642-29782-3_71,

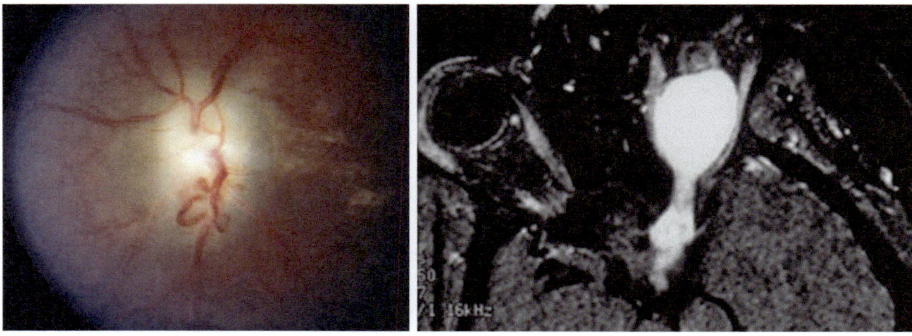

Fig. 71.1 Optic nerve glioma clinical. *Left*: swollen disc with dilated, tortuous vessels. *Right*: MRI with gadolinium shows fusiform enlargement of optic nerve

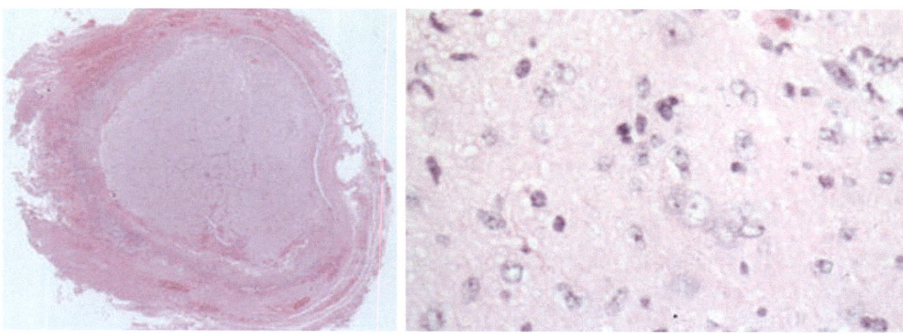

Fig. 71.2 Optic nerve glioma pathology. *Left*: The optic nerve is enlarged and there is perineural hyperplasia (arachnoidal gliosis) present. *Right*: The nerve fiber bundles are hypercellular and contain glial cells with large nuclei (*Left*, hematoxylin and eosin, ×25; *right*, hematoxylin and eosin, ×100)

Diagnostics

Optic nerve glioma: On MRI imaging, the tumor may be fusiform (sausage shaped) or saccular (balloon shaped); look for radiographic evidence of serial enlargement of optic foramen; chiasmal gliomas may cause death with raised intracranial pressure and interfere with pituitary/hypothalamic function. The optic nerve may also appear kinked.

Pathology

Optic nerve glioma (Fig. 71.2) with a thick perineural cuff and circumferential extension is a sign of neurofibromatosis. Intraneural growth with intact pial boundaries is a sign of an isolated glioma. Microscopically, the tumors spindle-shaped, cohesive astrocytes, pilocytic (hairlike astrocytes), oval/astrocytic nuclei, absence of mitosis, clusters of oligodendroglia (if majority is these cells, it is a oligodendroglioma), reactive area where tumor merges with normal; variants are myxomatous (mucopolysaccharide from astrocytes in extracellular matrix) and ancient (fibrotic, lipoid histiocytes, thick-walled fibrotic blood vessels suggestive of angiomatous lesion). Rosenthal fibers (degenerated glial filaments, eosinophilic intracellular electron dense granular material and glial filaments) may be present. Granular eosinophilic bodies may also be present. Arachnoidal gliomatosis (meningothelial cells, fibroblasts, neoplastic astrocytes) may be present and constitutes perineural cuff of cells. Malignant glioma of optic nerve and chiasm rarely occurs and includes numerous mitoses, atypical astrocytes, disruption of myelin/axons, and cellular pleomorphism.

Differential Diagnosis

The differential diagnosis of optic nerve glioma includes meningioma, vascular tumors, melanocytic tumors (melanocytoma), medulloepithelioma, and secondary optic disc/nerve tumors—melanoma, retinoblastoma, metastatic carcinoma, juxtapapillary RPE adenoma/adenocarcinoma, and combined hamartoma of RPE/retina. Inflammatory processes including pseudotumor and arachnoidal cysts may mimic primary optic nerve tumors. Other entities in the differential diagnosis include sarcoidosis, optic neuritis, and anterior ischemic optic neuropathy.

Prophylaxis

Optic nerve glioma may be found during routine screening of children with NF1.

Therapy

Options include observation, medical therapy, radiation, and surgical therapy. A biopsy may be performed to establish the diagnosis. The indications for medical or radiation therapy include documented progression with vision loss. Vincristine and cisplatin are most commonly used, although other agents have been used in various protocols. Radiation therapy may include: external beam radiation, intensity-modulated x-ray therapy, three-dimensional conformal radiation therapy, Gamma Knife, proton beam, or linear accelerator-based stereotactic multifraction radiotherapy. Surgical therapy is controversial and there is 5% recurrence if the tumor is incompletely excised. These excisions are usually transcranial in conjunction with neurosurgery. With optic nerve resection, there is a 92% 15-year survival rate. There are complications for any of these therapies.

Prognosis

Visual loss tends to stabilize in 80% of cases. Long-term survival without intervention is high.

Epidemiology

Optic nerve glioma may be associated with neurofibromatosis (NF) type 1. The incidence of NF1 is 1:3,500. The tumor usually presents during the first decade of life, with a mean age of diagnosis of 4.5 years in NF1 patients and 5.1 years in sporadic cases. This tumor represents 5% of intracranial tumors in children.

Cross-References

Optic nerve meningioma, phakomatoses, surgical techniques

Further Reading

Dutton JJ (2007) Chapter 92: Tumors of the optic nerve. In: Singh AD (ed) Clinical ophthalmic oncology. Saunders-Elsevier, Philadelphia, pp 549–554

Egan RE (2008) Tumors of the anterior visual pathways. In: Albert DA, Jakobiec FA (eds) Principles and practice of ophthalmology. Sauders-Elsevier, Philadelphia, pp 3898–3905

Packer RJ, Ater AJ, Phillips P et al (1997) Carboplatin and vincristine chemotherapy for children with newly diagnosed progressive low-grade gliomas. J Neurosurg 86(5):747–754

Optic Nerve Meningioma

72

Hans E. Grossniklaus

Synonyms

Meningotheliomatous meningioma

Definition

A tumor that arises from meningothelium in the arachnoid of the meninges surrounding the optic nerve

Etiology

Optic nerve meningioma occurs in 9% of patient with neurofibromatosis type 2.

Clinical Presentation

Optic nerve meningioma (Figs. 72.1 and 72.2). Patients will have decreased vision and an afferent papillary defect in the affected eye. The classic triad of optic nerve meningioma is optic atrophy, an optociliary shunt, and decreased vision. This optic disc may be swollen (early) or atrophic (late). There may be axial proptosis, diplopia, transient visual obscurations, orbital pain, or headache present. Visual fields may show a central scotoma or enlarged blind spot.

H.E. Grossniklaus, M.D.
Emory University School of Medicine, Emory Eye Center,
Department of Ophthalmology,
Atlanta, GA, USA
e-mail: ophtheg@emory.edu

H.E. Grossniklaus (ed.), *Pocket Guide to Ocular Oncology and Pathology*,
DOI 10.1007/978-3-642-29782-3_72,

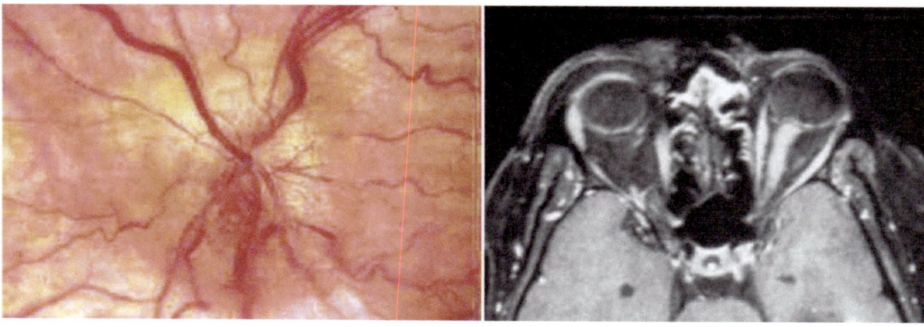

Fig. 72.1 Optic nerve meningioma clinical. *Left*: The optic disc is hyperemic and there are associated small vascular channels. *Right*: MRI with gadolinium shows enhancement of the enlarged left optic nerve

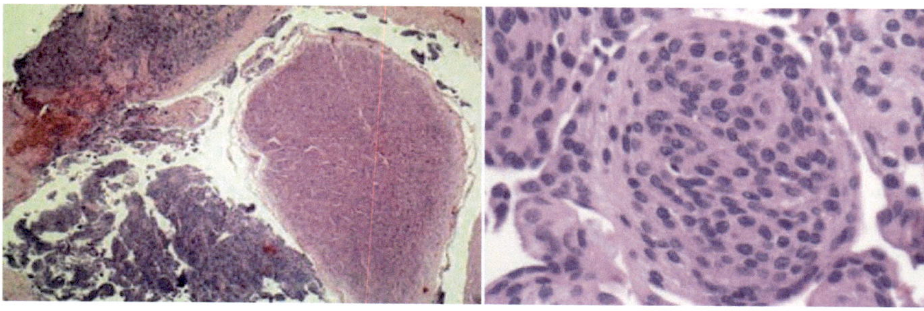

Fig. 72.2 Optic nerve meningioma pathology. *Left*: The optic nerve is atrophic and there is a cellular proliferation in the subdural space and extending into the dura. *Right*: The tumor contains whorls of epithelial-like cells that contain pseudonuclear inclusions (*left*, hematoxylin and eosin, ×25; *right*, hematoxylin and eosin, x100)

Diagnostics

The classic MRI image includes a "tram track" appearance, with enlargement of the nerve, thickening of the meninges (rails of the track), and vessels crossing the nerve (rails of the track). There may be fusiform or plaque-shaped enlargement of the optic nerve. A biopsy may be performed for diagnostic purposes in difficult cases This procedure is shown in Chapter 10, Figure 10.8

Pathology

Optic nerve meningioma may be ectopic/secondary and exhibit meningothelial, fibroblastic, angioblastic, or transitional subtypes. Primary optic nerve meningioma is invariably a meningotheliomatous meningioma, composed of sheets and nests of cells of arachnoid origin. These cells resemble epithelial cells, contain bland round to oval nuclei, and often display intranuclear pseudoinclusions. These cells interdigitate and form a syncytium. Unlike gliomas, meningiomas may extend through the dura and may display an intradural "sleevelike" growth pattern, which appears as toothpaste-like material on gross examination.

Differential Diagnosis

The differential diagnosis of optic nerve meningioma includes glioma, vascular tumors, melanocytic tumors (melanocytoma), medulloepithelioma, and secondary optic disc/nerve tumors—melanoma, retinoblastoma, metastatic carcinoma, juxtapapillary RPE adenoma/adenocarcinoma, and combined hamartoma of RPE/retina the list of primary and secondary optic disc/nerve tumors. Inflammatory processes including pseudotumor and arachnoidal cysts may mimic primary optic nerve tumors. Other entities in the differential diagnosis include sarcoidosis, optic neuritis, and anterior ischemic optic neuropathy.

Prophylaxis

Optic nerve meningioma may be found during routine screening of patients with NF2.

Therapy

Options include observation, radiation, medical therapy, and surgical therapy. Systemic steroids may be used for stabilization prior to observation. In order to establish the diagnosis, a biopsy may be performed. Radiation is the mainstay of therapy and may include fractionated external beam (5,000–5,500 Gy in daily fractions of 180–200 Gy), stereotactic radiation, 11-cobalt Gamma Knife (15–18 Gy to tumor margin), and proton beam. Medical therapy may include hydroxyurea, mifepristone, alpha interferon, bevacizumab, tamoxifen, cyclophosphamide, doxorubicin, vincristine, and other agents with corticosteroids given to decrease inflammation. Surgical therapy is not utilized if vision preservation is the goal. Resection may be used in poorly sighted eyes to decrease proptosis, relieve discomfort, and decrease the risk of intracranial spread. These resections are usually transcranial with orbital unroofing in conjunction with neurosurgery.

Prognosis

If the meningioma is confined to the optic nerve, the long-term prognosis for survival is high, although the chances of maintaining useful vision are low.

Epidemiology

The incidence of optic nerve meningioma increases with age, with 20% of patients diagnosed at 10 years old or younger and 20% of patients diagnosed at 20 years or younger. Two thirds of cases occur on females. This tumor comprises 10% of optic nerve tumors and 2% of orbital tumors.

Cross-References

Optic nerve glioma, phakomatoses, surgical techniques

Further Reading

Dutton JJ (2007) Tumors of the optic nerve. In: Singh AD (ed) Chapter 92 clinical ophthalmic oncology. Saunders-Elsevier, Philadelphia, pp 549–554

Egan RE (2008) Tumors of the anterior visual pathways. In: Albert DA, Jakobiec FA (eds) Principles and practice of ophthalmology. Saunders-Elsevier, Philadelphia, pp 3898–3905

Turbin RE, Thompson CR, Kenerdell JS, Cockerham KP, Kupersmith MJ (2002) A long-term visual outcome comparison in patients with optic nerve sheath meningioma managed with observation, surgery, radiotherapy or surgery and radiotherapy. Ophthalmology 109:890–899

Optic Nerve Head Melanocytoma 73

Martina C. Herwig and Hans E. Grossniklaus

Synonyms

Magnocellular nevus

Definition

Melanocytoma is a benign, pigmented hamartoma of the optic nerve head with typical clinical and histological features. Previously considered to be primary malignant melanomas of the optic disc, Zimmerman established the entity of "melanocytoma" indicating its benign nature.

Etiology

Melanocytoma of the optic nerve head is a congenital lesion thought to develop from proliferating uveal melanocytes normally found in the optic nerve and in the lamina cribrosa.

M.C. Herwig, M.D. (✉)
Department of Ophthalmology, Emory University School of Medicine,
Atlanta, GA, USA

Department of Ophthalmology, University of Bonn,
Bonn, Germany
e-mail: martina.c.herwig@emory.edu, martina.herwig@ukb.uni-bonn.de

H.E. Grossniklaus, M.D.
Emory University School of Medicine,
Emory Eye Center,
Department of Ophthalmology,
Atlanta, GA, USA
e-mail: ophtheg@emory.edu

H.E. Grossniklaus (ed.), *Pocket Guide to Ocular Oncology and Pathology*,
DOI 10.1007/978-3-642-29782-3_73, © Springer-Verlag Berlin Heidelberg 2013

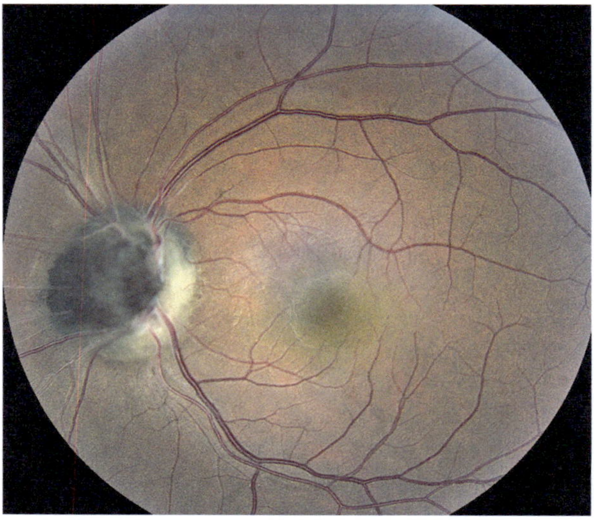

Fig. 73.1 Fundus photography of a left eye displaying a melanocytoma of the optic nerve head appearing as a pigmented lesion in the nasal part of the optic disc

Clinical Presentation

Melanocytoma of the optic disc is commonly seen in blacks and darker pigmented races although it occurs in all races. Most patients are asymptomatic, and the lesion is found on routine fundus examination.

Diagnostics

The diagnosis is usually made by the typical clinical appearance on funduscopic examination (Fig. 73.1). Melanocytomas of the optic disc are solitary, slightly elevated, dark-brown or black tumors usually involving the inferotemporal aspect of the optic disc. They may partially or totally obscure the optic disc and may have contiguous involvement of the choroid and retina. They tend to be stable or slowly growing tumors.

Pathology

Histologically, the tumor consists of uniform deeply pigmented cells containing numerous melanosomes. Bleaching by potassium permanganate is required to reveal the cytologic features of a melanocytoma: round or slightly polyhedral plump, densely pigmented cells with abundant cytoplasm and small uniform nuclei with inconspicuous nucleoli (type I cells) (Fig. 73.2), and small, sparingly pigmented spindle-shaped cells (type II cells). Type II tumor cells are accounted for the growth potential of melanocytomas and are more frequently found in areas of local invasion. Mitotic figures are uncommon. Melanomacrophages can

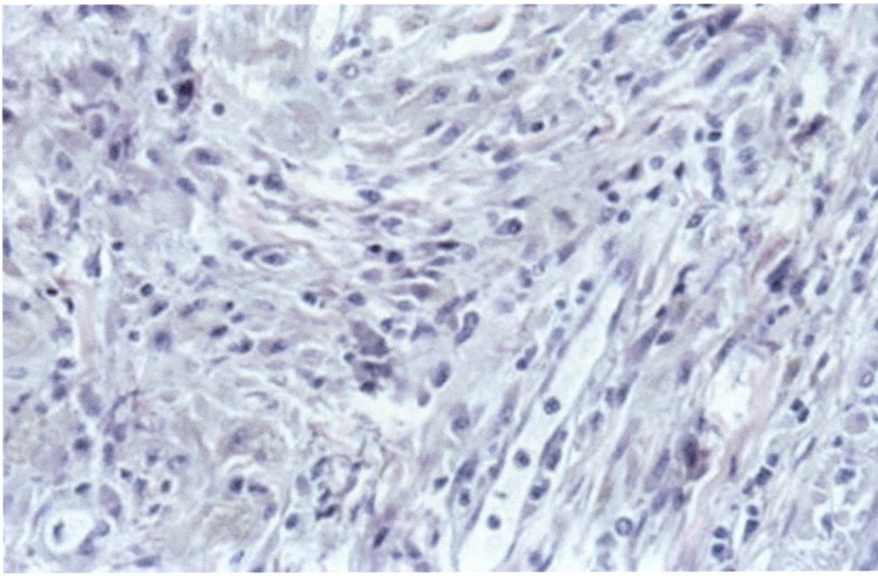

Fig. 73.2 The pathology of optic nerve head melanocytoma shows predominantly polyhedral cells with abundant cytoplasm and sparsely spindle-shaped cells (hematoxylin and eosin, bleached, ×100)

be observed in a scattered pattern. Albeit rare, malignant transformation into or coexistence of a malignant melanoma is characterized by the presence of melanoma cells with larger nuclei (spindle-shaped or epithelioid cell type) and prominent nucleoli.

Electron Microscopy

By electron microscopy, the two different cell types can be further distinguished: Type I cells contain giant melanosomes within their abundant cytoplasm and reveal a relative sparsity of other cytoplasmic organelles indicating metabolic inactivity. Type II cells consist of immature melanosomes and a markedly infolded nuclear membrane with a more prominent nucleoli (compared to type I cells) and reveal many cytoplasmic organelles suggesting an active metabolic rate. Common features of both cell types include occasional desmosome-like attachment, fine cytoplasmic filaments, and focal basement membrane production.

Differential Diagnosis

Differential diagnosis includes a juxtapapillary malignant melanoma of the choroid invading the optic disc, combined hamartoma of the retina and RPE, and adenoma of the RPE.

Prophylaxis

None

Therapy

Annual examination and fundus photography

Prognosis

The majority of optic nerve head melanocytomas remain stable over many years. Slight enlargement occurs in approximately 10% of cases. Optic nerve dysfunction and vascular occlusions have been associated with these tumors. Malignant transformation is rare but can occur in 1–2% of cases.

Cross-References

Choroidal melanoma

Further Reading

Juarez CP, Tso MOM (1980) An ultrastructural study of melanocytomas (magnocellular nevi) of the optic disk and uvea. Am J Ophthalmol 90:48–62

Loeffler KU, Tecklenborg H (1992) Melanocytoma-like growth of a juxtapapillary malignant melanoma. Retina 12:29–34

Rao NA, Spencer WH (1996) Optic nerve. In: Spender WH (ed) Ophthalmic pathology: an atlas and textbook, 4th edn. WB Saunders Company, Philadelphia, pp 584–588

Reidy JJ, Apple DJ, Steinmetz RL, Craythorn JM, Loftfield K, Gieser SC, Brady SE (1985) Melanocytoma: nomenclature, pathogenesis, natural history and treatment. Surv Ophthalmol 29:319–327

Zimmerman LE, Garron LK (1962) Melanocytoma of the optic disc. Int Ophthalmol Clin 2:431–440

Optic Nerve Metastasis

74

Hans E. Grossniklaus

Synonyms

None

Definition

Malignant neoplasm that spreads to the optic nerve via hematogenous dissemination or dissemination via the cerebrospinal fluid

Etiology

The etiology of this condition is metastasis from a primary malignancy at a distant site. It is possible for an intraocular tumor, such as melanoma or retinoblastoma, to directly extend into the optic nerve. Orbital tumors, such as meningioma, may also invade the optic nerve by direct extension. These two latter instances are direct extension and not metastases.

H.E. Grossniklaus, M.D.
Emory University School of Medicine,
Emory Eye Center,
Department of Ophthalmology,
Atlanta, GA, USA
e-mail: ophtheg@emory.edu

H.E. Grossniklaus (ed.), *Pocket Guide to Ocular Oncology and Pathology*,
DOI 10.1007/978-3-642-29782-3_74, © Springer-Verlag Berlin Heidelberg 2013

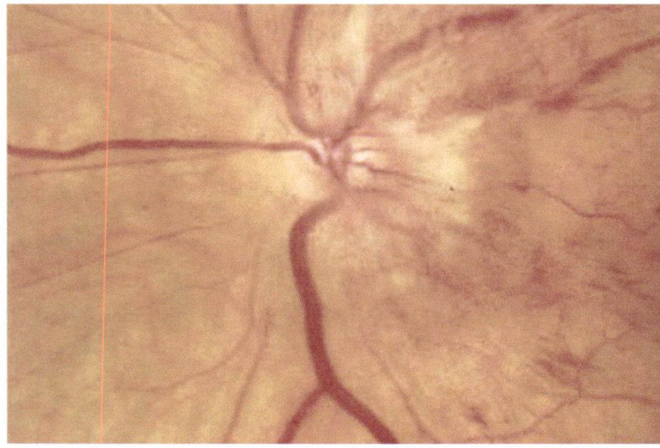

Fig. 74.1 There is disc edema of this patient who has metastatic breast carcinoma

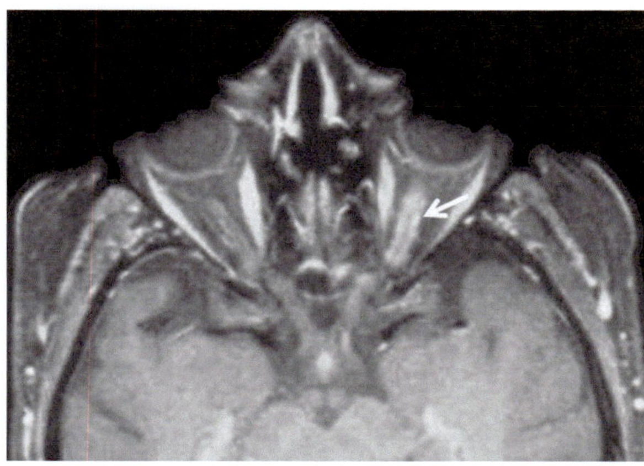

Fig. 74.2 MRI shows enlargement and enhancement of the left optic nerve (*arrow*) in a tram track sign configuration

Clinical Presentation

Optic nerve metastases may appear as swelling of the optic nerve head (Fig. 74.1) or atrophy of the optic nerve head. Neuroimaging will reveal an optic nerve mass that usually enhances. The mass may cause enlargement of the nerve or a tram track sign, similar to meningioma (Fig. 74.2).

Diagnosis

The diagnosis may be made on a clinical presumptive basis if there is already known widespread metastasis. An optic nerve biopsy may also be performed. The diagnosis then may also be made by histologic examination of an optic nerve biopsy.

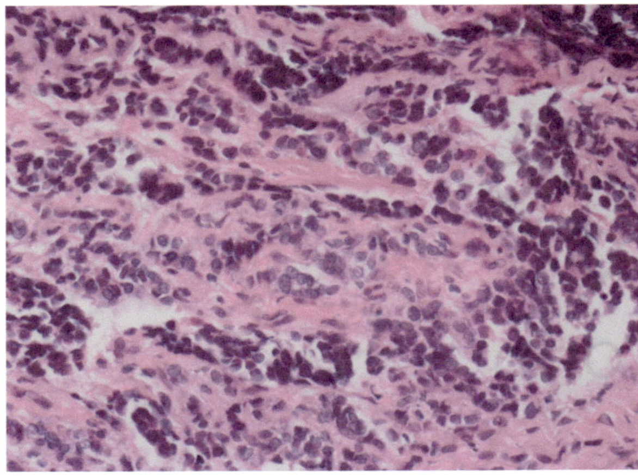

Fig. 74.3 A biopsy shows malignant cells with hyperchromatic nuclei arranged in single files (hematoxylin and eosin, ×100)

Pathology

The pathology of the metastatic tumor depends on the primary site. Carcinomas, such as metastatic breast carcinoma (Fig. 74.3), will grow in chords and sheets. Lymphoma and leukemia will grow in loosely coherent sheets. Sarcomas will generally be spindle cell tumors growing in tightly coherent sheets. Immunohistochemical stains, such as cytokeratins for carcinoma (Fig. 74.4), will assist in identifying the tumor.

Differential Diagnosis

The differential diagnosis includes primary optic nerve tumors, most commonly glioma and meningioma, and other infiltrative processes, such as sarcoidosis.

Prophylaxis

Adequate treatment of the primary tumor. If the primary tumor is a high risk for metastasis, there is no prophylactic treatment to prevent optic nerve metastasis.

Therapy

Therapy is treatment of the metastatic disease, either with chemotherapy, radiation therapy, or a combination of both. This will depend on the type and staging of the primary cancer. Coordination with the medical oncologist and radiation oncologist is recommended.

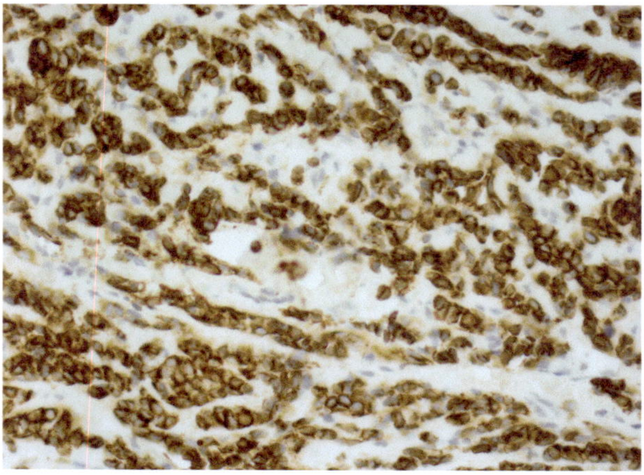

Fig. 74.4 Immunohistochemical stains for cytokeratins are positive in the malignant cells (peroxidase anti-peroxidase, ×100)

Prognosis

The prognosis is generally poor for vision and long-term survival.

Epidemiology

The epidemiology depends on the primary cancer. For instance, breast cancer is far more common in women than men, and lung cancer is more common in men.

Cross-References

Optic nerve glioma, optic nerve meningioma, surgical techniques

Further Reading

Christmas NJ, Mead MD, Richardson EP, Albert DM (1991) Secondary optic nerve tumors. Surv Ophthalmol 36:196–206

Newman NJ, Grossniklaus HE, Wojno TH (1996) Breast carcinoma metastatic to the optic nerve. Arch Ophthalmol 114:102–103

Phakomatoses

75

Hans E. Grossniklaus

General Considerations

Van der Hoeve coined the term "phakoma" (mother spot or birthmark) to describe this group of patients in 1932. A hamartia is a nontumorous normal tissue at its usual site; a hamartoma is a tumor of normal tissue at its usual site; a choristia is a nontumorous normal tissue at an abnormal site; a choristoma is a tumor composed of normal tissue at an abnormal site. Most of the phakomatoses are inherited in an autosomal dominant manner while Sturge-Weber and Wyburn-Mason are nonheritable. Most phakomatoses involve the eye, brain, and skin. Examples of involved tissue are glia (retina/brain in tuberous sclerosis) and hemangioblast (retina/cerebellum in von Hippel-Lindau). Most tumors in phakomatoses are benign, although there may be malignant variants such as malignant peripheral nerve sheath tumor. A forme fruste lesion lacks complete expressivity of the condition.

Tuberous Sclerosis (Bourneville Syndrome)

In 1880, Bourneville described a triad of adenoma sebaceum, epilepsy, and mental deficiency.

The tuberous sclerosis complex is caused by loss of function in one of two genes: *TSC1* on chromosome 9q34 or *TSC2* on 16p13. *TSC*1 and *TSC*2 code for hamartin and tuberin, respectively; TSC complex is caused by locus heterogeneity; hamartin and tuberin interact to suppress PI3K signal transduction pathway and integrate two

H.E. Grossniklaus, M.D.
Emory University School of Medicine,
Emory Eye Center,
Department of Ophthalmology,
Atlanta, GA, USA
e-mail: ophtheg@emory.edu

H.E. Grossniklaus (ed.), *Pocket Guide to Ocular Oncology and Pathology*,
DOI 10.1007/978-3-642-29782-3_75, © Springer-Verlag Berlin Heidelberg 2013

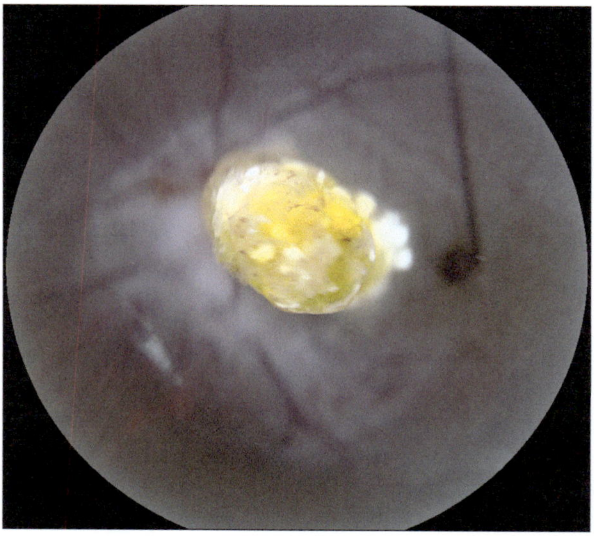

Fig. 75.1 A solitary mulberry-like astrocytic hamartoma arises in the retina in a patient with tuberous sclerosis

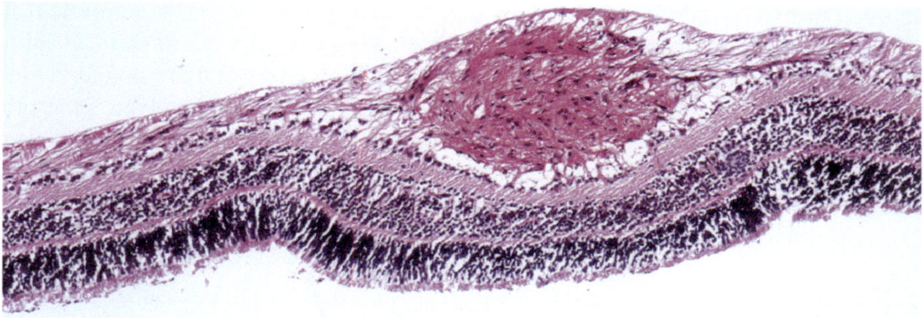

Fig. 75.2 Astrocytic hamartoma in inner retina in a patient with tuberous sclerosis. The astrocytic hamartoma is composed of glial cells forming a mass (H&E 100×)

important signals governing cell growth: growth factors and nutrients. The clinical features of tuberous sclerosis are as follows.

Three types of lesions may form in the brain: (1) cortical tubers (fascicles of neurons, astrocytes, and giant cells), (2) subependymal nodule (resembles tubers but has higher cellular packing density), and (3) subependymal giant cell astrocytoma (cells with prominent nuclei and abundant glassy eosinophilic cytoplasm). In the retina, an astrocytic hamartoma—sessile or slightly elevated lesion—may be unilateral, bilateral, solitary, multifocal, transparent, opaque, noncalcified, or calcified; giant cell hamartomas may be locally aggressive and contain areas of necrosis and calcospherites (Figs. 75.1 and 75.2). Skin lesions include adenoma sebaceum (angiofibroma) which may occur under fingernails (subungual fibroma), shagreen patches, depigmented macules, and café au lait spots

Neurofibromatosis (von Recklinghausen's Syndrome)

While isolated reports of this condition occurred during the nineteenth century, von Recklinghausen published the classic monograph in 1882. More recently, neurofibromatosis (NF) types 1 and 2 have been described. In NF type 1, 17q11.2 encodes a 350-kD protein "neurofibromin," a GTPase (GAP)-like protein that downregulates the ras oncogene. In NF type 2, 22q11.2–22q13.1 encodes "merlin," a tumor suppressor gene. The clinical criteria for diagnosing NF1 and NF2 are shown in Tables 75.1 and 75.2.

Ophthalmic tissue involvement in neurofibromatosis is as follows: (1) eyelid – peripheral nerve sheath tumors, fibroma molluscum, plexiform neurofibroma (Figs. 75.3 and 75.4); (2) conjunctiva/cornea – peripheral nerve sheath tumor, enlarged corneal nerves; (3) TM – diffuse thickening and secondary glaucoma, angle closure 2° forward displacement of iris by cb tumor, NVI, and secondary glaucoma; (4) lens – early onset PSC; (5) uveal tract – Lisch nodules (Figs. 75.5 and 75.6) and diffuse hamartoma (neurofibroma) of uveal tract; (6) increased incidence of nevi and melanoma and neurilemmoma (schwannoma); (7) retina – astrocytic hamartoma, myelinated nerve fibers, CHRPE, combined hamartoma; (8) optic nerve/orbit ON – astrocytic hamartoma, myelinated nerve fibers, juvenile

Table 75.1 Diagnostic Criteria for Type 1 Neurofibromatosis

NF type 1
NF type 1 (peripheral) 17q11.2
At least two of the following
At least six major café au lait macules (>1.5 cm)
2+ neurofibromas any type or one plexiform
Multiple axillary/inguinal freckles
Distinctive osseous lesion
Optic nerve glioma
Two or more Lisch nodules
First degree relative with NF type 1

Table 75.2 Diagnostic Criteria for Type 2 Neurofibromatosis

NF type 2
NF type 2 (central) 22q11.2–13.1
Each criterion:
1. CT/MRI evidence of acoustic neuroma
2. First degree relative with NF type 2 and either:
(a) Unilateral eighth nerve mass
(b) Two of the following:
(i) Neurofibroma
(ii) Meningioma
(iii) Schwannoma
(iv) Juvenile lens opacity

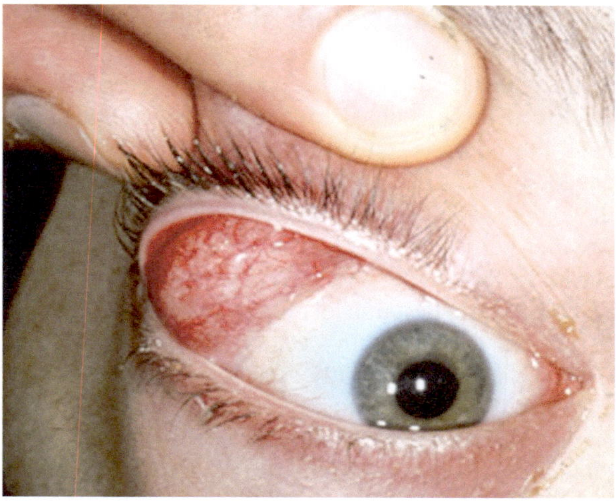

Fig. 75.3 Plexiform neurofibroma in upper eyelid/orbit of patient with neurofibromatosis

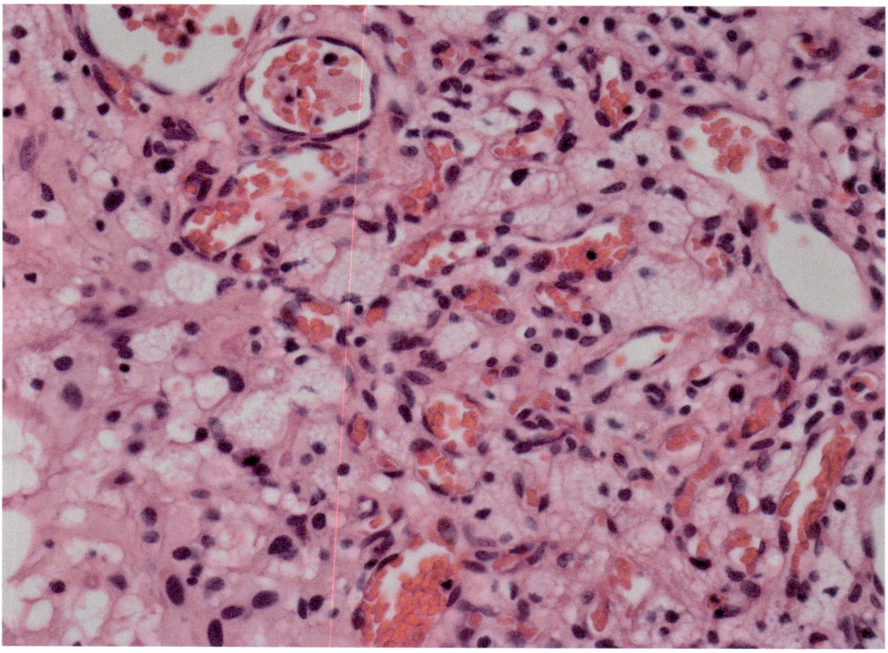

Fig. 75.4 The plexiform neurofibroma of the patient shown in Fig. 75.3 is composed of a proliferation of nerve fiber bundles with associated perineural cells (H&E × 10)

pilocytic astrocytoma (glioma), or meningioma and orbital plexiform neurofibroma, meningioma, pulsating exophthalmos; (9) skin – café au lait spots, nevi, peripheral nerve sheath tumors; and (10) brain/spinal cord – gliomas in area of 3 rd ventricle, pituitary tumors, spinal cord meningiomas, acoustic neuromas (bilateral) in NF type 2, syringomyelia.

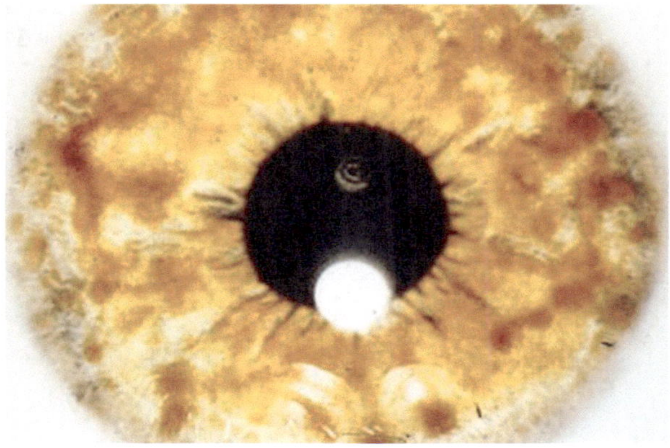

Fig. 75.5 Multiple Lisch nodules on the surface of the iris in a patient with neurofibromatosis

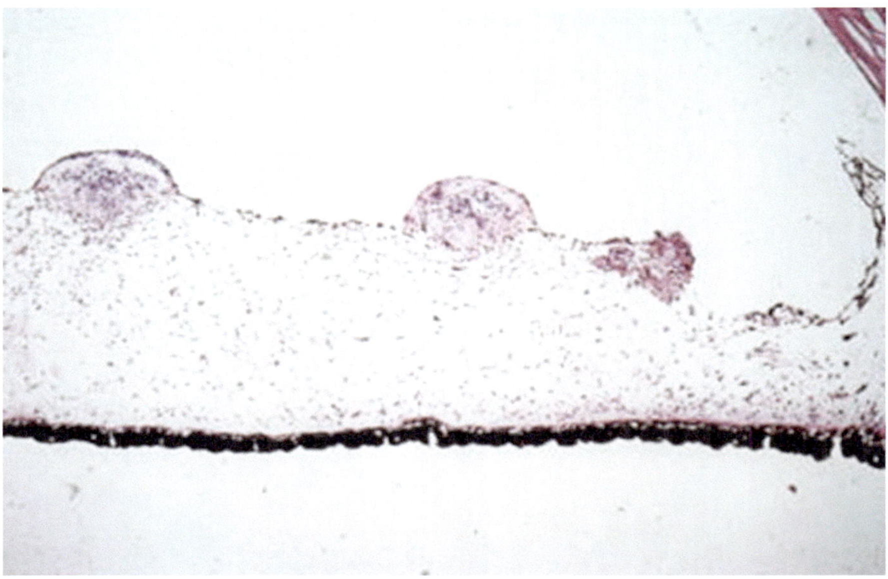

Fig. 75.6 The Lisch nodules are melanocytic hamartomas on and near the anterior border layer of the iris (H&E × 25)

Retinocerebellar Capillary Hemangiomatosis (von Hippel-Lindau Syndrome)

von Hippel reported retinal "angiomatosis" in 1926, and Lindau added cerebellar lesions to the syndrome. A mutation on 3p25.5, codes for VHL protein; VHL binds to ubiquitin ligase and ubiquitinates HIF1α by hydroxylation; if there is a mutation in VHL, HIF1α is not ubiquitinated and results in nuclear transcription of VEGF; the stromal cells in the angioblastoma are the tumor cells; the vascular component

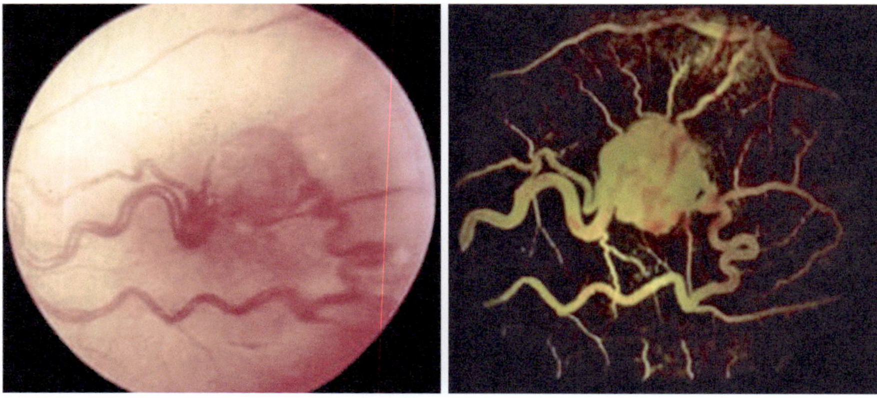

Fig. 75.7 A retinal hemangioblastoma is supplied by a feeder vessel; it appears as a *pink* to *reddish* mass and leaks fluorescein on angiography

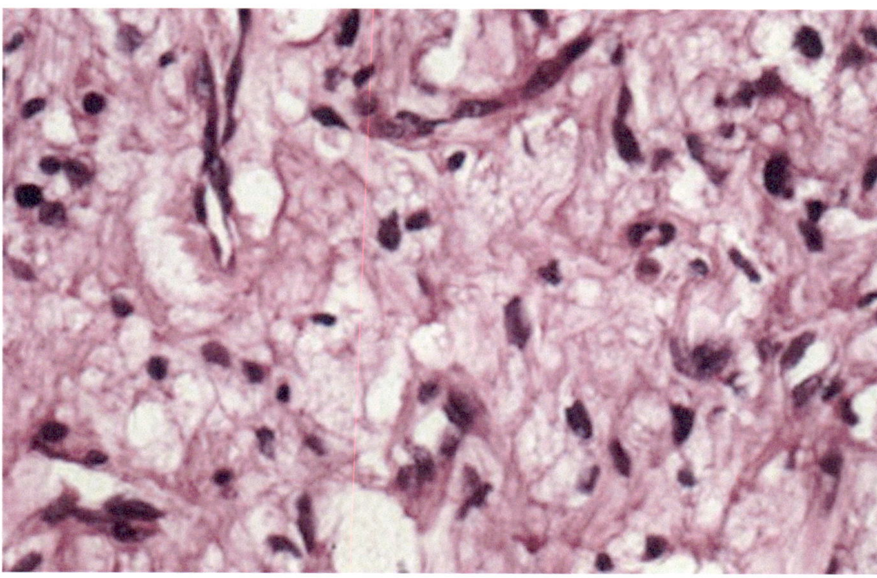

Fig. 75.8 The retinal hemangioblastoma is composed of stromal cells, some of which with intracytoplasmic vacuolations, and scattered vascular channels (H&E × 100)

of the tumor is secondary to VEGF production; thus, the tumor is not an "angioma." Inheritance is in a classic "two hit" fashions. The clinical features of this condition include: in the eye, a retinal hemangioblastoma with foamy stromal cells and secondary endothelial-lined vascular channels, which leak fluorescein, may be associated with subretinal exudates (Figs. 75.7 and 75.8); in the skin, rare angiomas, nevi, café au lait spots; in the brain/spinal cord, cerebellar hemangioblastoma; and other manifestations including renal cell carcinoma, pancreatic cysts, epididymis cystadenoma, and pheochromocytoma.

Encephalofacial Cavernous Hemangiomatosis (Sturge-Weber Syndrome)

Sturge described ipsilateral buphthalmos and contralateral seizures in 1879 and in 1922. Weber described the clinical manifestations in more detail in the first descriptions of this entity. There is no recognizable hereditary pattern for this condition. The clinical features of Sturge-Weber syndrome are as follows: (1) eyelid – nevus flammeus involving eyelid, involvement of upper eyelid associated with glaucoma; (2) conjunctiva/episclera – tortuous epibulbar vessels; (3) glaucoma – several types: anterior chamber abnormalities with buphthalmos, open angle type, NVI with angle involvement type; (4) choroid – diffuse choroidal hemangioma (tomato catsup fundus); (5) retina – retinal vascular changes; (6) others – hyperchromic heterochromia, RPE pigment changes; (7) skin – nevus flammeus or "port-wine" stain, vascular hamartoma; and (8) brain/spinal cord – diffuse leptomeningeal hemangioma with secondary calcification of cerebral cortex ("railroad track" sign).

Racemose Hemangiomatosis (Wyburn-Mason Syndrome)

Wyburn-Mason first described this condition in 1943. This condition is not heritable. The clinical features include: (1) retina – racemose hemangioma (AV malformation); (2) orbit – rarely vascular malformations; (3) skin – rarely small facial angiomas; and (4) brain/spinal cord – vascular malformation with associated seizures, spontaneous hemorrhages; may also involve maxilla/mandible precluding to bleeding during dental procedures.

Retinal Cavernous Hemangiomatosis with Cutaneous and CNS Vascular Malformations

This condition is more common in women than men and often displays an AD inheritance pattern. Clinical features include: (1) retina – cavernous hemangioma; (2) skin – vascular lesions most often on back of neck, eyelid involvement rare; (3) brain/spinal cord – vascular malformations, may be associated with seizures, diplopia, bleeding; may be subclinical.

Other Conditions Related to Phakomatoses

Ataxia Telangiectasia (Louis-Bar Syndrome)

This condition was first described by Madame Louis-Bar in 1941. It displays an AD inheritance pattern and has been mapped to 11q23, near CD3, THY1, and NCAM genes. Clinical features include: (1) conjunctival and cutaneous telangiectasia; (2) CNS – decreased reflexes, choreoathetosis, dysarthria; (3) immune incompetence – hypoplastic thymus, decreased IgA, lymphoma, leukemia.

Oculodermal Melanocytosis (Nevus of Ota)

This condition is manifest by hyperpigmentation of periocular skin along distribution of CN V, episcleral hyperpigmentation, and melanocytosis of uvea with an increased incidence of melanoma.

Klippel-Trenaunay-Weber Syndrome

This condition is associated with cutaneous hemangiomas/varicosities, soft tissue hemangiomas, hypertrophy of bone, and ophthalmic manifestations including orbital hemangioma, conjunctival vascular abnormalities, choroidal hemangioma, and congenital/acquired glaucoma.

Diffuse Neonatal Hemangiomatosis

This condition includes vascular hamartomas of skin, iris, conjunctiva, and CNS.

Nevus Sebaceous of Jadassohn

Patients with this condition exhibit geographic linear cutaneous nevus with alopecia and epibulbar complex choristoma and choroidal/scleral choristomas.

Combined Systemic Hamartomatosis

These include neurofibromatosis/von Hippel or Sturge-Weber/nevus of Ota; tuberous sclerosis/retinal vascular hamartoma.

Further Reading

Chan CC, Collins AB, Chew EY (2007) Molecular pathology of eyes with von Hippel-Lindau (VHL) disease: a review. Retina 27:1–7

Chang JH, Spraul CW, Lynn ML, Drack A, Grossniklaus HE (1998) The two-stage mutation model in retinal hemangioblastoma. Ophthalmic Genet 19:123–130

Ferner RE (2010) The neurofibromatoses. Pract Neurol 10:82–93

Friedman JM (1993) Neurofibromatosis 1. In: Pagon RA, Bird TD, Dolan CR, Stephens K (eds) GeneReviews [internet]. University of Washington, Seattle, 1998 Oct 02 [updated 2009 Jun 02]

Grossniklaus HE, Thomas JW, Vigneswaran N, Jarrett WH (1992) Retinal hemangioblastoma. A histologic, immunohistochemical, and ultrastructural evaluation. Ophthalmology 99:140–145

Jett K, Friedman JM (2010) Clinical and genetic aspects of neurofibromatosis 1. Genet Med 12:1–11

McGlaughlin ME, Pepin SM, Maccolin M, Choopong P, Lessell S (2007) Ocular pathologic findings in neurofibromatosis type 2. Arch Ophthalmol 125:389–394

Rowley SA, O'Callaghan FJ, Osborne JP (2001) Ophthalmic manifestations of tuberous sclerosis: a population based study. Br J Ophthalmol 85:420–423

Ruggieri M, Pavone P, Polizzi A, Di Pietro M, Scuderi A, Gabriele A, Spalice A, Iannetti P (2004) Ophthalmological manifestations in segmental neurofibromatosis type 1. Br J Ophthalmol 88:1429–1433

Wee SA, Fangman B (2007) Tuberous sclerosis. Dermatol Online J 13:22

MIX
Papier aus verantwortungsvollen Quellen
Paper from responsible sources
FSC® C105338

If you have any concerns about our products,
you can contact us on
ProductSafety@springernature.com

In case Publisher is established outside the EU,
the EU authorized representative is:
Springer Nature Customer Service Center GmbH
Europaplatz 3, 69115 Heidelberg, Germany

Printed by Libri Plureos GmbH
in Hamburg, Germany